Tarascon Pocket Pharmacopoeia®

2013 Classic for Nurses

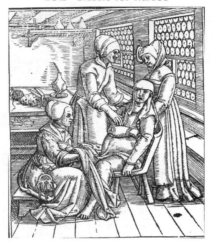

2ND EDITION

Albert Anthony Rundio, Jr., PhD, DNP, RN, APRN, NEA-BC
Associate Dean and Clinical Professor,
Drexel University College of Nursing and Health Professions,
Philadelphia, PA

Gloria F. Donnelly, PhD, RN, FAAN
Dean and Professor,
Drexel University College of Nursing and Health Professions,
Philadelphia, PA

JONES & BARTLETT
LEARNING

World Headquarters
Jones & Bartlett
  Learning
5 Wall Street
Burlington, MA 01803
978-443-5000
info@jblearning.com
www.jblearning.com

Jones & Bartlett Learning books and products are available through most bookstores and online booksellers. To contact Jones & Bartlett Learning directly, call 800-832-0034, fax 978-443-8000, or visit our website www.jblearning.com.

ISSN: 1945-9076
ISBN: 978-1-4496-7409-0
6048
Printed in the United States of America
16 15 14 13 12   10 9 8 7 6 5 4 3 2 1

Production Credits

Chief Executive Officer: Ty Field
President: James Homer
SVP, Chief Marketing Officer: Alison M. Pendergast
V.P., Design and Production: Anne Spencer
V.P., Manufacturing and Inventory Control: Therese Connell
Manufacturing and Inventory Control Supervisor: Amy Bacus
Executive Publisher: Christopher Davis
Senior Acquisitions Editor: Nancy Anastasi Duffy

Editorial Assistant: Marisa LaFleur
Production Editor: Daniel Stone
Medicine Marketing Manager: Rebecca Leitch
Composition: Newgen
Text and Cover Design: Anne Spencer
Printing and Binding: Cenveo
Cover Printing: Cenveo

If you obtained your Pocket Pharmacopoeia for Nurses from a bookstore, please send your address to info@tarascon.com. This allows you to be the first to hear of updates! (We don't sell or distribute our mailing lists, by the way.)

The cover woodcut courtesy of National Library of Medicine.

CONTENTS

PAGE INDEX FOR TABLES

TARASCON POCKET PHARMACOPOEIA EDITORIAL STAFF*

EDITOR IN CHIEF

Richard J. Hamilton, MD, FAAEM,FACMT, Professor and Chair, Department of Emergency Medicine, Drexel University College of Medicine, Philadelphia, PA

NURSING EDITORS

Elizabeth Blunt, PhD, RN, APN-BC, Assistant Professor & Director NP Programs, College of Nursing, Villanova University, Villanova, PA

Rosemary Dunn DrNP MBA RN, Chief Nursing Officer, Hahnemann University Hospital, Philadelphia, PA

Brian J. Fasolka, MSN, RN, CEN, Assistant Clinical Professor, College of Nursing & Health Professions, Drexel University, Philadelphia, PA

Rodney W. Hicks, PhD, RN, FNP-BC, FAANP, FAAN, Professor and Assistant DNP Program Director, College of Graduate Nursing, Western University of Health Sciences, Pomona, CA

H. Lynn Kane, RN, MSN, MBA, CCRN, Clinical Nurse Specialist, Thomas Jefferson University Hospital, Philadelphia, PA

Cindy Marino, MSN, RN, Senior Director of Nursing, Hahnemann University Hospital, Philadelphia, PA

Jennifer Olszewski, MSN, CRNP, Assistant Clinical Professor, College of Nursing and Health Professions, Drexel University, Philadelphia, PA

Linda Wilson, RN, PhD, CPAN, CAPA, BC, CNE, Assistant Dean & Associate Clinical Professor, College of Nursing & Health Professions, Drexel University, Philadelphia, PA

*Affiliations are given for information purposes only, and no affiliation sponsorship is claimed.

PREFACE TO THE TARASCON POCKET PHARMACOPOEIA®

The *Tarascon Pharmacopoeia Classic for Nurses* was especially designed for nurses who work in hospitals. The drugs listed are the most frequently ordered and commonly administered drugs in acute care settings. The nursing implications are especially designed with patient safety and drug efficacy in mind. Drugs are arranged by clinical class with a comprehensive index in the back. Trade names are italicized and capitalized. Drug doses shown in mg/kg are generally intended for children, while fixed doses represent typical adult recommendations. Brackets indicate currently available formulations, although not all pharmacies stock all formulations. The availability of generic, over-the-counter, and scored formulations is mentioned. Codes are as follows:

▶ **METABOLISM & EXCRETION: L** = primarily liver, **K** = primarily kidney, **LK** = both, but liver > kidney, **KL** = both, but kidney > liver.

♀ **SAFETY IN PREGNANCY: A** = Safety established using human studies, **B** = Presumed safety based on animal studies, **C** = Uncertain safety; no human studies and animal studies show an adverse effect, **D** = Unsafe - evidence of risk that may in certain clinical circumstances be justifiable, **X** = Highly unsafe - risk of use outweighs any possible benefit. For drugs that have not been assigned a category: **+** Generally accepted as safe, **?** Safety unknown or controversial, **−** Generally regarded as unsafe.

▶ **SAFETY IN LACTATION: +** Generally accepted as safe, **?** Safety unknown or controversial, **−** Generally regarded as unsafe. Many of our "+" listings are from the AAP policy "The Transfer of Drugs and Other Chemicals Into Human Milk" (see www.aap.org) and may differ from those recommended by the manufacturer.

© **DEA CONTROLLED SUBSTANCES: I** = High abuse potential, no accepted use (eg, heroin, marijuana), **II** = High abuse potential and severe dependence liability (eg, morphine, codeine, hydromorphone, cocaine, amphetamines, methylphenidate, secobarbital). Some states require triplicates. **III** = Moderate dependence liability (eg, *Tylenol #3*, *Vicodin*), **IV** = Limited dependence liability (benzodiazepines, propoxyphene, phentermine), **V** = Limited abuse potential (eg, *Lomotil*).

$ **RELATIVE COST:** Cost codes used are "per month" of maintenance therapy (eg, antihypertensives) or "per course" of short-term therapy (eg, antibiotics). Codes are calculated using average wholesale prices (at press time in US dollars) for the most common indication and route of each drug at a typical adult dosage. For maintenance therapy, costs are calculated based upon a 30-day supply or the quantity that might typically be used in a given month. For short-term therapy (ie, 10 days or less), costs are calculated on a single treatment course. When multiple forms are available (eg, generics), these codes reflect the least expensive generally available product. When drugs don't neatly fit into the classification scheme above, we have assigned codes based upon the relative cost of other similar drugs. *These codes should be used as a rough guide only*, as (1) they reflect cost, not charges, (2) pricing often varies substantially from location to location and time to time, and (3) HMOs, Medicaid, and buying groups often negotiate quite different pricing. Check with your local pharmacy if you have any questions.

Code	Cost
$	< $25
$$	$25 to $49
$$$	$50 to $99
$$$$	$100 to $199
$$$$$	≥ $200

🍁 **CANADIAN TRADE NAMES:** Unique common Canadian trade names not used in the US are listed after a maple leaf symbol. Trade names used in both nations or only in the US are displayed without such notation.

Ⓜ Drug contains more than one drug compound. See drug monograph for additional information.

ABBREVIATIONS IN TEXT

AAP – American Academy of Pediatrics
ac – before meals
ACCP – American College of Chest Physicians
ACT – activated clotting time
ADHD – attention deficit hyperactivity disorder
AHA – American Heart Association
Al – aluminum
ANC – absolute neutrophil count
ASA – aspirin
bid – twice per day
BP – blood pressure
BPH – benign prostatic hyperplasia
BUN – blood urea nitrogen
Ca – calcium
CAD – coronary artery disease
cap – capsule
cm – centimeter
CMV – cytomegalovirus
CNS – central nervous system
COPD – chronic obstructive pulmonary disease
CrCl – creatinine clearance
CVA – stroke
CYP – cytochrome P450

D5W – 5% dextrose
dL – deciliter
DM – diabetes mellitus
DPI – dry powder inhaler
ECG – electrocardiogram
EPS – extrapyramidal symptoms
ET – endotracheal
g – gram
GERD. – gastroesophageal reflux disease
gtts – drops
GU – genitourinary
h – hour
HAART – highly active antiretroviral therapy
Hb – hemoglobin
HCTZ – hydrochlorothiazide
HIT – heparin-induced thrombocytopenia
hs – bedtime
HSV – herpes simplex virus
HTN – hypertension
IM – intramuscular
INR – international normalized ratio
IU – international units
IV – intravenous
JRA – juvenile rheumatoid arthritis
kg – kilogram

lbs – pounds
LFT – liver function test
LV – left ventricular
LVEF – left ventricular ejection fraction
m^2 – sqaure meters
MAOI – monoamine oxidase inhibitor
mcg – microgram
MDI – metered dose inhaler
mEq – milliequivalent
mg – milligram
Mg – magnesium
MI – myocardial infarction
min – minute
mL – milliliter
mm – millimeter
mo – months old
MRSA – methicillin-resistant *Staphylococcus aureus*
ng – nanogram
NHLBI – National Heart, Lung, and Blood Institute
NS – normal saline
NPH – neutral protamine hagedorn
N/V – nausea/vomiting
NYHA – New York Heart Association
OA – osteoarthritis
oz – ounces
pc – after meals

PO – by mouth
PR – by rectum
prn – as needed
PTT – partial thromboplastin time
q – every
qam – every morning
qhs – at bedtime
qid – four times/day
qod – every other day
qpm – every evening
RA – rheumatoid arthritis
RSV – respiratory synctial virus
SC – subcutaneous
sec – second
soln – solution
supp – suppository
susp – suspension
tab – tablet
TB – tuberculosis
TCA – tricyclic antidepressant
tid – three times/day
TNF – tumor necrosis factor
TPN – total parenteral nutrition
UTI – urinary tract infection
wt – weight
y – year
yo – years old

THERAPEUTIC DRUG LEVELS

Drug	Level	Optimal Timing
amikacin peak	20–35 mcg/mL	30 minutes after infusion
amikacin trough	<5 mcg/mL	Just prior to next dose
carbamazepine trough	4–12 mcg/mL	Just prior to next dose
cyclosporine trough	50–300 ng/mL	Just prior to next dose
digoxin	0.8–2.0 ng/mL	Just prior to next dose
ethosuximide trough	40–100 mcg/mL	Just prior to next dose
gentamicin peak	5–10 mcg/mL	30 minutes after infusion
gentamicin trough	<2 mcg/mL	Just prior to next dose
lidocaine	1.5–5 mcg/mL	12–24 hours after start of infusion
lithium trough	0.6–1.2 meq/L	Just prior to first morning dose
NAPA	10–30 mcg/mL	Just prior to next procainamide dose
phenobarbital trough	15–40 mcg/mL	Just prior to next dose
phenytoin trough	10–20 mcg/mL	Just prior to next dose
primidone trough	5–12 mcg/mL	Just prior to next dose
procainamide	4–10 mcg/mL	Just prior to next dose
quinidine	2–5 mcg/mL	Just prior to next dose
theophylline	5–15 mcg/mL	8–12 hours after once daily dose
tobramycin peak	5–10 mcg/mL	30 minutes after infusion
tobramycin trough	<2 mcg/mL	Just prior to next dose
valproate trough (epilepsy)	50–100 mcg/mL	Just prior to next dose
valproate trough (mania)	45–125 mcg/mL	Just prior to next dose
vancomycin trough[1]	10–20 mg/L	Just prior to next dose
zonisamide[2]	10–40 mcg/mL	Just prior to dose

[1] Maintain trough >10 mg/L to avoid resistance; optimal trough for complicated infections is 15–20 mg/L
[2] Ranges not firmly established but supported by clinical trial results

PEDIATRIC DRUGS		*Age*	*2mo*	*4mo*	*6mo*	*9mo*	*12mo*	*15mo*	*2yo*	*3yo*	*5yo*
		kg	5	6½	8	9	10	11	13	15	19
		lbs	11	15	17	20	22	24	28	33	42
med	***strength***	***freq***	***teaspoons of liquid per dose** (1 tsp= 5 mL)*								
Tylenol (mg)		q4h	80	80	120	120	160	160	200	240	280
Tylenol (tsp)	160/t	q4h	½	½	¾	¾	1	1	1¼	1½	1¾
ibuprofen (mg)		q6h	-	-	75†	75†	100	100	125	150	175
ibuprofen (tsp)	100/t	q6h	-	-	¾†	¾†	1	1	1¼	1½	1¾
amoxicillin or	125/t	bid	1	1¼	1½	1¾	1¾	2	2¼	2¾	3½
Augmentin	200/t	bid	½	¾	1	1	1¼	1¼	1½	1¾	2¼
(not otitis media)	250/t	bid	½	½	¾	¾	1	1	1¼	1¼	1¾
	400/t	bid	¼	½	½	½	¾	¾	¾	1	1
amoxicillin,	200/t	bid	1	1¼	1¾	2	2	2¼	2¾	3	4
(otitis media)‡	250/t	bid	¾	1¼	1½	1½	1¾	1¾	2¼	2½	3¼
	400/t	bid	½	¾	¾	1	1	1¼	1½	1½	2
Augmentin ES‡	600/t	bid	?	½	½	¾	¾	¾	1	1¼	1½
azithromycin·§	100/t	qd	¼†	½†	½	½	½	½	¾	¾	1
(5-day Rx)	200/t	qd	--	¼†	¼	¼	¼	¼	½	½	½
Bactrim/Septra	---	bid	½	¾	1	1	1	1¼	1½	1½	2
cefaclor·	125/t	bid	1	1	1¼	1½	1½	1¾	2	2½	3
"	250/t	bid	½	½	¾	¾	¾	1	1	1¼	1½
cefadroxil	125/t	bid	½	¾	1	1	1¼	1¼	1½	1¾	2¼
"	250/t	bid	¼	½	½	½	¾	¾	¾	1	1
cefdinir	125/t	qd	--	¾†	1	1	1	1¼	1½	1¾	2
cefixime	100/t	qd	½	½	¾	¾	¾	1	1	1¼	1½
cefprozil*	125/t	bid	--	¾†	1	1	1¼	1½	1½	2	2¼
"	250/t	bid	--	½†	½	½	¾	¾	¾	1	1¼
cefuroxime	125/t	bid	-	¾	¾	1	1	1	1½	1¾	2¼
cephalexin	125/t	qid	--	½	¾	¾	1	1	1¼	1½	1¾
"	250/t	qid	-	¼	¼	½	½	½	¾	¾	1
clarithromycin	125/t	bid	½†	½†	½	½	¾	¾	¾	1	1¼
"	250/t	bid	--	--	--	¼	½	½	½	½	¾
dicloxacillin	62½/t	qid	½	¾	1	1	1¼	1¼	1½	1¾	2
nitrofurantoin	25/t	qid	¼	½	½	½	½	¾	¾	¾	1
Pediazole	---	tid	½	½	¾	¾	1	1	1	1¼	1½
penicillin V**	250/t	bid-tid	--	1	1	1	1	1	1	1	1
cetirizine	5/t	qd	-	-	½	½	½	½	½	½	½
Benadryl	12.5/t	q6h	½	½	¾	¾	1	1	1¼	1½	2
prednisolone	15/t	qd	¼	½	½	¾	¾	¾	1	1	1¼
prednisone	5/t	qd	1	1¼	1½	1¾	2	2¼	2½	3	3¾
Robitussin	---	q4h	-	-	¼†	¼†	½	½	¾	¾	1
Tylenol w/ codeine		q4h	-	-	-	-	-	-		1	1

*Dose shown is for otitis media only; see dosing in text for alternative indications.
†Dosing at this age/weight not recommended by manufacturer.
‡AAP now recommends high dose (80-90 mg/kg/d) for all otitis media in children; with Augmentin used as ES only.
§Give a double dose of azithromycin the first day.
**AHA dosing for streptococcal pharyngitis. Treat for 10 days.
tsp=teaspoon; t=teaspoon; q=every; h=hour; kg=kilogram; Lbs=pounds; mL=mililiter; bid=two times per day; tid=three times per day; qid=four times per day; qd=every day.

PEDIATRIC VITAL SIGNS AND INTRAVENOUS DRUGS		Pre-matr	New-born	2m	4m	6m	9m	12m	15m	2y	3y	5y
Age												
Weight	*(Kg)*	2	3½	5	6½	8	9	10	11	13	15	19
	(Lbs)	4½	7½	11	15	17	20	22	24	28	33	42
Maint fluids	*(mL/h)*	8	14	20	26	32	36	40	42	46	50	58
ET tube	*(mm)*	2½	3/3½	3½	3½	3½	4	4	4½	4½	4½	5
Defib	*(Joules)*	4	7	10	13	16	18	20	22	26	30	38
Systolic BP	*(high)*	70	80	85	90	95	100	103	104	106	109	114
	(low)	40	60	70	70	70	70	70	70	75	75	80
Pulse rate	*(high)*	145	145	180	180	180	160	160	160	150	150	135
	(low)	100	100	110	110	110	100	100	100	90	90	65
Resp rate	*(high)*	60	60	50	50	50	46	46	30	30	25	25
	(low)	35	30	30	30	24	24	20	20	20	20	20
adenosine	*(mg)*	0.2	0.3	0.5	0.6	0.8	0.9	1	1.1	1.3	1.5	1.9
atropine	*(mg)*	0.1	0.1	0.1	0.13	0.16	0.18	0.2	0.22	0.26	0.30	0.38
Benadryl	*(mg)*	-	-	-5	6½	8	9	10	11	13	15	19
Bicarbonate	(meq)	2	3½	5	6½	8	9	10	11	13	15	19
dextrose	*(g)*	1	2	5	6½	8	9	10	11	13	15	19
epinephrine	*(mg)*	.02	.04	.05	.07	.08	.09	0.1	0.11	0.13	0.15	0.19
lidocaine	*(mg)*	2	3½	5	6½	8	9	10	11	13	15	19
morphine	*(mg)*	0.2	0.3	0.5	0.6	0.8	0.9	1	1.1	1.3	1.5	1.9
mannitol	*(g)*	2	3½	5	6½	8	9	10	11	13	15	19
naloxone	*(mg)*	.02	.04	.05	.07	.08	.09	0.1	0.11	0.13	0.15	0.19
diazepam	*(mg)*	0.6	1	1.5	2	2.5	2.7	3	3.3	3.9	4.5	5
fosphenytoin*	*(PE)*	40	70	100	130	160	180	200	220	260	300	380
lorazepam	*(mg)*	0.1	0.2	0.3	0.35	0.4	0.5	0.5	0.6	0.7	0.8	1.0
phenobarb	*(mg)*	30	60	75	100	125	125	150	175	200	225	275
phenytoin*	*(mg)*	40	70	100	130	160	180	200	220	260	300	380
ampicillin	*(mg)*	100	175	250	325	400	450	500	550	650	750	1000
ceftriaxone	*(mg)*	-	-	250	325	400	450	500	550	650	750	1000
cefotaxime	*(mg)*	100	175	250	325	400	450	500	550	650	750	1000
gentamicin	*(mg)*	5	8	12	16	20	22	25	27	32	37	47

*Loading doses; fosphenytoin dosed in "phenytoin equivalents."

CONVERSIONS	*Liquid:*	*Weight:*
Temperature:	1 fluid ounce = 30 mL	1 kilogram = 2.2 lbs
F = (1.8) C + 32	1 teaspoon = 5 mL	1 ounce = 30 g
C = (F – 32)/1.8	1 tablespoon = 15 mL	1 grain = 65 mg

FORMULAS

Alveolar-arterial oxygen gradient = A-a = 148 − 1.2(PaCO2) − PaO2
  [normal = 10-20 mmHg, breathing room air at sea level]

Calculated osmolality = 2Na + glucose/18 + BUN/2.8 + ethanol/4.6
  [norm 280-295 meq/L. Na in meq/L; all others in mg/dL]

Pediatric IV maintenance fluids (see table on page xi)
  4 mL/kg/hr **or** 100 mL/kg/day for first 10 kg, plus
  2 mL/kg/hr **or** 50 mL/kg/day for second 10 kg, plus
  1 mL/kg/hr **or** 20 mL/kg/day for all further kg

$$mcg/kg/min = \frac{16.7 \times \text{drug conc [mg/mL]} \times \text{infusion rate [mL/h]}}{\text{weight [kg]}}$$

$$\text{Infusion rate [mL/h]} = \frac{\text{desired mcg/kg/min} \times \text{weight [kg]} \times 60}{\text{drug concentration [mcg/mL]}}$$

Fractional excretion of sodium =
[Pre-renal, etc <1%; ATN, etc >1%] $\left[\dfrac{\text{urine Na / plasma Na}}{\text{urine creat / plasma creat}} \right] \times 100\%$

Anion gap = Na − (Cl + HCO3)   [normal = 10-14 meq/L]

Creatinine clearance = $\dfrac{(\text{lean kg})(140 - \text{age})(0.85 \text{ if female})}{(72)(\text{stable creatinine [mg/dL]})}$
  [normal >80]

Glomerular filtration rate using MDRD equation (mL/min/1.73 m^2)
= 186 × (creatinine)$^{-1.154}$ × (age)$^{-0.203}$ × (0.742 if ♀) × (1.210 if African American)

Body surface area (BSA) = square root of: $\left[\dfrac{\text{height (cm)} \times \text{weight (kg)}}{3600} \right]$
  [in m^2]

DRUG THERAPY REFERENCE WEBSITES FORMULAS (selected)

Professional societies or governmental agencies with drug therapy guidelines		
AAP	American Academy of Pediatrics	www.aap.org
ACC	American College of Cardiology	www.acc.org
ACCP	American College of Chest Physicians	www.chestnet.org
ACCP	American College of Clinical Pharmacy	www.accp.com
ADA	American Diabetes Association	www.diabetes.org
AHA	American Heart Association	www.americanheart.org
AHRQ	Agency for Healthcare Research and Quality	www.ahcpr.gov
AMA	American Medical Association	www.ama-assn.org
APA	American Psychiatric Association	www.psych.org
APA	American Psychological Association	www.apa.org
ASHP	Amer. Society Health-Systems Pharmacists	www.ashp.org
ATS	American Thoracic Society	www.thoracic.org
CDC	Centers for Disease Control and Prevention	www.cdc.gov
CDC	CDC bioterrorism and radiation exposures	www.bt.cdc.gov
IDSA	Infectious Diseases Society of America	www.idsociety.org
MHA	Malignant Hyperthermia Association	www.mhaus.org
NHLBI	National Heart, Lung, and Blood Institute	www.nhlbi.nih.gov
Other therapy reference sites		
Cochrane library		www.cochrane.org
Emergency Contraception Website		www.not-2-late.com
Immunization Action Coalition		www.immunize.org
Int'l Registry for Drug-Induced Arrhythmias		www.qtdrugs.org
Managing Contraception		www.managingcontraception.com
Nephrology Pharmacy Associates		www.nephrologypharmacy.com

ANALGESICS

Antirheumatic Agents—Biologic Response Modifiers

NOTE: *Death, sepsis, and serious infections (eg, TB and invasive fungal infections) have been reported.*

ABATACEPT   (*Orencia*) ▶Serum ♀C ▶? © $$$$$ Inhibits production of tumor necrosis factor-alpha, interleukin-2, and interferon-gamma. Serious: Infection, malignancies, hypersensitivity. Frequent: Headache, pharyngitis, nausea.

> Nursing Implications   Administer by subcutaneous injection at rotated sites or by IV infusion. Monitor for severe allergic reaction/anaphylaxis. Closely monitor pt when drug is first injected into vein. Do not infuse with other drugs; do not shake bag or bottle; store at room temp and discard if not used in 24 h. With proper instruction, pt may self-inject. Infections are common, serious adverse reactions. Monitor pt for upper respiratory and urinary tract infections. Headache, high BP, and dizziness may occur within 1 h of first IV infusion. Orencia can reactivate hepatitis B or latent TB; screen pts for both since safe use of Orencia in these conditions is not determined.

ADALIMUMAB   (*Humira*) RA, psoriatic arthritis, ankylosing spondylitis: 40 mg SC every 2 weeks, alone or in combination with methotrexate or other disease-modifying antirheumatic drugs (DMARDs). May increase frequency to once a week if not on methotrexate. Crohn's disease: 160 mg SC at week 0, 80 mg at week 2, then 40 mg every other week starting with week 4. ▶Serum ♀B ▶? © $$$$$ Trade only: 40-mg prefilled glass syringes or vials with needles, 2 per pack. Monoclonal antibody that blocks tumor necrosis factor-alpha. Serious: Hypersensitivity, infection, lymphoma, lupus-like syndrome, aplastic anemia, thrombocytopenia, and leukopenia. Frequent: Injection site reaction.

> Nursing Implications   TB skin test prior to administration.

INFLIXIMAB   (*Remicade*) RA: 3 mg/kg IV in combination with methotrexate at 0, 2, and 6 weeks. Ankylosing spondylitis: 5 mg/kg IV at 0, 2, and 6 weeks. Plaque psoriasis, psoriatic arthritis, moderately to severely active Crohn's disease, ulcerative colitis, or fistulizing disease: 5 mg/kg IV infusion at 0, 2, and 6 weeks, then q 8 weeks. ▶Serum ♀B ▶? © $$$$$ Monoclonal antibody that blocks tumor necrosis factor-alpha. Serious: Anaphylaxis, disseminated TB, sepsis, worsening heart failure, lupus-like syndrome, optic neuropathy. Frequent: Infusion reaction.

> Nursing Implications   Do not give if pt is suffering from a serious or severe infection, such as TB. Pts need to be assessed and tested for TB and other infections prior to administration of this medication. The CBC, especially the WBC, should be monitored frequently. Observe pts for signs and symptoms of infection (fever, chills, flu symptoms, confusion, pain, or warmth or redness of skin). Pts may be prone to other medical conditions (eg, lymphoma) while on this medication.

Antirheumatic Agents—Disease-Modifying Antirheumatic Drugs (DMARDs)

GOLD SODIUM THIOMALATE   (*Myochrysine*) ▶K ♀C ▶+ © $$$$$ Decreases synovial inflammation; slows cartilage/bone destruction. Serious: Anaphylaxis, bone marrow suppression, proteinuria. Frequent: Diarrhea, dermatitis, stomatitis.

> Nursing Implications   Inform provider immediately if signs of toxicity occur including: rash, itching, bruising, metallic taste, sore mouth, nosebleed or bloody diarrhea. Instruct patient to avoid sun or wear sunscreen. Instruct patient to report allergy to gold, kidney, liver or heart disease, blood disorders, inflammatory bowel, diabetes or serious lung condition. Teach patient to lie down after each dose, to comply with blood and urine tests pre-injection and to report all prescription and OTC medications taken.

HYDROXYCHLOROQUINE   (*Plaquenil*) RA: Start 400 to 600 mg PO daily, then taper to 200 to 400 mg daily. SLE: 400 mg PO one to two times per day to start, then taper to 200 to 400 mg daily. ▶K ♀C ▶+ © $ Generic/Trade: Tabs 200 mg, scored. Unclear in the treatment of RA. Serious: Retinopathy, angioedema, bronchospasm. Frequent: Anorexia, nausea.

Nursing Implications Caution in pts with liver and/or kidney disease, alcoholism, obesity, pregnancy, or breastfeeding. Monitor for confusion, mood and behavior changes, seizures, low blood pressure, vision disturbances, ringing in ears, blood dyscrasias including bleeding and bruising, jaundice, weight loss, rashes, and skin eruptions. Teach pt to self-monitor and report any of the above. With long term-treatment, regular blood studies and eye checks may be warranted.

LEFLUNOMIDE (*Arava*) RA: Loading dose: 100 mg PO daily for 3 days. Maintenance dose: 10 to 20 mg PO daily. ▶LK ♀X ▶– © $$$$$ Generic/Trade: Tabs 10, 20 mg. Trade only: Tabs 100 mg. Immunosuppressant. Serious: Lymphoma, pancytopenia, Stevens-Johnson syndrome, hepatotoxicity, interstitial lung disease, cutaneous necrotizing vasculitis. Frequent: Diarrhea.

Nursing Implications Administer by mouth with or without food. Instruct patient to take medication regularly according to dosing instructions. Inform provider immediately if signs of infection occur or if patient experiences serious side effects such as: rapid heart rate, hair loss, chest pain, numbness in extremities, rash, itching, swelling or other allergic signs. Assess patient for previous immune disorders, kidney, liver or heart disease, alcoholism or lung disease. Test for pregnancy before starting drug. Store at room temperature in dry place, not in a bathroom.

METHOTREXATE—RHEUMATOLOGY (*Rheumatrex, Trexall*) RA, psoriasis: Start with 7.5 mg PO single dose once a week or 2.5 mg PO q 12 h for 3 doses given once a week. Max dose 20 mg/week. Supplement with 1 mg/day of folic acid. Chemotherapy doses vary by indication. ▶LK ♀X ▶– © $$ Trade only (Trexall): Tabs 5, 7.5, 10, 15 mg. Dose Pak (Rheumatrex) 2.5 mg (# 8, 12, 16, 20, 24). Generic/Trade: Tabs 2.5 mg, scored. Immunosuppressant, antimetabolite. Serious: Hepatotoxicity, pulmonary disease, lymphoma, bone marrow suppression, intestinal perforation. Frequent: Increased LFTs, diarrhea, stomatitis, bone marrow suppression.

Nursing Implications Administer by mouth and advise patient to drink liquids with medication to avoid side effects. Caution patient that medication benefit may take several months to occur. Report persistent side effects such as: nausea and vomiting, GI pain, dizziness or drowsiness, low urine output, yellowing skin or eye whites, chest pain, seizures or mood changes. Assess for any diseases that may contraindicate use of this drug, particularly immune disorders. Teach patient to avoid direct sunlight, alcohol, and to use caution while driving or operating machinery until full effects of the medication are known. Do not use during pregnancy.

Muscle Relaxants

BACLOFEN (*Lioresal, Kemstro*) Spasticity related to MS or spinal cord disease/injury: Start 5 mg PO three times per day, then increase by 5 mg/dose q 3 days until 20 mg PO three times per day. Max dose 20 mg four times per day. ▶K ♀C ▶+ © $$ Generic only: Tabs 10, 20 mg. Trade only (Kemstro): Tabs, orally disintegrating 10, 20 mg. Skeletal muscle relaxant. Serious: Hallucinations and seizures with abrupt withdrawal. Frequent: Hypotonia, somnolence, dizziness.

Nursing Implications To minimize side effects, instruct patient to take with food or milk. (For orally disintegrating tabs: Place on tongue w/dry hands. Once tab disintegrates, swallow with saliva or water.) IM: Screening phase; prior to use, test dose (50 mcg/ml) should be administered over 1 min, observe for decrease in muscle tone or frequency or severity of spasm. If response is inadequate, administer 2 additional test doses, each 24 h apart (75 mcg/1.5 mL and 100 mcg/2 mL respectively).

CARISOPRODOL (*Soma*) Acute musculoskeletal pain: 350 mg PO three to four times per day. Abuse potential. ▶LK ♀? ▶– © $ Generic/Trade: Tabs 350 mg. Trade only: Tabs 250 mg. Skeletal muscle relaxant. Serious: Idiosyncratic reaction with angioedema, hypotension, and anaphylactoid shock. Frequent: Dizziness and drowsiness.

Nursing Implications Do not confuse Soma with Soma Compound. Give dose at bedtime.

CYCLOBENZAPRINE (*Amrix, Flexeril, Fexmid*) Musculoskeletal pain: Start 5 to 10 mg PO three times per day, max 30 mg/day or 15 to 30 mg (extended-release) PO daily. Not recommended in elderly. ▶LK ♀B ▶? © $ Generic/Trade: Tab 5, 10 mg. Generic only: Tabs 7.5 mg. Trade only: (Amrix $$$$$): Extended-release caps 15, 30 mg. Skeletal muscle relaxant. Serious: Arrhythmia. Frequent: Drowsiness, dizziness, dry mouth, blurred vision.

| Nursing Implications | Extended-release form should be taken at same time each day; avoid driving until used to the drug; no alcohol, sedatives, OTC drugs; MAOs must be discontinued 14 days before use. Caution patient not to take for more than 3 weeks, can cause a CVA; low BP, MI, blurred vision, wide range of GI symptoms including paralytic ileus and bone marrow depression. Monitor patient closely for drug interactions. |

DANTROLENE (*Dantrium*) Chronic spasticity related to spinal cord injury, CVA, cerebral palsy, MS: 25 mg PO daily to start, up to max of 100 mg two to four times per day if necessary. Malignant hyperthermia: 2.5 mg/kg rapid IV push q 5 to 10 min continuing until symptoms subside or to a maximum total dose of 10 mg/kg. ▶LK ♀C ▶– © $$$$ Generic/Trade: Caps 25, 50, 100 mg. Skeletal muscle relaxant. Serious: Hepatotoxicity. Frequent: Drowsiness, dizziness, and weakness.

| Nursing Implications | Administer by mouth. Assess patient for liver disease as drug can be hepatotoxic. Avoid use in patients with pulmonary and cardiac disease. Transient side effects include: drowsiness, dizziness, general malaise and diarrhea. If diarrhea persists, inform provider to assess if medication should be discontinued. Patient should not drive or operate machinery until effects of medication are known. As Dantrolene interacts with many other drugs, check all patient's medications for possible drug interactions. |

METAXALONE (*Skelaxin*) Musculoskeletal pain: 800 mg PO three to four times per day. ▶LK ♀? ▶? © $$$$ Generic/Trade: Tabs 800 mg, scored. Skeletal muscle relaxant. Serious: Hypersensitivity, jaundice. Frequent: Drowsiness, dizziness, nausea.

| Nursing Implications | Administer PO and advise patient that medication can cause drowsiness or dizziness. |

METHOCARBAMOL (*Robaxin, Robaxin-750*) Acute musculoskeletal pain: 1500 mg PO four times per day or 1000 mg IM/IV three times per day for 48 to 72 h. Maintenance: 1000 mg PO four times per day, 750 mg PO q 4 h, or 1500 mg PO three times per day. Tetanus: Specialized dosing. ▶LK ♀C ▶? © $$ Generic/Trade: Tabs 500 and 750 mg. OTC in Canada. Skeletal muscle relaxant. Serious: Syncope, hypotension. Frequent: Drowsiness, dizziness, discolored urine (brown, black, green).

| Nursing Implications | IV or IM administration only. Do not give to patients allergic to this drug or those with myasthenia gravis. Teach patient to avoid alcohol and not to drive or operate machinery until effects of drug are known. Inform provider of serious side effects such as: flu like symptoms, faintness, decreased HR, seizures or yellowing of skin or eye whites. Pregnant women or those who may become pregnant should not use. Interacts with many drugs. Check all patient's medications to avoid drug interactions. |

ORPHENADRINE (*Norflex*) Musculoskeletal pain: 100 mg PO two times per day. 60 mg IV/IM two times per day. ▶LK ♀C ▶? © $$ Generic only: 100 mg extended-release. OTC in Canada. Skeletal muscle relaxant. Serious: Hypersensitivity, syncope. Frequent: Dry mouth, dizziness, constipation.

| Nursing Implications | Administer by mouth by extended release tablet. Do not give to patients experiencing enlarged prostate, difficult urination, GI blockage (including swallowing difficulties), glaucoma or myasthenia gravis. This drug is potentially habit forming and harmful to those with substance abuse/addictions. Do not drive or operate machinery until full effects of drug are known. Assess patient for cardiac disease prior to administration. Teach patient to swallow pill whole with 8 oz. of water and to report serious side effects such as irregular HF, confusion, agitation, hallucinations, seizures or decreased urination. Check all current medications for possible interactions. |

TIZANIDINE (*Zanaflex*) Muscle spasticity due to MS or spinal cord injury: 4 to 8 mg PO q 6 to 8 h prn, max 36 mg/day. ▶LK ♀C ▶? © $$$$ Generic/Trade: Tabs 4 mg, scored. Trade only: Caps 2, 4, 6 mg. Generic only: Tabs 2 mg. Skeletal muscle relaxant. Serious: Hypotension, hepatotoxicity. Frequent: Dry mouth, somnolence, asthenia, and dizziness.

| Nursing Implications | Do not confuse tizanidine with tiagabine. Administer with or without food. Titrate carefully to prevent side effects. Monitor hepatic and renal function for first 6 months of treatment. |

Non-Opioid Analgesic Combinations

ASCRIPTIN (acetylsalicylic acid + aluminum hydroxide + magnesium hydroxide + calcium carbonate, *Aspir-Mox*) Multiple strengths. 1 to 2 tabs PO q 4 h. ▶K ♀D ▶? © $ OTC Trade only: Tabs 325 mg aspirin/50 mg Mg hydroxide/50 mg Al hydroxide/50 mg Ca carbonate (Ascriptin and Aspir-Mox). 500 mg aspirin/33 mg Mg hydroxide/33 mg Al hydroxide/237 mg Ca carbonate (Ascriptin Maximum Strength). Anti-inflammatory, analgesic. Serious: Hypersensitivity, Reye's syndrome, GI bleeding, nephrotoxicity. Frequent: Nausea, dyspepsia.

> Nursing Implications Monitor hepatic functions.

BUFFERIN (acetylsalicylic acid + calcium carbonate + magnesium oxide + magnesium carbonate) 1 to 2 tabs/caps PO q 4 h. Max 12 in 24 h. ▶K ♀D ▶? © $ OTC Trade only: Tabs/caps 325 mg aspirin/158 mg Ca carbonate/63 mg of Mg oxide/34 mg of Mg carbonate. Bufferin ES: 500 mg aspirin/222.3 mg Ca carbonate/88.9 mg of Mg oxide/55.6 mg of Mg carbonate. Anti-inflammatory, analgesic. Serious: Hypersensitivity, Reye's syndrome, GI bleeding, nephrotoxicity. Frequent: Nausea, dyspepsia.

> Nursing Implications Teach patient to always take with a full glass of water. Take only the lowest effective dose and only as needed. Food will absorb more slowly but to its full extent.

ESGIC (acetaminophen + butalbital + caffeine) 1 to 2 tabs or caps PO q 4 h. Max 6 in 24 h. ▶LK ♀C ▶? © $ Generic only: Tabs/caps, 325 mg acetaminophen/50 mg butalbital/40 mg caffeine. Oral soln 325/50/40 mg per 15 mL. Generic/Trade: Tabs, Esgic Plus is 500/50/40 mg. Serious: Hepatotoxicity. Frequent: Drowsiness and dizziness.

> Nursing Implications Administer pill or capsule my mouth with food or milk. Do not give to patients on MAO inhibitors or those with cirrhosis of the liver. Patient should avoid alcohol and other medications containing acetaminophen such as cold medications. Butalbital can be habit forming, so carefully assess patient for history of substance abuse, mental illness or suicidal ideation. Avoid if pregnant. Teach patient to report serious side effects such as rapid, irregular HR, SOB, faintness, GI symptoms such as pain, clay colored stools, yellowing of skin and eye whites, or flu like symptoms. Teach patient to avoid using with other prescribed or OTC drugs that may cause drowsiness.

EXCEDRIN MIGRAINE (acetaminophen + acetylsalicylic acid + caffeine) 2 tabs/caps/geltabs PO q 6 h while symptoms persist. Max 8 tabs/caps/geltabs in 24 h. ▶LK ♀D ▶? © $ OTC Generic/Trade: Tabs/caps/geltabs 250 mg acetaminophen/250 mg aspirin/65 mg caffeine. Combination analgesic. Serious: Hepatotoxicity, hypersensitivity, Reye's syndrome, GI bleeding, nephrotoxicity. Frequent: Dyspepsia, nervousness, insomnia.

> Nursing Implications Refer to individual components for further information. Light and noise reduction may increase therapeutic effect. Use lowest effective dose for shortest period of time.

FIORICET (acetaminophen + butalbital + caffeine) 1 to 2 caps PO q 4 h. Max 6 caps in 24 h. ▶LK ♀C ▶? © $ Generic/Trade: Tabs 325 mg acetaminophen/50 mg butalbital/40 mg caffeine. Serious: Hepatotoxicity. Frequent: Drowsiness and dizziness.

> Nursing Implications Administer pill or capsule by mouth with food or milk. Do not give to patients on MAO inhibitors or those with cirrhosis of the liver. Patient should avoid alcohol and other medications containing acetaminophen such as cold medications. Butalbital can be habit forming, so carefully assess patient for history of substance abuse, mental illness or suicidal ideation. Avoid if pregnant. Teach patient to report serious side effects such as rapid, irregular HR, SOB, faintness, GI symptoms such as pain, clay colored stools, yellowing of skin and eye whites, or flu like symptoms. Teach patient to avoid using with other prescribed or OTC drugs that cause drowsiness.

FIORINAL (acetylsalicylic acid + butalbital + caffeine, ✛ *Trianal*) 1 to 2 tabs PO q 4 h. Max 6 tabs in 24 h. ▶LK ♀D ▶– ©III $ Generic/Trade: Caps 325 mg aspirin/ 50 mg butalbital/40 mg caffeine. Combination analgesic. Serious: Hypersensitivity, Reye's syndrome, GI bleeding, nephrotoxicity. Frequent: Drowsiness and dizziness.

> Nursing Implications Use lowest effective dose for shortest period of time. Explain therapeutic effect prior to administration to enhance analgesic effect. Regularly timed doses may be more effective than prn. Analgesic is more effective if given before pain becomes severe. Discontinue gradually after long-term use to prevent withdrawal symptoms. To minimize side effects, instruct patient to take medication with water, milk or food. Ⓜ

GOODY'S EXTRA STRENGTH HEADACHE POWDER (acetaminophen + acetylsalicylic acid + caffeine) 1 powder PO followed with liquid, or stir powder into a glass of water or other liquid. Repeat in 4 to 6 h prn. Max 4 powders in 24 h. ▶LK ♀D ▶? © $ OTC trade only: 260 mg acetaminophen/520 mg aspirin/32.5 mg caffeine per powder paper. Combination analgesic. Serious: Hepatotoxicity, hypersensitivity, Reye's syndrome, GI bleeding, nephrotoxicity. Frequent: Dyspepsia.

> Nursing Implications Explain therapeutic effect prior to administration to enhance analgesic effect. Regularly timed doses may be more effective than prn. Analgesic is more effective if given before pain becomes severe. To minimize side effects, instruct patient to take with water, milk, or food. Ⓜ

NORGESIC (orphenadrine + acetylsalicylic acid + caffeine) Multiple strengths; write specific product on Rx. Norgesic: 1 to 2 tabs PO three to four times per day. Norgesic Forte, 1 tab PO three to four times per day. ▶KL ♀D ▶? © $$ Generic/Trade: Tabs, Norgesic 25 mg orphenadrine/385 mg aspirin/30 mg caffeine. Norgesic Forte 50/770/60 mg. Combination analgesic/muscle relaxant. Serious: Hypersensitivity, Reye's syndrome, GI bleeding, nephrotoxicity, syncope. Frequent: Dry mouth, dizziness, constipation.

> Nursing Implications Do not confuse Norgesic (orphenadrine) with norfloxacin (Noroxin). Instruct patient to always swallow pills whole. Ⓜ

PHRENILIN (acetaminophen + butalbital) Tension or muscle contraction headache: 1 to 2 tabs PO q 4 h. Max 6 in 24 h. ▶LK ♀C ▶? © $ Generic/Trade: Tabs, Phrenilin 325 mg acetaminophen/50 mg butalbital. Caps, Phrenilin Forte 650/50 mg. Serious: Hepatotoxicity. Frequent: Drowsiness and dizziness.

> Nursing Implications Administer by mouth with or without food. Teach patient to take at first sign of headache. Drug can be habit forming and should be weaned. Avoid alcohol and other addictive substances. Call provider if serious side effects occur such as: SOB, rapid HR, seizures, mood changes, flu like symptoms, bruising/bleeding, signs of liver damage such as n/v, GI pain, discolored/dark urine, yellow skin or eye whites. Assess patient for history of kidney, liver disease or substance abuse. Cautionary use in elderly because of increased sensitivity. Do not drive or operate machinery until full effects of medication are known. Cautionary use with prescribed and OTC drugs that cause drowsiness. Check all possible drug interactions. Advise patient that drug may interfere with action of birth control pills. Store in a dark, dry place - not in a bathroom. Ⓜ

SEDAPAP (acetaminophen + butalbital) 1 to 2 tabs PO q 4 h. Max 6 tabs in 24 h. ▶LK ♀C ▶? © $ Generic only: Tabs 650 mg acetaminophen/50 mg butalbital. Serious: Hepatotoxicity. Frequent: Drowsiness and dizziness.

> Nursing Implications Administer by mouth with or without food. Teach patient to take at first sign of headache. Drug can be habit forming and should be weaned. Avoid alcohol and other addictive substances. Call provider if serious side effects occur such as SOB, rapid HR, seizures, mood changes, flu like symptoms, bruising/bleeding, signs of liver damage such as n/v, GI pain, discolored/dark urine, yellow skin or eye whites. Assess patient for history of kidney, liver disease or substance abuse. Cautionary use in elderly because of increased sensitivity. Do not drive or operate machinery until full effects of medication are known. Cautionary use with prescribed and OTC drugs that cause drowsiness. Check all possible drug interactions. Teach patient that drug may interfere with action of birth control pills. Store in a dark, dry place-not in a bathroom. Ⓜ

SOMA COMPOUND (carisoprodol + acetylsalicylic acid) 1 to 2 tabs PO four times per day. Abuse potential. ▶LK ♀D ▶– © $$$ Generic/Trade: Tabs 200 mg carisoprodol/325 mg aspirin. Combination analgesic/muscle relaxant. Serious: Hypersensitivity, Reye's syndrome, GI bleeding, nephrotoxicity. Idiosyncratic reaction with angioedema, hypotension, and anaphylactoid shock. Frequent: Dizziness and drowsiness.

> Nursing Implications Do not confuse Soma with Soma Compound. Administer at bedtime. Can be taken with food to minimize side effects.

ULTRACET (tramadol + acetaminophen, ✚ *Tramacet*) Acute pain: 2 tabs PO q 4 to 6 h prn (up to 8 tabs/day for no more than 5 days). Adjust dose in elderly and renal dysfunction. Avoid in opioid-dependent patients. Seizures may occur if concurrent antidepressants or seizure disorder. ▶KL ♀C ▶– © $$ Generic/Trade: Tabs 37.5 mg tramadol/ 325 mg acetaminophen. Combination analgesic. Serious: Seizures, anaphylactoid reactions, hepatotoxicity. Frequent: Constipation, somnolence.

> Nursing Implications | Administer tablet by mouth. May be habit forming and should not be used with MAOI's and St. John's Wort. Patient must avoid alcohol, hypnotics, narcotics and tranquilizers when taking Ultracet. Drug should be gradually weaned. Assess patient for liver damage/disease as drug contains acetaminophen. Immediately report n/v, GI pain, discolored, dark urine, fatigue and yellow skin or eye whites. Assess patient for brain disorders including head injury, COPD, kidney and liver disease, sleep apnea, GI disorders and history of substance abuse before administering. Do not drive or operate heavy machinery until full effect of medication is known. ⓜ

Non-Steroidal Anti-Inflammatories—COX-2 Inhibitors

CELECOXIB   (*Celebrex*) OA, ankylosing spondylitis: 200 mg PO daily or 100 mg PO two times per day. RA: 100 to 200 mg PO two times per day. Familial adenomatous polyposis: 400 mg PO two times per day with food. Acute pain, dysmenorrhea: 400 mg single dose, then 200 mg two times per day prn. An additional 200 mg dose may be given on day 1 if needed. JRA: Give 50 mg PO two times per day for age 2 to 17 yo and wt 10 to 25 kg, give 100 mg PO two times per day for wt greater than 25 kg. Contraindicated in sulfonamide allergy. ▶L ♀C (D in 3rd trimester) ▶? © $$$$$ Trade only: Caps 50, 100, 200, 400 mg. Anti-inflammatory, analgesic. Serious: Nephrotoxicity, hepatotoxicity, Stevens-Johnson syndrome. Frequent: Fluid retention.

> Nursing Implications | Administer PO by capsule. All risks associated with NSAIDs are present including serious cardiovascular events such as MI and stroke, clotting, serious GI problems including bleeding and perforation. Teach pt to call prescriber immediately if experiencing chest pain; breathing, vision, or speech difficulties; bloody stools, "coffee ground" vomit, or bloody sputum; swelling; and wt gain. Do not give to pt with asthma who is aspirin sensitive, pts allergic to other NSAIDs, or pts who have had recent heart surgery. Monitor pt for most common adverse reactions such as GI disturbances, headache, and infection. Pts on lithium may experience potentiation of lithium effects as a result of taking celecoxib.

Non-Steroidal Anti-Inflammatories—Salicylic Acid Derivatives

ACETYLSALICYLIC ACID   (*Ecotrin, Empirin, Halfprin, Bayer, Anacin, ZORprin*, aspirin, ✦ *Asaphen, Entrophen, Novasen*) Analgesia: 325 to 650 mg PO/PR q 4 to 6 h. Platelet aggregation inhibition: 81 to 325 mg PO daily. ▶K ♀D ▶? © $ Generic/Trade (OTC): Tabs, 325, 500 mg; chewable 81 mg; enteric-coated 81, 162 mg (Halfprin), 81, 325, 500 mg (Ecotrin), 650, 975 mg. Trade only: Tabs, controlled-release 650, 800 mg (ZORprin, Rx). Generic only (OTC): Supps 60, 120, 200, 300, 600 mg. Anti-inflammatory, antipyretic, analgesic. Inhibits prostaglandin synthesis and platelet aggregation by inactivating the enzyme cyclooxygenase. Serious: Hypersensitivity, Reye's syndrome, GI bleeding, nephrotoxicity. Frequent: Nausea, dyspepsia, tinnitus (large doses), dizziness (large doses).

> Nursing Implications | Do not use in children or adolescents with fever, flu-like symptoms, or chicken pox. Do not use in patients allergic to aspirin drugs. Do not use in patients with a history of stomach, intestinal bleeding, or other bleeding disorders. Caution in patients with history of renal or liver dysfunction, stomach conditions, congestive heart failure, asthma or allergies, bleeding or clotting disorders, gout, or nasal polyps. Use as prescribed by healthcare provider and assess for any other medications or herbal supplements that patient may be taking in conjunction with aspirin.

DIFLUNISAL   (*Dolobid*) Pain: 500 to 1000 mg initially, then 250 to 500 mg PO q 8 to 12 h. RA/OA: 500 mg to 1 g PO divided two times per day. ▶K ♀C (D in 3rd trimester) ▶– © $$$ Generic/Trade: Tabs 250, 500 mg. Anti-inflammatory, analgesic. Serious: Hypersensitivity, Reye's syndrome, GI bleeding, nephrotoxicity. Frequent: Nausea, dyspepsia.

> Nursing Implications | Administer tablets by mouth with 8 oz. of water. Patient should remain upright for 30 minutes after taking medication. Cautionary use in elderly who may be prone to GI bleeding and in patients with heart disease. Patient must report serious side effects such as: GI pain, coffee ground vomit, tarry/black stools, SOB, one sided weakness, pain in chest, slurred speech or vision changes. Cautionary use in combination with ACE inhibitors, lithium, methotrexate or warfarin. Advise patient that full effect of medication may take up to 2 weeks. Assess for allergies to aspirin compounds, asthma, diabetes, heart disease, blood disorders including clotting tendencies. Patient should not drink alcohol or smoke and should not drive or operate machinery until full effect of medication is known. Store in dark, dry place - not in a bathroom.

SALSALATE (*Salflex, Disalcid, Amigesic*) RA/OA: 3000 mg/day PO divided q 8 to 12 h. ▶K ♀C (D in 3rd trimester) ▶? © $$ Generic only: Tabs 500, 750 mg, scored. Serious: Hypersensitivity, Reye's syndrome, GI bleeding, nephrotoxicity. Frequent: Nausea, dyspepsia.

> **Nursing Implications** Administer tablet by mouth with food. Cautionary use in combination with lithium, other NSAIDS and blood thinners. Assess patient for aspirin allergy, CHG, high BP, asthma, diabetes, stroke and fluid retention problems before administering. Serious side effects are more common at higher dosages and can include GI problems: stomach ulcers, n/v, GI bleeding, tarry black stools, orthostatic hypotension, ringing in ears, heart problems including high BP and failure and kidney problems. Teach patient to avoid alcohol and smoking and not to drive or operate machinery until full effect of medication is known. Assess all other medications for possible drug interactions.

Non-Steroidal Anti-Inflammatories—Other

ARTHROTEC (diclofenac + misoprostol) OA: One 50/200 tab PO three times per day. RA: One 50/200 tab PO three to four times per day. If intolerant, may use 50/200 or 75/200 PO two times per day. Misoprostol is an abortifacient. ▶LK ♀X ▶– © $$$$$ Trade only: Tabs 50 mg/200 mcg, 75 mg/200 mcg, diclofenac/misoprostol. Anti-inflammatory/mucosal protectant, analgesic. Serious: Fetal death, nephrotoxicity, gastritis, peptic ulcer disease, GI bleeds. Frequent: Diarrhea, abdominal pain, nausea, dyspepsia.

> **Nursing Implications** Administer tablet by mouth. Cautionary use in elderly, in patients with ulcers, asthma, CV or renal disease. Advise patient to take medication on an empty stomach 1 hour before or after meals and to remain upright for at least 30 minutes. Observe for bleeding. Weigh patient for fluid retention. Stop drug if dizziness, tinnitus, GI symptoms or bleeding ulcers develop, avoid OTC analgesics. Store tablets at room temperature. Cautionary use in patients taking blood thinners, lithium, methotrexate, BP lowering drugs, antacids and angiotensin receptor blockers. If patient is also on digoxin, blood levels must be monitored. Drug should not be used by pregnant women, as misoprostol has been known to cause miscarriages and birth defects. Ⓜ

DICLOFENAC (*Voltaren, Voltaren XR, Cataflam, Flector, Zipsor, Cambia, ✦ Voltaren Rapide*) Multiple strengths; write specific product on Rx. Immediate- or delayed-release 50 mg PO two to three times per day or 75 mg PO two times per day. Extended-release (Voltaren XR): 100 to 200 mg PO daily. Patch (Flector): Apply 1 patch to painful area two times per day. Gel: 2 to 4 g to affected area four times per day. Acute migraine with or without aura: 50 mg single dose (Cambia) ▶L ♀B (D in 3rd trimester) ▶– © $$$ Generic/Trade: Tabs, immediate-release (Cataflam) 50 mg, extended-release (Voltaren XR) 100 mg. Generic only: Tabs, delayed-release 25, 50, 75 mg. Trade only: Patch (Flector), 1.3% diclofenac epolamine. Topical gel (Voltaren), 1%, 100 g tube. Trade only: Caps, liquid-filled (Zipsor) 25 mg. Trade only: Powder for oral soln (Cambia) 50 mg. Anti-inflammatory, analgesic. Serious: Hypersensitivity, GI bleeding, hepato-/nephrotoxicity. Frequent: Nausea, dyspepsia, pruritus, and dermatitis with patch and gel.

> **Nursing Implications** Cautionary use in elderly; pts with ulcers, asthma, CV, or renal disease. Observe for bleeding; take on empty stomach I h pre- or post-meal and remain upright for at least 30 minutes; weigh pt for fluid retention; stop drug if dizziness, tinnitus, GI symptoms, or bleeding ulcers; avoid OTC analgesics.

Analgesics—NSAIDs

Salicylic acid derivatives	ASA, diflunisal, salsalate, Trilisate
Propionic acids	flurbiprofen, ibuprofen, ketoprofen, naproxen, oxaprozin
Acetic acids	diclofenac, etodolac, indomethacin, ketorolac, nabumetone, sulindac, tolmetin
Fenamates	meclofenamate
Oxicams	meloxicam, piroxicam
COX-2 inhibitors	celecoxib

Note: If one class fails, consider another.

ETODOLAC Lodine Multiple strengths; write specific product on Rx. Immediate-release 200 to 400 mg PO two to three times per day. Extended-release: 400 to 1200 mg PO daily. ▶L ♀C (D in 3rd trimester) ▶– © $$$ Generic only: Caps immediate-release 200, 300 mg, Tabs immediate-release 400, 500 mg, Tabs extended-release 400, 500, 600 mg. Anti-inflammatory, analgesic. Serious: Hypersensitivity, GI bleeding, nephrotoxicity, toxic epidermal necrolysis. Frequent: Nausea, dyspepsia.

> Nursing Implications This medication is contraindicated in patients with an aspirin allergy or an allergy to another NSAID, patients who are pregnant, lactating, and those with severe renal impairment. This medication should be used cautiously in patients with impaired hearing, hepatic dysfunction, hypertension, and CV and GI problems. Increased risk of GI bleeding can occur if this medication is administered with aspirin and other anticoagulants. Patient should be advised to take this medication with food or milk, especially if GI upset results when on this medication. Patient should be advised to report black and /or tarry stools promptly to their health care provider. Patients on long term therapy should have periodic ophthalmologic examinations. Patients of child bearing age should be advised to utilize contraceptives when on this medication.

FENOPROFEN   (*Nalfon*) ▶L ♀C (D in 3rd trimester) ▶– © $ Generic/Trade: Caps 200 and 300 mg. Generic only: Tab 600 mg. Anti-inflammatory, analgesic. Serious: Hypersensitivity, GI bleeding, nephrotoxicity. Frequent: Nausea, dyspepsia.

> Nursing Implications This medication is contraindicated in patients with an aspirin allergy or an allergy to another NSAID, patients who are pregnant, lactating, and those with severe renal impairment. This medication should be used cautiously in patients with impaired hearing, hepatic dysfunction, hypertension, and CV and GI problems.Increased risk of GI bleeding can occur if this medication is administered with aspirin and other anticoagulants. Patients should be advised to take this medication with food or milk, especially if GI upset results when on this medication. Patients should be advised to report black and /or tarry stools promptly to their health care provider. Patients on long term therapy should have periodic ophthalmologic examinations. Patients of child bearing age should be advised to utilize contraceptives when on this medication.

FLURBIPROFEN   (*Ansaid*, ✦ *Froben, Froben SR*) 200 to 300 mg/day PO divided two to four times per day. ▶L ♀B (D in 3rd trimester) ▶+ © $$$ Generic/Trade: Tabs immediate-release 50, 100 mg. Serious: Hypersensitivity, GI bleeding, nephrotoxicity. Frequent: Nausea, dyspepsia.

> Nursing Implications This medication is contraindicated in patients with an aspirin allergy or an allergy to another NSAID, patients who are pregnant, lactating, and those with severe renal impairment. This medication should be used cautiously in patients with impaired hearing, hepatic dysfunction, hypertension, and CV and GI problems. Increased risk of GI bleeding can occur if this medication is administered with aspirin and other anticoagulants. Patients should be advised to take this medication with food or milk, especially if GI upset results when on this medication. Patients should be advised to report black and /or tarry stools promptly to their health care provider. Patients on long term therapy should have periodic ophthalmologic examinations. Patients of child bearing age should be advised to utilize contraceptives when on this medication.

IBUPROFEN   (*Motrin, Advil, Nuprin, Rufen, NeoProfen, Caldolor*) 200 to 800 mg PO three to four times per day. Peds older than 6 mo: 5 to 10 mg/kg PO q 6 to 8 h. GI perforation and necrotizing enterocolitis have been reported with NeoProfen. ▶L ♀B (D in 3rd trimester) ▶+ © $ OTC: Caps/Liqui-Gel Caps 200 mg. Tabs 100, 200 mg. Chewable tabs 50, 100 mg. Susp (infant gtts) 50 mg/1.25 mL (with calibrated dropper), 100 mg/5 mL. Rx Generic/Trade: Tabs 300, 400, 600, 800 mg. Vials: 400 mg/4 mL or 800 mg/8 mL. Anti-inflammatory/antipyretic, analgesic. Serious: Hypersensitivity, GI bleeding, nephrotoxicity. Frequent: Nausea, dyspepsia.

> Nursing Implications Observe patients for severe allergic reactions such as hives, urticaria, shortness of breath, tightness in the chest, and swelling of the mouth, face, lips, or tongue. Patients should be assessed for a history of GI and other bleeding as this medication would be contraindicated in such patients. The most common side effects are allergic reaction (as described above); swelling usually of the lower extremities, but may also include the hands; and gastrointestinal bleeding. Patients need to be educated not to exceed the dosing recommendations. Ideally, this medication should be taken with food and/or milk. This medication can affect the hepatic and renal systems.

INDOMETHACIN   (*Indocin, Indocin SR, Indocin IV, ✦ Indocid-P.D.A.*) Multiple strengths; write specific product on Rx. Immediate-release preparations 25 to 50 mg cap PO three times per day. Sustained-release: 75 mg cap PO one to two times per day. ▶L ♀B (D in 3rd trimester) ▶+ © $ Generic/Trade: Caps, sustained-release 75 mg. Generic only: Caps, immediate-release 25, 50 mg. Suppository 50 mg. Trade only: Oral susp 25 mg/5 mL (237 mL) Anti-inflammatory, analgesic. Prostaglandin inhibition leads to closure of a patent ductus arteriosus. Tocolytic. Serious: Hypersensitivity, GI bleeding, nephrotoxicity. During labor: Premature closure of the ductus arteriosus and fetal pulmonary hypertension, oligohydramnios, postpartum hemorrhage. Frequent: Nausea, dyspepsia, dizziness, drowsiness.

Nursing Implications This medication is contraindicated in patients with an aspirin allergy or an allergy to another NSAID, patients who are pregnant (especially during the 3rd trimester), lactating, who have proctitis or rectal bleeding, pain associated with coronary bypass graft surgery, and severe renal impairment. This medication should be used cautiously in patients with impaired hearing, hepatic dysfunction, renal dysfunction, peptic ulcers, GI bleeding, hypertension, CV and GI problems. Increased risk of GI bleeding can occur if this medication is administered with aspirin and other anticoagulants. Patients should be advised to take this medication with food or milk, especially if GI upset results when on this medication. Patients should be advised to report black and /or tarry stools promptly to their health care provider. Patients on long term therapy should have periodic ophthalmologic examinations. Patients of child bearing age should be advised to utilize contraceptives when on this medication.

KETOPROFEN   (*Orudis, Orudis KT, Actron, Oruvail, ✦ Orudis SR*) Immediate-release: 25 to 75 mg PO three to four times per day. Extended-release: 100 to 200 mg cap PO daily. ▶L ♀B (D in 3rd trimester) ▶– © $$$ OTC: Tabs, immediate-release 12.5 mg. Rx Generic only: Caps, extended-release 100, 150, 200 mg. Caps, immediate-release 25, 50, 75 mg. Serious: Hypersensitivity, GI bleeding, nephrotoxicity. Frequent: Nausea, dyspepsia.

Nursing Implications This medication is contraindicated in patients with an aspirin allergy or an allergy to another NSAID, patients who are pregnant, lactating, and those with severe renal impairment. This medication should be used cautiously in patients with impaired hearing, hepatic dysfunction, hypertension, and CV and GI problems. Increased risk of GI bleeding can occur if this medication is administered with aspirin and other anticoagulants. Patients should be advised to take this medication with food or milk, especially if GI upset results when on this medication. Patients should be advised to report black and /or tarry stools promptly to their health care provider. Patients on long term therapy should have periodic ophthalmologic examinations. Patients of child bearing age should be advised to utilize contraceptives when on this medication.

KETOROLAC   (*Toradol*) Moderately severe acute pain: 15 to 30 mg IV/IM q 6 h or 10 mg PO q 4 to 6 h prn. Combined duration IV/IM and PO is not to exceed 5 days. ▶L ♀C (D in 3rd trimester) ▶+ © $ Generic only: Tabs 10 mg. Serious: Hypersensitivity, GI bleeding, nephrotoxicity. Frequent: Nausea, dyspepsia.

Nursing Implications This medication is intended for short-term use of 3 -5 days. This medication is contraindicated in patients with an aspirin allergy or an allergy to another NSAID, patients who are pregnant, lactating, and those with severe renal impairment. This medication should be used cautiously in patients with impaired hearing, hepatic dysfunction, hypertension, and CV and GI problems. Increased risk of GI bleeding can occur if this medication is administered with aspirin and other anticoagulants. Patients should be advised to take this medication with food or milk, especially if GI upset results when on this medication. Patients should be advised to report black and /or tarry stools promptly to their health care provider. Patients on long term therapy should have periodic ophthalmologic examinations. Patients of child bearing age should be advised to utilize contraceptives when on this medication.

MECLOFENAMATE   Mild to moderate pain: 50 mg PO q 4 to 6 h prn. Max dose 400 mg/day. Menorrhagia and primary dysmenorrhea: 100 mg PO three times per day for up to 6 days. RA/OA: 200 to 400 mg/day PO divided three to four times per day. ▶L ♀B (D in 3rd trimester) ▶– © $$$ Generic only: Caps 50, 100 mg. Anti-inflammatory, analgesic. Serious: Hypersensitivity, GI bleeding, nephrotoxicity, autoimmune hemolytic anemia. Frequent: Nausea, dyspepsia.

Nursing Implications This medication is contraindicated in patients with an aspirin allergy or an allergy to another NSAID, patients who are pregnant, lactating, have coronary bypass graft surgical pain, and severe renal impairment. This medication should be used cautiously in patients with impaired hearing, hepatic dysfunction, hypertension, CV and GI problems. Increased risk of GI bleeding can occur if this medication is administered with aspirin and other anticoagulants. Patients should be advised to take this medication with food or milk, especially if GI upset results when on this medication. Patients should be advised to report black and /or tarry stools promptly to their health care provider. Patients of child bearing age should be advised to utilize contraceptives when on this medication.

MELOXICAM   (**Mobic**, ◆ **Mobicox**) RA/OA: 7.5 mg PO daily. JRA age 2 yo or older: 0.125 mg/kg PO daily. ▶L ♀C (D in 3rd trimester) ▶? © $ Generic/Trade: Tabs 7.5, 15 mg. Susp 7.5 mg/5 mL (1.5 mg/mL). Anti-inflammatory, analgesic. Serious: Hypersensitivity, GI bleeding, nephrotoxicity. Frequent: Nausea, dyspepsia.

Nursing Implications This medication is contraindicated in patients with an aspirin allergy or an allergy to another NSAID, patients who are pregnant, lactating, have coronary bypass graft surgical pain, and severe renal impairment. This medication should be used cautiously in patients with impaired hearing, hepatic dysfunction, hypertension, CV and GI problems. Increased risk of GI bleeding can occur if this medication is administered with aspirin and other anticoagulants. Patients should be advised to take this medication with food or milk, especially if GI upset results when on this medication. Patients should be advised to report black and /or tarry stools promptly to their health care provider. Patients of child bearing age should be advised to utilize contraceptives when on this medication.

NABUMETONE   (**Relafen**) RA/OA: Initial: Two 500 mg tabs (1000 mg) PO daily. May increase to 1500 to 2000 mg PO daily or divided two times per day. ▶L ♀C (D in 3rd trimester) ▶– © $$$ Generic only: Tabs 500, 750 mg. Serious: Hypersensitivity, GI bleeding, nephrotoxicity, hepatotoxicity, Stevens-Johnson syndrome, erythema multiforme, toxic epidermal necrolysis, eosinophilic pneumonia. Frequent: Nausea, dyspepsia.

Nursing Implications Observe for severe allergic reactions such as hives, urticaria, shortness of breath, tightness in the chest, and swelling of the mouth, face, lips, or tongue. Observe for signs of bleeding such as blood in a patient's vomitus, coffee ground vomitus, or tarry (dark colored) stools. There is an increased risk of life-threatening heart or circulation problems such as heart attack or stroke.

NAPROXEN   (**Naprosyn, Aleve, Anaprox, EC-Naprosyn, Naprelan, Prevacid, NapraPac**) Immediate-release: 250 to 500 mg PO two times per day. Delayed-release: 375 to 500 mg PO two times per day (do not crush or chew). Controlled-release: 750 to 1000 mg PO daily. JRA: Give 2.5 mL PO two times per day for wt 13 kg or less, give 5 mL PO two times per day for 14 to 25 kg, Give 7.5 mL PO two times per day for 26 to 38 kg. 500 mg naproxen equivalent to 550 mg naproxen sodium. ▶L ♀B (D in 3rd trimester) ▶+ © $$$ OTC Generic/Trade (Aleve): Tabs immediate-release 200 mg. OTC Trade only (Aleve): Caps, Gelcaps immediate-release 200 mg. Rx Generic/Trade: Tabs immediate-release (Naprosyn) 250, 375, 500 mg, (Anaprox) 275, 550 mg. Tabs delayed-release, enteric-coated (EC-Naprosyn) 375, 500 mg. Tabs, controlled-release (Naprelan) 375, 500, 750 mg. Susp (Naprosyn) 125 mg/5 mL. Prevacid NapraPac: 7 lansoprazole 15 mg caps packaged with 14 naproxen tabs 375 mg or 500 mg. Anti-inflammatory, analgesic. Serious: Hypersensitivity, GI bleeding, nephrotoxicity. Frequent: Nausea, dyspepsia.

Nursing Implications Observe patients for severe allergic reactions such as hives, urticaria, shortness of breath, tightness in the chest, and swelling of the mouth, face, lips, or tongue. Patients need to be advised that this medication should be taken with food and/or milk. This medication needs to be used cautiously in elderly patients. It is best not to take this medication on a routine basis. Nursing needs to observe patients for gastrointestinal side effects such as gastrointestinal bleeding—either bloody vomitus or tarry (dark colored) stools. Patients need to be advised not to take aspirin while on this medication. Pregnant woman should be advised not to take this medication as it may harm the fetus. This medication may affect the renal system so periodic monitoring of the serum creatinine and blood urea nitrogen levels are warranted. A common side effect of this medication is joint swelling, especially at the ankles.

OXAPROZIN   (*Daypro*) 1200 mg PO daily. ▶L ♀C (D in 3rd trimester) ▶– © $$$ Generic/Trade: Tabs 600 mg, trade scored. Serious: Hypersensitivity, GI bleeding, nephrotoxicity. Frequent: Nausea, dyspepsia.

> Nursing Implications. This medication is contraindicated in patients with an aspirin allergy or an allergy to another NSAID, patients who are pregnant, lactating, and those with severe renal impairment. This medication should be used cautiously in patients with impaired hearing, hepatic dysfunction, hypertension, and CV and GI problems. Increased risk of GI bleeding can occur if this medication is administered with aspirin and other anticoagulants. Patients should be advised to take this medication with food or milk, especially if GI upset results when on this medication. Patients should be advised to report black and /or tarry stools promptly to their health care provider. Patients on long term therapy should have periodic ophthalmologic examinations. Patients of child bearing age should be advised to utilize contraceptives when on this medication.

PIROXICAM   (*Feldene, Fexicam*) 20 mg PO daily. ▶L ♀B (D in 3rd trimester) ▶+ © $$$ Generic/Trade: Caps 10, 20 mg. Serious: Hypersensitivity, GI bleeding, nephrotoxicity. Frequent: Nausea, dyspepsia.

> Nursing Implications. Patients need to be observed for severe allergic reactions (rash; hives; difficulty breathing; tightness in the chest; swelling of the mouth, face, lips, or tongue). Common side effects of this medication are gastrointestinal such as nausea, vomiting, and diarrhea. This medication may lower the seizure threshold. This medication may cause edema of the hands, feet, and legs. Some patients have experienced bruising and bleeding. Nursing should observe for these signs and symptoms.

SULINDAC   (*Clinoril*) 150 to 200 mg PO two times per day. ▶L ♀B (D in 3rd trimester) ▶– © $$$ Generic/Trade: Tabs 200 mg. Generic only: Tabs 150 mg. Anti-inflammatory, analgesic. Serious: Hypersensitivity, GI bleeding, nephrotoxicity, pancreatitis. Frequent: Nausea, dyspepsia.

> Nursing Implications. This medication is contraindicated in patients with an aspirin allergy or an allergy to another NSAID, patients who are pregnant, lactating, and those with severe renal impairment. This medication should be used cautiously in patients with impaired hearing, hepatic dysfunction, hypertension, and CV and GI problems. Increased risk of GI bleeding can occur if this medication is administered with aspirin and other anticoagulants. Patients should be advised to take this medication with food or milk, especially if GI upset results when on this medication. Patients should be advised to report black and /or tarry stools promptly to their health care provider. Patients on long term therapy should have periodic ophthalmologic examinations. Patients of child bearing age should be advised to utilize contraceptives when on this medication.

TOLMETIN   (*Tolectin*) 200 to 600 mg PO three times per day. ▶L ♀C (D in 3rd trimester) ▶+ © $$$$ Generic/Trade: Tabs 200 (trade scored), 600 mg. Caps 400 mg. Anti-inflammatory, analgesic. Serious: Hypersensitivity, GI bleeding, nephrotoxicity. Frequent: Nausea, dyspepsia.

> Nursing Implications. This medication is contraindicated in patients with an aspirin allergy or an allergy to another NSAID, patients who are pregnant, lactating, and those with severe renal impairment. This medication should be used cautiously in patients with impaired hearing, hepatic dysfunction, hypertension, and CV and GI problems. Increased risk of GI bleeding can occur if this medication is administered with aspirin and other anticoagulants. Patients should be advised to take this medication with food or milk, especially if GI upset results when on this medication. Patients should be advised to report black and /or tarry stools promptly to their health care provider. Patients on long term therapy should have periodic ophthalmologic examinations. Patients of child bearing age should be advised to utilize contraceptives when on this medication.

Opioid Agonist-Antagonists

BUPRENORPHINE   (*Buprenex, Butrans, Subutex*) Analgesia: 0.3 to 0.6 mg IV/IM q 6 h prn. Treatment of opioid dependence (must undergo special training and be registered to prescribe for this indication): Induction 8 mg SL on day 1, 16 mg SL on day 2. Maintenance: 16 mg SL daily. Can individualize to range of 4 to 24 mg SL daily. Moderate to severe chronic pain: 5 to 20 mcg/h patch changed q 7 days. ▶L ♀C ▶– ©III $ IV, $$$$$ SL Generic/Trade (Subutex): SL Tabs 2, 8 mg. Trade only (Butrans): transdermal patches 5, 10, 20 mcg/h. Opioid agonist-antagonist analgesic. Serious: Respiratory depression, hepatitis, hypersensitivity. Frequent: Sedation, dizziness, nausea, headache, constipation.

> **Nursing Implications** This is a Schedule III opioid agonist medication that is utilized for chronic pain management as well as for relapse prevention in opioid dependent patients. Patients need to be monitored during the induction phase of this medication. Once the effective dose schedule is established, this medication is either administered once daily or BID (split dose manner). The safety profile of this medication is much better than other opioid medications. This medication is utilized in OBOT (Office Based Opioid Treatment) centers. This medication is also available as a delayed patch (Butrans) for chronic pain management. The most common adverse effects of this medication are respiratory depression and constipation.

NALBUPHINE (*Nubain*) 10 to 20 mg IV/IM/SC q 3 to 6 h prn. ▶LK ♀? ▶? © $ Serious: Respiratory depression. Frequent: Sedation, dizziness, nausea.

> **Nursing Implications** Patients need to be monitored when this medication is administered. Vital signs inclusive of an accurate respiratory rate should be taken prior to and after the administration of this medication. A validated pain assessment scale should be utilized and documented prior to and after administration of this medication. Patients need to be observed for potential abuse of this medication as it can create dependency problems. The most common adverse effects of this medication are respiratory depression and constipation.

PENTAZOCINE (*Talwin NX*) 30 mg IV/IM q 3 to 4 h prn (Talwin). 1 tab PO q 3 to 4 h. (Talwin NX = 50 mg pentazocine/0.5 mg naloxone). ▶LK ♀C ▶? ©IV $$$ Generic/Trade: Tabs 50 mg with 0.5 mg naloxone, trade scored. Opioid agonist-antagonist analgesic. Serious: Respiratory depression, seizures, hallucinations, hypersensitivity. Frequent: Sedation, dizziness, nausea.

> **Nursing Implications** Patients need to be monitored when this medication is administered. Vital signs inclusive of an accurate respiratory rate should be taken prior to and after the administration of this medication. A validated pain assessment scale should be utilized and documented prior to and after administration of this medication. Patients need to be observed for potential abuse of this medication as it can create dependency problems. The most common adverse effects of this medication are respiratory depression and constipation.

Opioid Agonists

CODEINE 0.5 to 1 mg/kg up to 15 to 60 mg PO/IM/IV/SC q 4 to 6 h. Do not use IV in children. ▶LK ♀C ▶– ©II $$ Generic only: Tabs 15, 30, 60 mg. Oral soln: 15 mg/5 mL. Opioid agonist analgesic. Serious: Respiratory depression/arrest. Frequent: N/V, constipation, sedation.

> **Nursing Implications** Monitor respiratory rate and density of respirations, notify prescriber if respiratory rate decreases to 10 breaths/min or if shortness of breath occurs. Assess for dependence. Teach pt to consume plenty of fluids and increase fiber-rich foods; monitor for hypostatic response.

FENTANYL (*Duragesic, Actiq, Fentora, Sublimaze, IONSYS, Abstral, Subsys, Lazanda*) Transdermal (Duragesic): 1 patch q 72 h (some with chronic pain may require q 48 h dosing). May wear more than 1 patch to achieve the correct analgesic effect. Transmucosal lozenge (Actiq) for breakthrough cancer pain: 200 to 1600 mcg, goal is 4 lozenges on a stick per day in conjunction with long-acting opioid. Buccal tab (Fentora) for breakthrough cancer pain: 100 to 800 mcg, titrated to pain relief. Buccal soluble film (Onsolis) for breakthrough cancer pain: 200 to 1200 mcg, titrated to pain relief. Sublingual tab (Abstral) for breakthrough cancer pain: 100 mcg, may repeat once after 30 minutes. Sublingual spray (Subsys) for breakthrough cancer pain: 100 mcg, may repeat once after 30 minutes. Nasal spray (Lazanda) for breakthrough cancer pain: 100 mcg. Adult analgesia/procedural sedation: 50 to 100 mcg slow IV over 1 to 2 min; carefully titrate to effect. Analgesia: 50 to 100 mcg IM q 1 to 2 h prn. ▶L ♀C ▶+ ©II $$$$$$ Generic/Trade: Transdermal patches 12, 25, 50, 75, 100 mcg/h. Actiq lozenges on a stick, berry flavored 200, 400, 600, 800, 1200, 1600 mcg. Trade only: IONSYS: Iontophoretic transdermal system: 40 mcg fentanyl per activation; max 6 doses/h. Max per system is eighty 40 mcg doses over 24 h. Trade only: (Fentora) buccal tab 100, 200, 300, 400, 600, 800 mcg. Trade only: (Onsolis) buccal soluble film 200, 400, 600, 800, 1200 mcg in child-resistant, protective foil. Trade only: (Abstral) sublingual tab: 100, 200, 300, 400, 600, 800 mcg, packs of 12 or 32 (32 only for 600 and 800 mcg). Trade only: (Subsys) sublingual spray: 100, 200, 400, 600, 800 mcg blister packs in cartons of 6, 14, and 28. Trade only: (Lazanda) nasal spray: 100, 400 mcg/spray, 8 sprays/bottle, cartons of 1 or 4. Opioid agonist analgesic. Serious: Respiratory depression/arrest, chest wall rigidity. Frequent: N/V, constipation, sedation, skin irritation, dental decay with Actiq.

FENTANYL TRANSDERMAL DOSE (Dosing based on ongoing morphine requirement.)

Morphine (IV/IM)	Morphine (PO)	Transdermal fentanyl
10–22 mg/day	60–134 mg/day	25 mcg/h
23–37 mg/day	135–224 mg/day	50 mcg/h
38–52 mg/day	225–314 mg/day	75 mcg/h
53–67 mg/day	315–404 mg/day	100 mcg/h

For higher morphine doses, see product insert for transdermal fentanyl equivalencies.

Nursing Implications Administer intact skin patch to dry, clean flat surface of skin. A potent, Schedule II drug with high abuse potential and risk of overdose. Use only in opioid-tolerant pts. Monitor pt for hypoventilation even at 20 to 72 h after initial administration and beyond. Pts should be assessed for prior substance abuse. Site of patch should not be exposed to heat such as hot baths, sun bathing, heat lamps, electric blankets. Monitor pt for adverse reactions such as rapid HR, vision problems, loss of wt, and edema. Check all other drugs pts is taking because fatal respiratory depression can occur. Teach pt that if patch falls off, a new one must be applied at a different site. Edges of patch may be taped if adhesion is a problem. Pt must avoid alcohol or other CNS depressants. Drug must be weaned.

HYDROMORPHONE　(*Dilaudid, Dilaudid-5, Exalgo,* ✦ *Hydromorph Contin*) Adults: 2 to 4 mg PO q 4 to 6 h. 0.5 to 2 mg IM/SC or slow IV q 4 to 6 h. 3 mg PR q 6 to 8 h. Titrate dose as high as necessary to relieve cancer or nonmalignant pain where chronic opioids are necessary. Peds age 12 yo or younger: 0.03 to 0.08 mg/kg PO q 4 to 6 h prn or give 0.015 mg/kg/dose IV q 4 to 6 h prn. Controlled-release tabs: 8 to 64 mg daily. ▶L ♀C ▶? ©II $$ Generic/Trade: Tabs 2, 4, 8 mg (8 mg trade scored). Oral soln 5 mg/5 mL. Suppository: 3 mg. Controlled-release tabs (Exalgo): 8, 12, 16 mg. Opioid agonist analgesic. Serious: Respiratory depression/arrest. Frequent: N/V, constipation, sedation.

Nursing Implications Observe patients for signs and symptoms of allergic reactions such as hives, urticaria, shortness of breath, tightness in the chest, and swelling of the mouth, face, lips, throat, or tongue; unusual hoarseness. The most significant system to observe is the respiratory system as narcotic medication can depress respiratory function. Improper dosing can result in accidental overdose and possible death. Narcotic use for prolonged time periods can cause constipation. Neonatal absintence syndrome may result from prolonged use of narcotics during pregnancy.

LEVORPHANOL　(*Levo-Dromoran*) 2 mg PO q 6 to 8 h prn. ▶L ♀C ▶? ©II $$$$ Generic only: Tabs 2 mg, scored. Serious: Respiratory depression/arrest. Frequent: N/V, constipation, sedation.

Nursing Implications Patients need to be monitored when this medication is administered. Vital signs inclusive of an accurate respiratory rate should be taken prior to and after the administration of this medication. A validated pain assessment scale should be utilized and documented prior to and after administration of this medication. Patients need to be observed for potential abuse of this medication as it can create dependency problems. The most common adverse effects of this medication are respiratory depression and constipation.

MEPERIDINE　(*Demerol,* pethidine) 1 to 1.8 mg/kg up to 150 mg IM/SC/PO or slow IV q 3 to 4 h. 75 mg meperidine IV/IM/SC is equivalent to 300 mg meperidine PO. ▶LK ♀C but + ▶+ ©II $$$ Generic/Trade: Tabs 50 (trade scored), 100 mg. Syrup 50 mg/5 mL (trade banana flavored). Opioid agonist analgesic. Serious: Respiratory depression/arrest, seizures, anaphylaxis. Frequent: N/V, constipation, sedation.

Nursing Implications Patients need to be monitored when this medication is administered. Vital signs inclusive of an accurate respiratory rate should be taken prior to and after the administration of this medication. A validated pain assessment scale should be utilized and documented prior to and after administration of this medication. Patients need to be observed for potential abuse of this medication as it can create dependency problems. The most common adverse effects of this medication are respiratory depression and constipation.

OPIOID EQUIVALENCY*

Opioid	PO	IV/SC/IM	Opioid	PO	IV/SC/IM
buprenorphine	n/a	0.3–0.4 mg	meperidine	300 mg	75 mg
butorphanol	n/a	2 mg	methadone	5–15 mg	2.5–10 mg
codeine	130 mg	75 mg	morphine	30 mg	10 mg
fentanyl	?	0.1 mg	nalbuphine	n/a	10 mg
hydrocodone	20 mg	n/a	oxycodone	20 mg	n/a
hydromorphone	7.5 mg	1.5 mg	oxymorphone	10 mg	1 mg
levorphanol	4 mg	2 mg	pentazocine	50 mg	30 mg

*Approximate equianalgesic doses as adapted from the 2003 American Pain Society (www.ampainsoc.org) guidelines and the 1992 AHCPR guidelines. Not available = "n/a." See drug entries for starting doses. Many recommend initially using lower than equivalent doses when switching between different opioids. IV doses should be titrated slowly with appropriate monitoring. All PO dosing is with immediate-release preparations. Individualize all dosing, especially in the elderly, children, and in those with chronic pain, opioid naïve, or hepatic/renal insufficiency.

METHADONE (*Diskets, Dolophine, Methadose, ✚ Metadol*) Severe pain in opioid-tolerant patients: 2.5 to 10 mg IM/SC/PO q 3 to 4 h prn. Titrate dose as high as necessary to relieve cancer or nonmalignant pain where chronic opioids are necessary. Opioid dependence: 20 to 100 mg PO daily. Treatment longer than 3 weeks is maintenance and only permitted in approved treatment programs. ▶L ♀C ▶? ©II $ Generic/Trade: Tabs 5, 10 mg. Dispersible tabs 40 mg (for opioid dependence only). Oral concentrate (Intensol): 10 mg/mL. Generic only: Oral soln 5, 10 mg/5 mL. Opioid agonist analgesic. Serious: Respiratory depression/cardiorespiratory arrest, dependence, withdrawal, seizures, bradycardia. Frequent: N/V, constipation, sedation, dry mouth, urinary retention, rash.

> **Nursing Implications** This medication is primarily utilized as a relapse prevention medication for opioid dependency. Methadone can also be utilized for chronic pain. This medication has a long half-life and a cumulative effect. Induction dosing should be low and slow and should always be guided by a clinical opiate withdrawal scale. At high dosages (above 100 milligrams) this medication may cause QT abnormalities and patients may develop lethal rhythms such as torsade's de pointes.

MORPHINE (*MS Contin, Kadian, Avinza, Roxanol, Oramorph SR, MSIR, DepoDur, ✚ Statex, M.O.S., Doloral*) Controlled-release tabs (MS Contin, Oramorph SR): Start at 30 mg PO q 8 to 12 h. Controlled-release caps (Kadian): 20 mg PO q 12 to 24 h. Extended-release caps (Avinza): Start at 30 mg PO daily. Do not break, chew, or crush MS Contin or Oramorph SR. Kadian and Avinza caps may be opened and sprinkled in applesauce for easier administration; however, the pellets should not be crushed or chewed. Give 0.1 to 0.2 mg/kg up to 15 mg IM/SC or slow IV q 4 h. Titrate dose as high as necessary to relieve cancer or nonmalignant pain where chronic opioids are necessary. ▶LK ♀C ▶+ ©II $$$$ Generic/Trade: Tabs, immediate-release 15, 30 mg. Oral soln: 10 mg/5 mL, 20 mg/5 mL, 20 mg/mL (concentrate). Rectal supps 5, 10, 20, 30 mg. Controlled-release tabs (MS Contin) 15, 30, 60, 100, 200 mg. Trade only: Controlled-release caps (Kadian) 10, 20, 30, 50, 60, 80, 100, 200 mg, Controlled-release tabs (Oramorph SR) 15, 30, 60, 100 mg. Extended-release caps (Avinza) 30, 45, 60, 75, 90, 120 mg. Opioid agonist analgesic. Serious: Respiratory depression/arrest. Frequent: N/V, constipation, sedation, hypotension.

> **Nursing Implications** Patients need to be monitored when this medication is administered. Vital signs inclusive of an accurate respiratory rate should be taken prior to and after the administration of this medication. A validated pain assessment scale should be utilized and documented prior to and after administration of this medication. Patients need to be observed for potential abuse of this medication as it can create dependency problems. The most common adverse effects of this medication are respiratory depression and constipation.

OXYCODONE (*Roxicodone, OxyContin, Percolone, OxyIR, OxyFAST, Oxecta, ✚ Endocodone, Supeudol*) Immediate-release preparations: 5 mg PO q 4 to 6 h prn. Controlled-release (OxyContin): 10 to 40 mg PO q 12 h (no supporting data for shorter dosing intervals for controlled-release tabs). Titrate dose as high as necessary to relieve cancer or nonmalignant pain where chronic opioids are necessary. Do not break, chew, or crush controlled-release preparations or Oxecta. ▶L ♀B ▶– ©II $$$$$ Generic/Trade: Immediate-release: Tabs 5 mg, scored. Caps 5 mg. Tabs 15, 30 mg. Oral soln 5 mg/5 mL. Oral concentrate 20 mg/mL. Generic only: Immediate-release tabs 10, 20 mg. Trade only: Immediate-release tabs: 7.5 mg. Controlled-release tabs: 10, 15, 20, 30, 40, 60, 80 mg. Opioid agonist analgesic. Serious: Respiratory depression/arrest. Frequent: N/V, constipation, sedation.

> Nursing Implications This medication is a controlled, dangerous substance with a high abuse potential. This medication is habit forming with continued use and may create a mental and physical dependence. The most common side effects to this medication are respiratory depression (especially in overdose) and constipation. Other side effects include dizziness, lightheadedness, and fainting. Patients should be educated to drink plenty of fluids such as water, and to increase the amount of fiber in their diet. Signs and symptoms of withdrawal from this medication include abdominal pain and cramping, nausea, general malaise, increased lacrimation, piloerection, tremors, sweating, and trouble sleeping.

Opioid Analgesic Combinations

NOTE: *Refer to individual components for further information. May cause drowsiness and/or sedation, which may be enhanced by alcohol and other CNS depressants. Opioids, carisoprodol, and butalbital may be habit forming. Avoid exceeding 4 g/day of acetaminophen in combination products. Caution people who drink 3 or more alcoholic drinks/day to limit acetaminophen use to 2.5 g/day due to additive liver toxicity. Opioids commonly cause constipation; concurrent laxatives are recommended. All opioids are pregnancy class D if used for prolonged periods or in high doses at term.*

ANEXSIA (hydrocodone + acetaminophen) Multiple strengths; write specific product on Rx. 1 tab PO q 4 to 6 h prn. ▶LK ♀C ▶– ©III $$ Generic/Trade: Tabs 5/325, 5/500, 7.5/325, 7.5/650, 10/750 mg hydrocodone/mg acetaminophen, scored. Serious: Respiratory depression/arrest, hepatotoxicity. Frequent: N/V, constipation, sedation.

> Nursing Implications To avoid side effects, instruct patient to take with milk or food.

FIORICET WITH CODEINE (acetaminophen + butalbital + caffeine + codeine) 1 to 2 caps PO q 4 h prn. Max 6 caps per day. ▶LK ♀C ▶– ©III $$$ Generic/Trade: Caps 325 mg acetaminophen/50 mg butalbital/40 mg caffeine/30 mg codeine. Serious: Respiratory depression/arrest, hepatotoxicity. Frequent: N/V, constipation, sedation.

> Nursing Implications Patients need to be monitored when this medication is administered. Vital signs inclusive of an accurate respiratory rate should be taken prior to and after the administration of this medication. A validated pain assessment scale should be utilized and documented prior to and after administration of this medication. Patients need to be observed for potential abuse of this medication as it can create dependency problems. The most common adverse effects of this medication are respiratory depression and constipation. **Ⓜ**

PERCOCET (oxycodone + acetaminophen, ✦ *Percocet-Demi, Oxycocet, Endocet*) Multiple strengths; write specific product on Rx. 1 to 2 tabs PO q 4 to 6 h prn (2.5/325 and 5/325). 1 tab PO q 4 to 6 h prn (7.5/500 and 10/650). ▶L ♀C ▶– ©II $ Trade only: Tabs 2.5/325 oxycodone/acetaminophen. Generic/Trade: Tabs 5/325, 7.5/325, 7.5/500, 10/325, 10/650 mg. Generic only: 2.5/300, 5/300, 7.5/300, 10/300, 2.5/400, 5/400, 7.5/400, 10/400, 10/500 mg. Serious: Respiratory depression/arrest, hepatotoxicity. Frequent: N/V, constipation, sedation.

> Nursing Implications This medication is a controlled, dangerous substance with a high abuse potential. This medication is habit forming with continued use and may create a mental and physical dependence. The most common side effects to this medication are respiratory depression (especially in overdose) and constipation. Other side effects include dizziness, lightheadedness, and fainting. Patients should be educated to drink plenty of fluids such as water, and to increase the amount of fiber in their diet. Signs and symptoms of withdrawal from this medication include abdominal pain and cramping, nausea, general malaise, increased lacrimation, piloerection, tremors, sweating, and trouble sleeping. Patients should be advised not to drink alcohol when taking this medication as alcohol may potentiate the side effects of this medication.

SOMA COMPOUND WITH CODEINE (carisoprodol + acetylsalicylic acid + codeine) Moderate to severe musculoskeletal pain: 1 to 2 tabs PO four times per day prn. ▶L ♀D ▶– ©III $$$ Generic/Trade: Tabs 200 mg carisoprodol/325 mg aspirin/16 mg codeine. Combination analgesic. Serious: Respiratory depression/arrest, hypersensitivity, Reye's syndrome, GI bleeding, nephrotoxicity, idiosyncratic reaction with angioedema, hypotension, and anaphylactoid shock. Frequent: N/V, dyspepsia, constipation, sedation.

> Nursing Implications Patients need to be monitored when this medication is administered. Vital signs inclusive of an accurate respiratory rate should be taken prior to and after the administration of this medication. A validated pain assessment scale should be utilized and documented prior to and after administration of this medication. Patients need to be observed for potential abuse of this medication as it can create dependency problems. The most common adverse effects of this medication are respiratory depression and constipation. Ⓜ

Other Analgesics

TAPENTADOL (*Nucynta, Nucynta ER*) Moderate to severe acute pain: Immediate replease: 50 to 100 mg PO q 4 to 6 h prn, max 600 mg/day. Moderate to severe chronic pain: Extended release: 50 to 250 mg PO twice daily. Adjust dose in elderly, renal and hepatic dysfunction. Avoid in opioid-dependent patients. Seizures may occur with concurrent antidepressants or seizure disorder. ▶LK ♀C ▶– ©II $$$$ Trade only: Immediate release: Tabs 50, 75, 100 mg. Extended release: Tabs 50, 100, 150, 200, 250 mg. Opioid agonist/norepinephrine reuptake inhibitor. Serious: Seizures, anaphylactoid reactions, respiratory depression. Frequent: Nausea, dizziness, vomiting, somnolence.

> Nursing Implications Patients should be advised to take this medication with a full glass of water, with or without food. Patients need to be aware that this medication can not be crushed or mixed with another liquid as death may result. This medication may impair thinking and reaction time. Patients need to be aware that alcohol is contraindicated as side effects can be fatal.

TRAMADOL (*Ultram, Ultram ER, Ryzolt*) Moderate to moderately severe pain: 50 to 100 mg PO q 4 to 6 h prn, max 400 mg/day. Chronic pain, extended-release: 100 to 300 mg PO daily. Adjust dose in elderly, renal and hepatic dysfunction. Avoid in opioid-dependent patients. Seizures may occur with concurrent serotonergic agents or seizure disorder. ▶KL ♀C ▶– © $$$ Generic/Trade: Tabs, immediate-release 50 mg. Trade only (Ultram ER, Ryzolt): Extended-release tabs 100, 200, 300 mg. Opioid agonist/ norepinephrine and serotonin reuptake inhibitor. Serious: Seizures, anaphylactoid reactions. Frequent: Constipation, nausea, somnolence.

> Nursing Implications Do not administer with sedatives, narcotics, or sleeping medicines. Do not use in patients with suicidal thoughts or history of suicidal actions, diabetes, liver, heart, kidney, COPD, siezures, or breathing issues. People allergic to codeine or other opioids should not take tramadol. Patients should be advised not to drink alcohol when taking this medication. Patients on carbamazepine, nefazodone, sodium oxybate (GHB), or a thioxanthene should not take tramadol. Patients who have a history of opioid dependency should not be prescribed tramadol as this may trigger relapse in such patients. This medication should not be used in pregnancy. There may be an increased risk of seizures in patients with a low seizure threshold.

ANESTHESIA

Anesthetics and Sedatives

DEXMEDETOMIDINE (*Precedex*) ICU sedation less than 24 h: Load 1 mcg/kg over 10 min followed by infusion 0.2 to 0.7 mcg/kg/h titrated to desired sedation endpoint. Beware of bradycardia and hypotension. ▶L ♀C ▶? © $$$$ Alpha-2 adrenergic agonist with sedative properties. Serious: Bradycardia, heart block, hypotension. Frequent: Sedation.

> Nursing Implications Administer by continuous IV infusion. Cautionary use in elderly pts or in those with liver disease. Do not administer with other drugs. Store at room temp. Monitor pt for serious reactions such as low BP, slow HR, or cardiac arrest. Transient hypertension may occur at loading dose. Monitor pt for GI disturbances, fever, or dry mouth. Precedex given in combination with other sedatives, opioids, or hypnotics may increase drug effects; dosages should be carefully monitored if coadministered.

ETOMIDATE (*Amidate*) Induction: Give 0.3 mg/kg IV. ▶L ♀C ▶? © $ Nonbarbiturate hypnotic without analgesic properties. Serious: Respiratory depression, hypotension, adrenal suppression. Frequent: Myoclonus, N/V.

Nursing Implications Should be given only by clinicians experienced in administering anesthetics. Solution must be clear; container undamaged. Discard unused amidate. Avoid injecting rapidly. Assess for venous pain post-administration, high or low BP, rapid or slow HR or arrhythmias, involuntary muscle movements, nausea and vomiting, problems breathing, and anaphylaxis. In elderly, closely monitor kidney function and cardiac symptoms.

MIDAZOLAM (*Versed*) Adult sedation/anxiolysis: 5 mg or 0.07 mg/kg IM; or 1 mg IV slowly q 2 to 3 min up to 5 mg. Peds: 0.25 to 1 mg/kg to max of 20 mg PO, or 0.1 to 0.15 mg/kg IM. IV route (6 mo to 5 yo): initial dose 0.05 to 0.1 mg/kg IV, then titrated to max 0.6 mg/kg. IV route (6 to 12 yo): initial dose 0.025 to 0.05 mg/kg IV, then titrated to max 0.4 mg/kg. Monitor for respiratory depression. ▶LK ♀D ▶–©IV $ Generic only: Oral liquid 2 mg/mL. Short-acting benzodiazepine sedative. Serious: Respiratory depression. Frequent: Sedation.

Nursing Implications Observe patients for severe allergic reactions such as hives, urticaria, shortness of breath, tightness in the chest, and swelling of the mouth, face, lips, or tongue. Common side effects include blurred vision; changes in blood pressure, breathing, and heart rate; coughing; dizziness; drowsiness; dry mouth; headache; hiccups; low blood pressure (children); nausea; short-term memory loss; slurred speech; and vomiting. Patients need to be educated about not drinking alcoholic beverages as this may exacerbate the sedative effects of this medication and can be potentially harmful.

PENTOBARBITAL (*Nembutal*) Pediatric sedation: 1 to 6 mg/kg IV, adjusted in increments of 1 to 2 mg/kg to desired effect, or 2 to 6 mg/kg IM, max 100 mg. ▶LK ♀D ▶? ©II $$ Serious: Respiratory depression, blood dyscrasias, anemia, thrombocytopenia, Stevens-Johnson syndrome, angioedema, dependence, withdrawal reactions. Frequent: Drowsiness, fatigue, N/V bradycardia, paradoxical CNS excitation.

Nursing Implications Administer by *slow* IV infusion or IM injection into large muscle. Monitor for severe allergic reaction/anaphylaxis. Drug dependence may occur with prolonged use of barbiturates and is similar to alcohol dependence. Call prescriber if pt experiences breathing problems; slow, weak pulse/HR; faintness; or confusion. Sleepiness/drowsiness is the most common adverse reaction. Pt should be protected from falls. If pt becomes dependent a planned withdrawal regimen must be employed. Assess pt for use of anticoagulants, steroids, griseofulvin, doxycycline, phenytoin, other CNS depressants, MAOIs, and steroidal hormones since barbiturates may interfere with the actions of these drugs.

PROPOFOL (*Diprivan*) Induction dose: 40 mg IV q 10 seconds until induction (2 to 2.5 mg/kg). ICU ventilator sedation: Infusion 5 to 50 mcg/kg/min. Deep sedation: 1 mg/kg IV over 20 to 30 seconds. Repeat 0.5 mg/kg IV prn. ▶L ♀B ▶– © $$$ Nonbarbiturate hypnotic without analgesic properties. Serious: Respiratory depression, hypotension, hypersensitivity. Frequent: Injection site pain, sedation.

Nursing Implications Observe for severe allergic reactions such as hives, urticaria, shortness of breath, tightness in the chest, and swelling of the mouth, face, lips, or tongue. This medication needs to be administered by an anesthesiologist and/or a Certified Registered Nurse Anesthetist. This medication is administered by IV drip. Patients need to be on a cardiac monitor, pulse oximetry and continuous wave form capnography that measures end tidal CO2. Nursing's role is to assist anesthesia in the monitoring of patients receiving this medication and to make certain that the IV remains patent. As this medication depresses respiratory function appropriate resuscitation equipment should always be available.

REMIFENTANIL (*Ultiva*) ▶L ♀C ▶? ©II $$ Serious: Respiratory depression, hypotension, bradycardia, chest wall rigidity, opiate dependence, hypersensitivity. Frequent: Sedation, N/V.

Nursing Implications Observe for signs and symptoms of severe allergic reactions such as hives, urticaria, shortness of breath, tightness in the chest, and swelling of the mouth, face, lips, or tongue. Do not use Ultiva in patients with a history of substance abuse or dependence problems or heart or breathing problems. Alcohol, amiodarone, benzodiazepines, cimetidine, and Naltrexone should not be used with Ultiva because of side effects. This medication is a controlled substance and may lead to an increase in tolerance, dependency, and abuse. Observe for signs and symptoms of withdrawal such as anxiety, diarrhea, fever, rhinorrhea, piloerection, nausea, vomiting, tremors, hallucinations both auditory and visual, and trouble sleeping.

Local Anesthetics

BUPIVACAINE (*Marcaine, Sensorcaine*) Local and regional anesthesia. ▶LK ♀C ▶? © $ 0.25%, 0.5%, 0.75%, all with or without epinephrine. Amide local anesthetic. Serious: Seizures, cardiovascular depression, bradycardia, hypersensitivity, methemoglobinemia. Frequent: None.

> Nursing Implications See drug insert.

LIDOCAINE—LOCAL ANESTHETIC (*Xylocaine*) 0.5 to 1% injection with and without epinephrine. ▶LK ♀B ▶? © $ 0.5, 1, 1.5, 2%. With epi: 0.5, 1, 1.5, 2%. Amide local anesthetic. Serious: Seizures, cardiovascular depression, bradycardia, hypersensitivity, methemoglobinemia. Frequent: None.

> Nursing Implications This medication has various uses including: use as an agent to anesthetize soft tissues prior to suturing a wound and as a cardiac antidysrhythmic medication for ventricular dysrhythmias. The product literature on this medication should be reviewed carefully prior to use. This medication can be administered at half the initial calculated dosage every 3 to 5 minutes not to exceed a total dosage of 3 milligrams per kilogram of body weight. A maintenance drip usually follows IV bolus dose administration. Each hospital's pharmacy and therapeutics committee should have established guidelines for maintenance drips. Overdose situations can result in seizures, coma and death.

ROPIVACAINE (*Naropin*) ▶LK ♀B ▶? © $ 0.2, 0.5, 0.75, 1%. Amide local anesthetic. Serious: Seizures, cardiovascular depression, bradycardia, hypersensitivity, methemoglobinemia. Frequent: None.

> Nursing Implications Administered for surgical, labor, and postsurgical pain by epidural or nerve block.

Neuromuscular Blockers

ROCURONIUM (*Zemuron*) Paralysis: 0.6 mg/kg IV. Duration 30 min. Rapid-sequence intubation: 0.6 to 1.2 mg/kg IV ▶L ♀B ▶? © $$ Nondepolarizing skeletal muscle relaxant. Serious: Apnea, bronchospasm. Frequent: Apnea.

> Nursing Implications Administer by IV infusion only by clinicians trained in uses, actions, and complications of the drug. Notify prescriber if pt experiences increased or uneven HR, breathing problems, muscle weakness, or inability to move. Assess pt for history of liver, kidney, or heart disease or circulation problems. Do not infuse with the many drugs with which Zemuron is incompatible. Check label before administering. Most common adverse reaction is change in BP. Analgesia and concurrent sedation are needed. Patients need to have cardiac and respiratory function monitored.

VECURONIUM (*Norcuron*) Paralysis: 0.08 to 0.1 mg/kg IV. Duration 15 to 30 min. ▶LK ♀C ▶? © $ Nondepolarizing skeletal muscle relaxant. Serious: Apnea. Frequent: Apnea.

> Nursing Implications This medication is administered intravenously. This medication should be administered by an anesthesiologist or certified registered nurse anesthetist in a monitored situation inclusive of continuous wave-form capnography for measurement of end-tidal carbon dioxide when the patient is intubated and continuous cardiac monitoring. Proper life support personnel with equipment on hand in case of an emergency. Neuroleptic malignant syndrome may result from use of this medication. Signs and symptoms of this condition include increased body heat, rigid muscles, altered mentation, lack of response to surroundings, cardiac dysrhythmias, and sweating. This can be a fatal condition and is a medical emergency situation. This medication contains benzyl alcohol, which is a preservative and should not be utilized in newborns.

ANTIMICROBIALS

Aminoglycosides

NOTE: *See also Dermatology and Ophthalmology. Can cause nephrotoxicity, ototoxicity.*

AMIKACIN 15 mg/kg/day (up to 1500 mg/day) IM/IV divided q 8 to 12 h. Peak 20 to 35 mcg/mL, trough is less than 5 mcg/mL. Alternative 15 mg/kg IV q 24 h. ▶K ♀D ▶? © $$$ Inhibits bacterial protein synthesis by interfering with function of ribosomal 30S subunit. Bactericidal. Serious and frequent: Nephrotoxicity, neuromuscular blockade, ototoxicity. Serious and rare: Vestibular toxicity.

Monitor renal function before and daily during therapy; monitor for: tinnitus, vertigo, and muscle weakness during prolonged therapy. Promote reporting of symptoms such as hearing changes, ringing in ears, headache, nausea, vomiting, and changes in urination. Maintain hydration. Avoid in patients with hypersensitivity to aminoglycosides. Avoid in patients with potent diuretics.

TOBRAMYCIN (***TOBI***) Adults: 3 to 5 mg/kg/day IM/IV divided q 8 h. Peak 5 to 10 mcg/mL, trough is less than 2 mcg/mL. Alternative 5 to 7 mg/kg IV q 24 h. Peds: 2 to 2.5 mg/kg q 8 h. Cystic fibrosis (TOBI): 300 mg nebulized two times per day 28 days on, then 28 days off. ▶K ♀D ▶? © Trade only: TOBI 300 mg ampules for nebulizer. Inhibits bacterial protein synthesis by interfering with function of ribosomal 30S subunit. Bactericidal. Serious and frequent: Nephrotoxicity, neuromuscular blockade, ototoxicity. Serious and rare: Vestibular toxicity.

Administer by inhalation through nebulizer. Call prescriber if allergic reaction, hearing problems, dizziness, breathing problems, or muscle weakness occurs. Pt should be assessed preadministration and prescriber called if pt has a history of hearing problems, Parkinson's, kidney disorders, or myasthenia gravis. Teach patient to inhale for 15 minutes through hand-held nebulizer for 28 days ONLY then 28 days off and on again; store out of direct light and in refrigerator. Pt may experience ringing in ears and voice alterations while on drug.

Antifungal Agents—Azoles

CLOTRIMAZOLE (***Mycelex***, ✦ ***Canesten, Clotrimaderm***) Oral troches 5 times per day for 14 days. ▶L ♀C ▶? © $$$$ Generic/Trade: Oral troches 10 mg. Serious: None.

Available OTC. Promote following prescriber's, or manufacturer's, recommendations. Promote reporting any allergic reaction.

FLUCONAZOLE (***Diflucan***) Vaginal candidiasis: 150 mg PO single dose ($). All other dosing regimens IV/PO. Oropharyngeal candidiasis: 100 to 200 mg daily for 7 to 14 days. Esophageal candidiasis: 200 to 400 mg daily for 14 to 21 days. Candidemia: 800 mg on first day, then 400 mg daily. Cryptococcal meningitis (per IDSA guideline): Amphotericin B preferably in combo with flucytosine for at least 2 weeks (induction), followed by fluconazole 400 mg PO once daily for 8 weeks (consolidation), then chronic suppression with fluconazole 200 mg PO once daily until immune system reconstitution. Peds: Oropharyngeal candidiasis: 6 mg/kg on first day, then 3 mg/kg daily for 7 to 14 days. Esophageal candidiasis: 12 mg/kg on first day, then 6 mg/kg daily for 14 to 21 days. Systemic candidiasis; cryptococcal meningitis in AIDS: 12 mg/kg on first day, then 6 to 12 mg/kg daily. ▶K ♀C for single-dose treatment of vaginal candidiasis, D for all other indications ▶+ © $$$$ Generic/Trade: Tabs 50, 100, 150, 200 mg. 150 mg tab in single-dose blister pack. Susp 10, 40 mg/mL (35 mL). Triazole that inhibits the synthesis of ergosterol (a sterol required for normal fungal cytoplasmic membrane). Serious: Hepatotoxicity (rare), anaphylaxis (rare), exfoliative skin disorders (rare). Frequent: Increased transaminase levels. Single-dose for vaginal candidiasis: Headache, nausea, abdominal pain.

Use cautiously in patients with heart arrhythmia conditions. Monitor liver and renal function during therapy—notify prescriber at signs of dysfunction. Monitor for skin rash, hallucinations, and paranoia. Promote completing entire course of therapy. In diabetic patients, frequent monitoring of blood glucose level. May increase prothrombin time.

ITRACONAZOLE (***Onmel, Sporanox***) Oral caps for onychomycosis "pulse dosing": 200 mg PO two times per day for 1st week of month for 2 months (fingernails) or 3 to 4 months (toenails). Standard regimen, toenail onychomycosis: 200 mg PO daily with full meal for 12 weeks. Fluconazole-refractory oropharyngeal or esophageal candidiasis: Oral soln 200 mg PO daily for 14 to 21 days. CYP3A4 inhibitor. Contraindicated with dofetilide, ergot alkaloids, lovastatin, PO midazolam, pimozide, quinidine, simvastatin, triazolam. Negative inotrope; do not use for onychomycosis if ventricular dysfunction. ▶L ♀C ▶– © $$$$$ Trade: Tabs 200 mg. Oral soln 10 mg/mL (150 mL). Generic/Trade: Caps 100 mg. Triazole that inhibits the synthesis of ergosterol (a sterol required for normal fungal cytoplasmic membrane). Serious: Negative inotrope, hepatotoxicity (even early in therapy), hypokalemia (with high doses). Frequent: GI complaints, allergic rash.

Use cautiously in patients with heart disease, COPD, renal or liver impairment, and hypersensitivity to other azole antifungals. Administer with a meal. Monitor renal and liver function. Discontinue if patient displays fatigue, dyspnea, and peripheral edema. Assess for rash every 8 h.

MICONAZOLE—BUCCAL   (*Oravig*) Oropharyngeal candidiasis: Apply 50 mg buccal tab to gums once daily for 14 days. Increased INR with warfarin. ▶L ♀C ▶? © $$$$$ Trade: Buccal tabs, 50 mg. Triazole that inhibits the synthesis of ergosterol (a sterol required for normal fungal cytoplasmic membrane). Severe: Hypersensitivity.

> **Nursing Implications** Instruct patient to let tablet dissolve—do not crush, chew, or swallow. Monitor for diarrhea, nausea, headache, dysgeusia, changes in taste, upper abdominal pain, and vomiting. Do not use in patients with hypersensitivity to miconazole or milk protein concentrate. Discontinue at first sign of allergic reaction. Monitor patients with hypersensitivity to other azole antifungals.

POSACONAZOLE   (*Noxafil*) Prevention of invasive Aspergillus or Candida infection, age 13 yo or older: 200 mg (5 mL) PO three times per day. Oropharyngeal candidiasis, age 13 yo or older: 100 mg (2.5 mL) PO twice on day 1, then 100 mg PO once daily for 13 days. Oropharyngeal candidiasis resistant to itraconazole/fluconazole, age 13 yo or older: 400 mg (10 mL) PO two times per day. Take with full meal or liquid nutritional supplement. CYP3A4 inhibitor. ▶Glucuronidation ♀C ▶– © $$$$$ Trade only: Oral susp 40 mg/mL, 105 mL bottle. Triazole that inhibits the synthesis of ergosterol (a sterol required for normal fungal cytoplasmic membrane). Possible hepatotoxicity.

> **Nursing Implications** Use cautiously in patients with liver and renal disease, hypersensitivity to other azole antifungals, or if family history of long QT syndrome. Follow directions for preparation provided by manufacturer. Promote taking drug with or within 20 minutes after a full meal or liquid nutritional supplement, or with ginger ale. Promote reporting of severe diarrhea or vomiting.

VORICONAZOLE   (*Vfend*) Aspergillosis, systemic Candida infections: 6 mg/kg IV q 12 h for 2 doses, then 3 to 4 mg/kg IV q 12 h (use 4 mg/kg for aspergillosis). Esophageal candidiasis or maintenance therapy of aspergillosis/candidiasis: 200 mg PO two times per day. For wt less than 40 kg, reduce to 100 mg PO two times per day. Dosage adjustment for efavirenz: Voriconazole 400 mg PO two times per day with efavirenz 300 mg PO once daily (use caps). Peds younger than 12 yo: 7 mg/kg IV q 12 h. Infuse IV over 2 h. Take tabs and/or susp 1 h before or after meals. CYP3A4 inhibitor. Many drug interactions. ▶L ♀D ▶? © $$$$$ Trade only: Tabs 50, 200 mg (contains lactose). Susp 40 mg/mL (75 mL). Triazole that inhibits the synthesis of ergosterol (a sterol required for normal fungal cytoplasmic membrane). Serious: Anaphylactoid reactions (IV only), QT interval prolongation, hepatotoxicity (rare), severe skin reactions and photosensitivity rarely, pancreatitis. Frequent: Mild transient visual disturbances, rash, elevated LFTs. Other: Hallucinations, confusion.

> **Nursing Implications** This medication is contraindicated in pregnancy, lactation, treatment with other medications that prolong the QTc interval, and severe hepatic impairment. This medication interacts with several other medications (refer to product literature). Patients should be advised to use barrier contraceptives when taking this medication. Patients may experience visual changes on this medication and should avoid potentially hazardous tasks while on this medication. Patients should have a CBC and LFTs done prior to starting this medication. An EKG should also be performed prior to starting this medication. Patients should be advised to take the oral form of this medication on an empty stomach either 1 hour prior to eating a meal or 2 hours after eating a meal.

Antifungal Agents—Echinocandins

CASPOFUNGIN   (*Cancidas*) Infuse over 1 h, give 70 mg IV loading dose on day 1, then 50 mg once daily. Peds: 70 mg/m^2 IV loading dose on day 1, then 50 mg/m^2 once daily (max of 70 mg/day). ▶KL ♀C ▶? © $$$$$ Echinocandin that blocks the synthesis of glucan, a fungal cell wall polysaccharide. Serious: Anaphylaxis (rare). Abnormal LFTs reported; possible risk of hepatitis. Frequent: Fever, rash, N/V, diarrhea, hypokalemia, phlebitis at injection site. Some infusion reactions (like facial flushing) caused by histamine release.

> **Nursing Implications** Follow prescriber's instructions for dosage exactly and infuse over at least 1 h. Do not mix with solutions containing dextrose or glucose. Promote completion of entire course of therapy. Use cautiously in patients with liver disease, or those who have recently had a kidney, heart, or liver transplant. Monitor for nausea, vomiting, pain at IV site. Report fever, flu-like symptoms, swelling in hands and feet, weakness, muscle cramps, or irregular heart rate.

MICAFUNGIN (*Mycamine*) Infuse IV over 1 h. Esophageal candidiasis: 150 mg once daily. Prevention of candidal infections in bone marrow transplant patients: 50 mg once daily. Candidemia, acute disseminated candidiasis, Candida peritonitis/abscess: 100 mg once daily. ▶L, feces ♀C ▶? ☺ $$$$$ Echinocandin that blocks the synthesis of glucan, a fungal cell wall polysaccharide. Serious: Anaphylaxis/anaphylactoid reactions (rare); renal/hepatic dysfunction; hemolysis/hemolytic anemia. Frequent: Rash. Injection site reactions more common with peripheral infusion.

> Nursing Implications Administer by IV infusion. Use cautiously in patients with liver and renal dysfunction. Follow directions for preparation provided by manufacturer. Infuse slowly over 1 h. Monitor for allergic reaction and notify prescriber if symptoms appear. Monitor liver and renal function during therapy. Promote reporting of discomfort at infusion site and any persistent signs and symptoms.

Antifungal Agents—Polyenes

AMPHOTERICIN B DEOXYCHOLATE (*Fungizone*) Test dose 0.1 mg/kg up to 1 mg slow IV. Wait 2 to 4 h, and if tolerated then begin 0.25 mg/kg IV daily and advance to 0.5 to 1.5 mg/kg/day depending on fungal type. Maximum dose 1.5 mg/kg/day. ▶Tissues ♀B ▶? ☺ $$$$ Polyene antifungal. Insertion into fungal cytoplasmic membrane increases membrane permeability. Serious for IV Fungizone: Anaphylaxis, anemia, nephrotoxicity. Frequent: Acute infusion reactions, nephrotoxicity (hypokalemia, hypomagnesemia, renal tubular acidosis).

> Nursing Implications Follow directions for preparation provided by manufacturer. Monitor renal function every other day, then twice weekly during therapy. Cumulative dose of more than 4 g may lead to irreversible renal dysfunction. Monitor CBC and platelet count weekly. Monitor for fever, shaking chills, chest pain, nausea, vomiting, abdominal pain, decrease in respiratory function, skin changes, and muscle spasms. Administer 1 h before or 3 h after meals.

AMPHOTERICIN B LIPID FORMULATIONS (*Amphotec, Abelcet, AmBisome*) Abelcet: 5 mg/kg/day IV at 2.5 mg/kg/h. AmBisome: 3 to 5 mg/kg/day IV over 2 h. Amphotec: Test dose of 10 mL over 15 to 30 min, observe for 30 min, then 3 to 4 mg/kg/day IV at 1 mg/kg/h. ▶? ♀B ▶? ☺ $$$$$ Polyene antifungal. Insertion into fungal cytoplasmic membrane increases membrane permeability. Serious: Anaphylaxis. Frequent: Acute infusion reactions, nephrotoxicity (hypokalemia, hypomagnesemia, renal tubular acidosis). Lipid formulations better tolerated than amphotericin deoxycholate.

> Nursing Implications This medication cannot be administered in the same IV line as other medications. The most common side effects are toxicity and nephrotoxicity. Patients should have their hearing assessed prior to administration of this medication. Serum creatinine, BUN and liver function studies (LFTs) should also be assessed prior to administration of this medication.

Antifungal Agents—Other

FLUCYTOSINE (*Ancobon*) 50 to 150 mg/kg/day PO divided four times per day. Myelosuppression. ▶K ♀C ▶– ☺ $$$$$ Generic/Trade: Caps 250, 500 mg. Deaminated to inhibitor of thymidylate synthetase, which interferes with DNA synthesis. Serious: Myelosuppression (frequent); anaphylaxis; hepatic, renal, cardiac, and CNS toxicity (all rare). Frequent: N/V, diarrhea, rash.

> Nursing Implications Use cautiously in patients with renal dysfunction, blood or bone marrow disease. Promote completing entire course of therapy. Monitor for nausea and vomiting.

GRISEOFULVIN (*Grifulvin V, ✚ Fulvicin*) Tinea capitis: 500 mg PO daily in adults; 15 to 20 mg/kg (up to 1 g) PO daily in peds. Treat for 4 to 6 weeks, continuing for 2 weeks past symptom resolution. ▶Skin ♀C ▶? ☺ $$$$ Generic/Trade: Susp 125 mg/5 mL (120 mL). Trade only: Tabs 250, 500 mg. Inhibits fungal mitosis by disrupting mitotic spindle. Serious: Photosensitivity, lupus-like syndrome/exacerbation of lupus, increased porphyrins (not for use by patients with porphyria). Frequent: Allergic skin reactions, headache.

> Nursing Implications This medication is contraindicated in pregnancy and lactation. Patients need to be advised to utilize birth control methods when taking this medication. The most common side effects are: diarrhea, dizziness, headache, nausea, upset stomach, tiredness, nausea and vomiting. Griseofulvin should be discontinued if signs/symptoms of severe allergic reaction occur, such as urticaria, hives, shortness of breath, difficulty breathing, and swelling of the lips, face, mouth and tongue.

GRISEOFULVIN ULTRAMICROSIZE   (**Gris-PEG**) ▶Skin ♀C ▶? © $$$$ Trade only: Tabs 125, 250 mg. Inhibits fungal mitosis by disrupting mitotic spindle. Serious: Photosensitivity, lupus-like syndrome/ exacerbation of lupus, increased porphyrins (not for use by patients with porphyria). Frequent: Allergic skin reactions, headache.

> Nursing Implications Do not administer to pregnant patients. Use with extreme caution in children under 3 yo. Possible interactions with barbiturates and anticoagulants. Do not chew or divide tablet—can be crushed, sprinkled over applesauce, and swallowed. Monitor for allergic reaction, confusion, fever, headache, joint pain, sore throat, and thrush. Promote completing entire course of therapy. Promote avoidance of prolonged exposure to sunlight.

NYSTATIN   (**◆ Nilstat**) Thrush: 4 to 6 mL PO, swish and swallow four times per day. Infants: 2 mL/dose with 1 mL in each cheek four times per day. ▶Not absorbed ♀B ▶? © $$ Generic only: Susp 100,000 units/mL (60, 480 mL). Troches 500,000 units/tab. Serious: None. Frequent: None.

> Nursing Implications The most common side effects of this medication are gastrointestinal upset such as nausea, vomiting and diarrhea. Uritcaria has been reported rarely as has Stevens-Johnson syndrome. Patients need to be aware that oral irritation and sensitization has been reported.

TERBINAFINE   (**Lamisil**) Onychomycosis: 250 mg PO daily for 6 weeks to treat fingernails, for 12 weeks to treat toenails. Tinea capitis, age 4 yo or older: Give granules PO once daily with food for 6 weeks: 125 mg for wt less than 25 kg, 187.5 mg for wt 25 to 35 kg, 250 mg for wt more than 35 kg. ▶LK ♀B ▶– © $ Generic/Trade: Tabs 250 mg. Trade only: Oral granules 125, 187.5 mg/packet. Inhibits squalene epoxidase, an enzyme involved in the synthesis of ergosterol (a sterol required for normal fungal cytoplasmic membrane). Serious: Hepatotoxicity, neutropenia, taste and smell disturbances. May rarely cause or exacerbate lupus. Frequent: N/V, rash.

> Nursing Implications Can be taken with or without food. Oral granules should be taken with food and may be sprinkled on a spoonful of pudding or other soft, nonacidic food, such as mashed potatoes, and swallowed in entirety. Applesauce or fruit-based foods should not be used.

Antimalarials

NOTE: For help treating malaria or getting antimalarials, see www.cdc.gov/malaria or call the CDC "malaria hotline" (770) 488–7788 Monday through Friday 9 am to 5 pm EST; after hours/weekend (770) 488–7100. Pediatric doses of antimalarials should never exceed adult doses.

CHLOROQUINE   (**Aralen**) Malaria prophylaxis, chloroquine-sensitive areas: 8 mg/kg up to 500 mg PO q week starting 1 to 2 weeks before exposure to 4 weeks after exposure. Chloroquine resistance is widespread. Can prolong QT interval and cause torsades de pointes. ▶KL ♀C but + ▶+ © $ Generic only: Tabs 250 mg. Generic/Trade: Tabs 500 mg (500 mg phosphate equivalent to 300 mg base). Plasmodicidal mechanism of action unknown, may inhibit heme polymerase or interact with DNA. Serious: Retinopathy with chronic/high doses; can cause torsades. Fatal malaria in patients receiving chloroquine prophylaxis in areas with chloroquine resistance.

> Nursing Implications Use cautiously in patients with glucose-6-phosphate dehydrogenase deficiency, psoriasis, porphyia, or liver disease. Promote caution when driving and avoidance of hazardous activities. Promote reporting of blurred or misty vision, difficulty focusing, and changes in hearing.

COARTEM   (artemether + lumefantrine, coartemether) Uncomplicated malaria: Take PO with food two times per day for 3 days. On day 1, give 2nd dose 8 h after 1st dose. Dose based on wt: 1 tab for 5 to 14 kg; 2 tabs for 15 to 24 kg; 3 tabs for 25 to 34 kg; 4 tabs for 35 kg or greater. Repeat dose if vomiting occurs within 1 to 2 h. Can prolong QT interval. ▶L ♀C ▶? © $$$ Trade only: Tabs, artemether 20 mg + lumefantrine 120 mg. Artemether and lumefantrine are blood schizonticides. Serious: Urticaria/ angioedema. Can prolong QT interval. Frequent: Headache, anorexia, dizziness, asthenia in adults. Fever, cough, vomiting, anorexia, headache in children.

> Nursing Implications Use only in the treatment of malaria. Do not use in patients allergic to artemether or lumefantrine. Use cautiously in patients with history of heart disease, liver or kidney disease, or long QT syndrome. Give dosage with food, milk, oatmeal, or broth. Promote reporting of symptoms such as vomiting or inability to eat to prescriber.

HALOFANTRINE ▶? ♀? ▶? © ? Not available in the United States or Canada. Plasmodicidal mechanism of action unknown. QT interval prolongation; fatal arrhythmias reported.

> Nursing Implications Do not use in patients with history of heart arrhythmia disorders, such as long QT syndrome. Use cautiously in patients with liver or kidney disease. Administer dosage on an empty stomach, at least 1 h before or 2 h after eating. Promote caution when driving and avoidance of hazardous activities. Promote reporting of dizziness.

MALARONE **(atovaquone + proguanil)** Prevention of malaria: Give the following dose PO once daily from 1 to 2 days before exposure until 7 days after. Dose based on wt: ½ ped tab for wt 5 to 8 kg; ¾ ped tab for wt 9 to 10 kg; 1 ped tab for wt 11 to 20 kg; 2 ped tabs for 21 to 30 kg; 3 ped tabs for 31 to 40 kg; 1 adult tab for all patients wt greater than 40 kg. Treatment of malaria: Give the following dose PO once daily for 3 days. Dose based on wt: 2 ped tabs for 5 to 8 kg; 3 ped tabs for 9 to 10 kg; 1 adult tab for 11 to 20 kg; 2 adult tabs for 21 to 30 kg; 3 adult tabs for 31 to 40 kg; 4 adult tabs for all patients wt greater than 40 kg. Take with food or milky drink. ▶Fecal excretion; LK ♀C ▶? © $$$$$ Generic or trade: Adult tabs atovaquone 250 mg plus proguanil 100 mg. Trade only: Pediatric tabs 62.5 mg plus 25 mg. Atovaquone and proguanil interfere with two different pyrimidine biosynthesis pathways. Atovaquone inhibits parasitic mitochondrial electron transport. A proguanil metabolite, cycloguanil, inhibits dihydrofolate reductase. Serious: Hepatitis/increased LFTs, anaphylaxis, Stevens-Johnson syndrome, photosensitivity. Frequent: Vomiting with malaria treatment doses, GI complaints, headache, asthenia, dizziness.

> Nursing Implications Do not use in patients allergic to atovaquone or proguanil. Do not use in patients with history of liver or kidney disease. Promote reporting of uncontrolled vomiting or diarrhea. Administer dosage at the same time daily with food or a milky drink.

MEFLOQUINE Malaria prophylaxis for chloroquine-resistant areas: 250 mg PO once a week from 1 week before exposure to 4 weeks after. Malaria treatment: 1250 mg PO single dose. Peds malaria prophylaxis: Give the following dose PO once a week starting 1 week before exposure to 4 weeks after: Dose based on wt: 5 mg/kg (prepared by pharmacist) for wt 9 kg or less; ¼ tab for wt greater than 9 kg to 19 kg; ½ tab for wt greater than 19 kg to 30 kg; ¾ tab for wt greater than 30 to 45 kg; 1 tab for wt 45 kg or greater. Peds malaria treatment: 20 to 25 mg/kg PO single dose or divided into 2 doses given 6 to 8 h apart. Take on full stomach. ▶L ♀B ▶? © $$ Generic only: Tabs 250 mg. Acts as blood schizonticide, exact mechanism of action is unknown. Serious: Cardiac conduction disturbances including QT prolongation, psychiatric reactions. Frequent: Dizziness, loss of balance, sleep disturbances (especially early in therapy and in women). Early vomiting in children with malaria treatment dose.

> Nursing Implications Do not use in patients allergic to quinine or quinidine. Do not use in patients with recent history of seizures, depression, anxiety, or schizophrenia. Do not use in patients with history of liver or kidney disease. Promote reporting of fever, uncontrolled vomiting, or diarrhea.

PRIMAQUINE Prevention of relapse, *P. vivax/ovale* malaria: 0.5 mg/kg (up to 30 mg) base PO daily for 14 days. Do not use unless normal G6PD level. ▶L ♀− ▶− © $$ Generic only: Tabs 26.3 mg (equivalent to 15 mg base). Unknown. May affect mitochondrial electron transport chain or pyrimidine synthesis. Active against all forms of malaria; only drug active against latent parasites in liver. Serious: Hemolytic anemia with G6PD deficiency, methemoglobinemia with NADH methemoglobin reductase deficiency.

> Nursing Implications Use cautiously in patients with glucose-6-phosphate dehydrogenase deficiency, rheumatoid arthritis, lupus, or a history of allergic reactions to previous primaquine therapy. Promote caution when driving and avoidance of hazardous activities. Promote reporting of blurred or misty vision, difficulty focusing, and changes in hearing.

QUININE (***Qualaquin***) Malaria: 648 mg PO three times per day. Peds: 25 to 30 mg/kg/day (up to 2 g/day) PO divided q 8 h. Treat for 3 days (Africa/South America) or 7 days (Southeast Asia). Also give 7-day course of doxycycline, tetracycline, or clindamycin. Nocturnal leg cramps: 325 mg PO at bedtime. FDA warns that risks exceed potential benefit for this indication. Can cause life-threatening adverse effects: Cinchonism with overdose, hemolysis with G6PD deficiency, hypersensitivity, thrombocytopenia, HUS/TTP, QT interval prolongation, many drug interactions. ▶L ♀C ▶+? © $$$$ Trade only: Caps 324 mg. Unknown, may have similar mechanism of action as chloroquine. Serious: Thrombocytopenia, hemolytic uremic syndrome/thrombotic thrombocytopenic purpura, cinchonism, hemolytic anemia with G6PD deficiency, cardiac conduction disturbances, hearing impairment with high levels, hypoglycemia (especially in pregnant women).

> **Nursing Implications** Monitor for blurred vision, confusion, diplopia, fever, headache, loss of hearing, and tinnitus. Do not crush or chew tablets. Administer with or after meals.

Antimycobacterial Agents

NOTE: *Treat active mycobacterial infection with at least 2 drugs. See guidelines at www.thoracic.org/statements/index.php and www.aidsinfo.nih.gov.*

CAPREOMYCIN (***Capastat***) ▶K ♀C ▶? © $$$$$ Polypeptide; mechanism of action unknown. Serious: Nephrotoxicity (frequent), ototoxicity (frequent), hypersensitivity, hypokalemia, hypomagnesemia, leukopenia, sterile abscess at injection site. Frequent: Eosinophilia, leukocytosis, injection site reactions, proteinuria.

> **Nursing Implications** Use cautiously in patients with renal dysfunction, impaired hearing, or history of hypersensitivity. Monitor serum and electrolyte levels during therapy. Promote reporting of any adverse side effects, such as bleeding at injection site, hearing loss, or tinnitus.

CLOFAZIMINE (***Lamprene***) ▶Fecal excretion ♀C ▶?– © Caps 50 mg. Distributed only through investigational new drug application. For leprosy, contact National Hansen's Disease Program (phone 800–642–2477). For nonleprosy indications, contact FDA Division of Special Pathogen and Transplant Drugs Program (phone 301–796–1600). Unknown. Serious: Rare reports of splenic infarction, bowel obstruction, and GI bleeding. Frequent: Abdominal pain, discoloration of urine and body secretions, pink to brownish-black skin pigmentation that may persist for months to years.

> **Nursing Implications** Do not use in patients with history of allergic reaction to clofazimine or allergies to other medicines. Use cautiously in pregnant patients. May cause reaction with the following medications—aluminum hydroxide, magnesium hydroxide, phenytoin. Do not give with orange juice. Promote reporting of kidney or liver dysfunction, stomach or intestinal problems.

CYCLOSERINE (***Seromycin***) ▶KL ♀C ▶– © $$$$$ Trade only: Caps 250 mg. Structural analog of d-alanine; inhibits steps in cell-wall synthesis that require d-alanine. Serious: Dose-related neurotoxicity including psychosis, seizures, depression, peripheral neuropathy. Frequent: Drowsiness (warn about hazardous tasks).

> **Nursing Implications** Monitor mental status, mood, LFT and CBC levels. Monitor for aggression, depression, suicidal thoughts, dizziness, or drowsiness. Promote avoidance of alcohol, driving, and hazardous activities during therapy. Advise patient to contact prescriber if no improvement shown in 2 to 3 weeks.

DAPSONE (***Aczone***) Pneumocystis prophylaxis, leprosy: 100 mg PO daily. Pneumocystis treatment: 100 mg PO daily with trimethoprim 5 mg/kg PO three times per day for 21 days. Acne (Aczone; $$$$): Apply two times per day. ▶LK ♀C ▶– © $ Generic only: Tabs 25, 100 mg. Trade only (Aczone): Topical gel 5% 30 or 60 g. Sulfone that inhibits dihydropteroate synthase and prevents bacterial folic acid synthesis. Serious: Blood dyscrasias, allergic skin reactions, sulfone syndrome, hemolysis in G6PD deficiency, hepatotoxicity, neuropathy, photosensitivity, leprosy reactional states. Frequent: Rash, headache, GI complaints, mononucleosis-like syndrome. Topical, frequent: dryness, pruritus, erythema, scaling.

> **Nursing Implications** Do not use in patients with history of glucose-6-phosphate dehydrogenase (G6PD) deficiency, methemoglobin reductase deficiency, or liver disease. Promote immediate reporting of symptoms such as sore throat, fever, pale skin, bruising, pinpoint red spots on skin or other rash, and yellowing of skin or eyes. Do not use in pregnant or breast feeding patients.

ETHAMBUTOL (***Myambutol***, ✚ ***Etibi***) 15 to 20 mg/kg PO daily. Dose with whole tabs: Give 800 mg PO daily for wt 40 to 55 kg, 1200 mg for wt 56 to 75 kg, 1600 mg for wt 76 to 90 kg. Base dose on estimated lean body wt. Peds: 15 to 20 mg/kg (up to 1 g) PO daily. ▶LK ♀C but + ▶+ © $$$$ Generic/Trade: Tabs 100, 400 mg. Inhibits arabinosyl transferase enzymes involved in synthesis of mycobacterial cell wall. Serious: Retrobulbar neuritis, peripheral neuropathy, anaphylactoid reactions.

> **Nursing Implications** Monitor and report any vision changes and stop therapy if they occur. Monitor liver, renal function, and increased uric acid level. Promote taking dose with food. Advise patient to contact prescriber if no improvement shown in 3 weeks.

ETHIONAMIDE (*Trecator*) ▶L ♀ ▶? © $$$$$ Trade only: Tab 250 mg. Isonicotinic acid derivative that may inhibit peptide synthesis. Serious: Hepatotoxicity, hypothyroidism, seizures, peripheral and optic neuritis, anxiety, depression, psychosis, hypothyroidism, exacerbation of diabetes. Frequent and serious: N/V, anorexia, abdominal pain, metallic taste.

> Nursing Implications Do not use in patients with history of allergic reaction to ethionamide, liver disease, or diabetes mellitus. Promote reporting to prescriber symptoms such as stomach upset, loss of appetite, metallic taste in the mouth, or excessive salivation. Promote completion of entire course of therapy.

ISONIAZID (*INH*, ✦ *Isotamine*) Adults: 5 mg/kg (up to 300 mg) PO daily. Peds: 10 to 15 mg/kg (up to 300 mg) PO daily. Hepatotoxicity. Consider supplemental pyridoxine up to 50 mg per day to prevent neuropathy. ▶LK ♀C but + ▶+ © $ Generic only: Tabs 100, 300 mg. Syrup 50 mg/5 mL. Inhibits synthesis of mycolic acid, a component of mycobacterial cell walls. Serious: Hepatotoxicity, peripheral neuropathy, lupus. Frequent: Increased LFTs, positive ANA.

> Nursing Implications Do not use in patients with history of allergic reaction to isoniazid, or persons with liver or kidney disease. Promote avoidance of alcohol during therapy. Promote reporting to prescriber symptoms such as numbness in hands and feet, weakness, fatigue, loss of appetite, nausea and vomiting, yellowing of the skin or eyes, and darkening of the urine. Usually Vitamin B6 is administered concurrently.

Antiparasitics

ATOVAQUONE (*Mepron*) Pneumocystis treatment: 750 mg PO two times per day for 21 days. Pneumocystis prevention: 1500 mg PO daily. Take with meals. ▶Fecal ♀C ▶? © $$$$$ Trade only: Susp 750 mg/5 mL (210 mL), foil pouch 750 mg/5 mL (5, 10 mL). Ubiquinone analog that may inhibit nucleic acid and ATP synthesis via effects on mitochondrial electron transport. Serious: Hepatotoxicity (rare). Frequent: Rash, nausea, fever, headache, insomnia, increased LFTs.

> Nursing Implications Administer PO ONLY with meals through a foil pouch or bottled susp. Monitor for serious allergic reaction. Call prescriber if bruising/bleeding, flu-like symptoms: oral white patches, problems breathing, and cough that worsens occurs. Assess pt for prior liver disease, GI or lung disorders. Teach pt not to drive or operate machinery until used to drug; alcohol should be avoided. Pt may experience the following adverse events: GI disturbances, rash, flu-like symptoms, breathing and upper respiratory problems. Do NOT use concurrently with rifampin.

Antiviral Agents—Anti-CMV

CIDOFOVIR (*Vistide*) CMV retinitis in AIDS: 5 mg/kg IV once a week for 2 weeks, then 5 mg/kg q 2 weeks. Severe nephrotoxicity. ▶K ♀C ▶– © $$$$$ Selectively inhibits cytomegalovirus DNA polymerase. Serious: Nephrotoxicity (also frequent), Fanconi syndrome, neutropenia (also frequent), metabolic acidosis, iritis/uveitis, ocular hypotony. Frequent: Nausea, fever, alopecia, myalgia.

> Nursing Implications Observe for signs and symptoms of severe allergic reactions such as hives, urticaria, shortness of breath, tightness in the chest, and swelling of the mouth, face, lips, or tongue. This medication may cause drowsiness and vertigo. Patients need to be advised that this medication may lower one's ability to fight infection. Diabetic patients should be advised to check their blood sugar more frequently as this medication may affect blood sugar levels. Other side effects include fever, tremors, change in wt, unusual bruising or bleeding, seizures, swelling, hallucinations, loss of cordination, and depression. Testing includes eye exam, CBC with differential, and renal function. This medication is teratogenic.

VALGANCICLOVIR (*Valcyte*) CMV retinitis: 900 mg PO two times per day for 21 days, then 900 mg PO daily. Prevention of CMV disease in high-risk transplant patients: 900 mg PO daily given within 10 days post transplant until 100 days post transplant for heart or kidney/pancreas or 200 days for kidney transplant. See prescribing information for peds dose. Greater bioavailability than oral ganciclovir. Give with food. Impaired fertility, myelosuppression, potential carcinogen and teratogen. ▶K ♀C ▶– © $$$$$ Trade only: Tabs 450 mg. Oral soln 50 mg/mL. Prodrug of ganciclovir. Similar to ganciclovir.

> **Nursing Implications** Patients on Valcyte should have their white blood cell and platelet levels checked. Patients need to be advised to take the tabs with food and to swallow whole. Patients should be advised not to drink alcohol while on this medication. It is important to maintain adequate hydration while on this medication. This medication lowers the ability for one to fight infection. Patients should observe and report signs and symptoms of infection. This medication is teratogenic.

Antiviral Agents—Anti-HIV—Integrase Strand Transfer Inhibitor

RALTEGRAVIR (*Isentress, RAL*) 400 mg PO two times per day. Increase to 800 mg PO two times per day if given with rifampin. Peds. Film-coated tabs, age 6 yo and older and wt 25 kg or greater: 400 mg PO two times per day. Chew tabs, 2 to 11 yo: Give PO two times per day at a dose of 75 mg for 10 kg to less than 14 kg; 100 mg for 14 kg to less than 20 kg; 150 mg for 20 kg to less than 28 kg; 200 mg for 28 kg to less than 40 kg; 300 mg for 40 kg or more. ▶Glucuronidation ♀C ▶– © $$$$$ Trade only: Film-coated tabs 400 mg. Chewable tabs (contain phenylalanine) 25 mg, 100 mg. Inhibits HIV-1 integrase, an enzyme required for insertion of virus into host genome. Inhibition of integrase prevents viral propagation. Serious: Myopathy and rhabdomyolysis (causality unclear). Severe skin and hypersensitivity reactions, including Stevens-Johnson syndrome, toxic epidermal necrolysis, and drug rash with eosinophilia and systemic symptoms (DRESS). Frequent: Insomnia, headache, increased CPK.

> **Nursing Implications** Administer with or without food.

Antiviral Agents—Anti-HIV—Non-Nucleoside Reverse Transcriptase Inhibitors

EFAVIRENZ (*Sustiva, EFV*) Adults and children wt 40 kg or greater: 600 mg PO at bedtime. With voriconazole: Use voriconazole 400 mg PO two times per day and efavirenz 300 mg PO once daily. With rifampin: Increase efavirenz to 800 mg PO at bedtime if wt is 50 kg or greater. Peds, age 3 yo or older: Give PO at bedtime 200 mg for wt 10 kg to less than 15 kg, 250 mg for wt 15 kg to less than 20 kg, 300 mg for wt 20 kg to less than 25 kg, 350 mg for wt 25 kg to less than 32.5 kg, 400 mg for wt 32.5 kg to less than 40 kg. Do not give with high-fat meal. ▶L ♀D ▶– © $$$$$ Trade only: Caps 50, 100, 200 mg. Tabs 600 mg. Inhibits HIV reverse transcriptase by different mechanism of action from NRTIs. Cross-resistance possible between efavirenz and nevirapine. Serious: Depression and other psychiatric reactions, convulsions, severe rash, Stevens-Johnson syndrome, lipoatrophy, hepatotoxicity (rare). Frequent: Rash (especially in children), CNS symptoms (dizziness, insomnia, vivid dreams, impaired concentration; warn about hazardous tasks).

> **Nursing Implications** This medication is contraindicated in patients who are pregnant and must be utilized cautiously in patients with hepatic impairment, psychiatric disorders, and hyperlipidemia. This medication interacts with several other medications (refer to product literature). Patients should be advised not to eat a high fat meal as a high fat meal will decrease the absorption of this medication. Patients should be advised that this medication can cause a false positive urine cannabinoid (THC) test. Patients should be advised not to use this medication with OTC St. John's Wort. Patients should be advised that this medication does not decrease the risk of transmission of the HIV virus and appropriate precautions need to be utilized to prevent the spread of HIV disease. Report any medications including over-the-counter medications and herbal supplements that they are taking to provider. Barrier contraceptive precautions should be utilized when patients are on this medication. Patients need to have a CBC and chemistry profile inclusive of lipid panel done prior to starting and after taking this medication.

Antiviral Agents—Anti-HIV—Nucleoside/Nucleotide Reverse Transcriptase Inhibitors

TENOFOVIR (*Viread, TDF*) Adults and adolescents: 300 mg PO daily. Peds, 2 yo and older: 8 mg/kg PO once daily (max 300 mg/day) as oral powder. Dosing scoop for oral powder delivers 40 mg tenofovir per scoop. Mix powder with 2 to 4 ounces of soft food that does not require chewing (applesauce, baby food, yogurt). Use immediately after mixing. Do not mix powder with liquid. Tabs for peds, wt 17 kg or greater: Give PO once daily at dose of 150 mg for wt 17 kg to less than 22 kg; 200 mg for wt 22 kg to less than 28 kg; 250 mg for wt 28 kg to less than 35 kg; 300 mg for wt 35 kg or greater. ▶K ♀B ▶– © $$$$$ Trade only: Tabs 150, 200, 250, 300 mg. Oral powder 40 mg tenofovir/g. Nucleotide reverse transcriptase inhibitor. Similar mechanism of action to NRTIs, but does not require phosphorylation step required to activate NRTIs. Reduces HIV replication within infected cells by inhibiting HIV reverse transcriptase. Has activity against hepatitis B. Serious: Lactic acidosis/hepatic steatosis, renal impairment including acute renal failure and Fanconi syndrome, hypophosphatemia. Immune reconstitution syndrome, including autoimmune disorders. Exacerbation of hepatitis B after discontinuation of tenofovir. Decreased bone mineral density in adults and children; fracture risk unknown. Reports of syncope, usually with vagal syndrome. Frequent: GI complaints, dizziness.

> **Nursing Implications** Fatal lactic acidosis and liver problems have been seen in patients on Viread. Viread patients with hepatitis B virus had severe reactions after taking Viread, close medical follow up should be maintained after stopping use. Patients should have HBV testing prior to taking Viread if HIV positive. Patients should be advised not to drink alcohol when on this medication. Patients need to be advised that this is not a cure for HIV or HBV infection. This medication may affect bone mineral density. Patients need to have periodic monitoring of renal, kidney, and bone density.

ZIDOVUDINE (*Retrovir, AZT, ZDV*) 600 mg/day PO divided two or three times per day for wt 30 kg or greater. Peds dose based on wt: Give 24 mg/kg/day PO divided two or three times per day for wt 4 to 8 kg, 18 mg/kg/day PO divided two or three times per day for wt 9 to 29 kg. ▶LK ♀C ▶– © $$$$$ Generic/Trade: Caps 100 mg. Tabs 300 mg. Syrup 50 mg/5 mL (240 mL). Decreases or inhibits HIV replication within infected cells by inhibiting HIV reverse transcriptase. Serious: Lactic acidosis/hepatic steatosis, lipoatrophy (possibly), hematologic toxicity, symptomatic myopathy, hepatic decompensation in HCV/HIV coinfected patients. Granulocytopenia more common in children receiving zidovudine and nevirapine. Frequent: GI intolerance, headache, insomnia, asthenia, anorexia.

> **Nursing Implications** Observe patients for signs and symptoms of severe allergic reactions such as hives, urticaria, shortness of breath, tightness in the chest, and swelling of the mouth, face, lips, or tongue. While on Zidovudine, do not take doxorubicin, ribavirin, stavudine, or any other zidovudine-containing medication. Doxorubicin or stavudine may reduce the drug's effectiveness. This medication is not a cure for HIV disease and does not prevent the spread of HIV to other individuals through blood and/or sexual contact. This medication may cause anemia in some patients. CBC and tests for renal and hepatic function need to be done periodically. Patients need to be educated that this medication should be taken at the same time each day and doses should not be missed.

Antiviral Agents—Anti-HIV—Protease Inhibitors

NOTE: *See www.aidsinfo.nih.gov for AIDS treatment guidelines and use of rifamycins with protease inhibitors. Many serious drug interactions: Always check before prescribing. Protease inhibitors inhibit CYP3A4. Contraindicated with most antiarrhythmics, alfuzosin, ergot alkaloids, lovastatin, pimozide, rifampin, salmeterol, high-dose sildenafil for pulmonary hypertension, simvastatin, St. John's wort, triazolam. Midazolam contraindicated in labeling, but can use single-dose IV cautiously with monitoring for procedural sedation. Monitor INR with warfarin. Avoid inhaled/nasal fluticasone with ritonavir if possible; increased fluticasone levels can cause Cushing's syndrome/adrenal suppression. Other protease inhibitors may increase fluticasone levels; find alternatives for long-term use. May need to reduce trazodone dose. Reduce colchicine dose; do not coadminister colchicine and protease inhibitors in patients with renal or hepatic dysfunction. Adjust dose of bosentan or tadalafil for pulmonary hypertension. Erectile dysfunction: Single dose of sildenafil 25 mg every 48 h, tadalafil 5 mg (not more than 10 mg) every 72 h, or vardenafil initially 2.5 mg every 72 h. Adverse effects include spontaneous bleeding in hemophiliacs, hyperglycemia, hyperlipidemia, immune reconstitution syndrome, and fat redistribution. Coinfection with hepatitis C or other liver disease increases the risk of hepatotoxicity with protease inhibitors; monitor LFTs at least twice in first month of therapy, then every 3 months.*

ATAZANAVIR (*Reyataz, ATV*) Adults, therapy-naive: 400 mg PO once daily (without ritonavir if ritonavir-intolerant) OR 300 mg + ritonavir 100 mg PO both once daily. With tenofovir, therapy-naive: 300 mg plus ritonavir 100 mg PO, both once daily. With efavirenz, therapy-naive: 400 mg plus ritonavir 100 mg PO both once daily. Do not give atazanavir with efavirenz in therapy-experienced patients. Therapy-experienced: 300 mg plus ritonavir 100 mg PO both once daily. Peds, age 6 yo or older: atazanavir/ritonavir PO once daily 150/100 mg for wt 15 kg to less than 20 kg; 200/100 mg for wt 20 kg to less than 40 kg; 300/100 mg for 40 kg or greater.Therapy-naive, ritonavir-intolerant, age 13 yo or older and wt 39 kg or greater:

400 mg PO once daily. Give caps with food. Give atazanavir 2 h before or 1 h after buffered didanosine. ▶L ♀B ▶– © $$$$$ Trade only: Caps 100, 150, 200, 300 mg. Prevents cleavage of protein precursors required for HIV maturation, reproduction, and infection of new cells. Serious: Can prolong PR interval; rare cases of second-degree AV block reported; serious skin reactions like Stevens-Johnson syndrome and DRESS. Frequent: Increased indirect bilirubin, jaundice/scleral icterus, nausea, rash. Nephrolithiasis. Class effects: Hyperglycemia, fat redistribution, spontaneous bleeding in hemophiliacs.

> **Nursing Implications** Monitor ECG and the cardiovascular system closely (ie, heart rate and blood pressure). Pay special attention to these stats while treating with other drugs that are known to prolong the PR interval. Check lab work on a regular basis. Check blood glucose levels with diabetic patients. Periodically check PT/INR, this is important with current warafin therapy. If patient is jaundiced, check their bilirubin. Also check LFTs at baseline and periodically thereafter. Patients need to be advised that HIV can still be transmitted while on this medication and universal precautions must be utilized. Patients need to be advised to take this medication with food and to swallow the tab whole. This medication must be taken on a regular schedule and at the same time each day. This medication should not be stopped. The exception would be an acute allergic reaction. Patients on hormonal birth control need to take additional precaution.

NELFINAVIR (*Viracept, NFV*) 750 mg PO three times per day or 1250 mg PO two times per day. Peds: 45 to 55 mg/kg PO two times per day (up to 2500 mg/day). Take with meals. ▶L ♀B ▶– © $$$$$ Trade only: Tabs 250, 625 mg. Oral powder 50 mg/g (114 g). Prevents cleavage of protein precursors required for HIV maturation, reproduction, and infection of new cells. Frequent: Diarrhea, transaminase elevation. Class effects: Hyperglycemia, fat redistribution, lipid abnormalities, spontaneous bleeding in hemophiliacs.

> **Nursing Implications** Observe for signs and symptoms of severe allergic reactions such as hives, urticaria, shortness of breath, tightness in the chest, and swelling of the mouth, face, lips, or tongue. People with liver issues should not use Viracept. Do not administer with alfuzosin, amiodarone, astemizole, carbamazepine, benzodiazepines, cisapride, an ergot derivative, HMG-CoA reductase inhibitors (eg, lovastatin, simvastatin), phenobarbital, pimozide, omeprazole, quinidine, rifampin, salmeterol, St. John's wort, terfenadin, or sildenafil. Patients should be advised to utilize alternate forms of birth control as this medication may lower the efficacy of hormonal birth control methods. Diabetic patients need to check blood sugars more regularly. Patients need to be educated that this medication is not a cure for HIV infection and does not prevent the spread of HIV to others through blood and/or sexual contact. Common side effects are gastrointestinal in nature such as nausea, stomach pain and cramping, and increased flatulence.

RITONAVIR (*Norvir, RTV*) Adult doses of 100 mg PO daily to 400 mg PO two times per day used to boost levels of other protease inhibitors. Full-dose regimen (600 mg PO two times per day) is poorly tolerated. Peds, full-dose regimen: Start with 250 mg/m^2 two times per day and increase q 2 to 3 days by 50 mg/m^2 two times per day to achieve usual dose of 350 to 400 mg/m^2 PO two times per day for age older than 1 mo (up to 600 mg/dose). If 400 mg/m^2 twice daily not tolerated, consider other alternatives. See specific protease inhibitor entries (atazanavir, darunavir, fosamprenavir, tipranavir) for pediatric boosting doses of ritonavir. ▶L ♀B ▶– © $$$$$ Trade only: Caps 100 mg, tabs 100 mg. Oral soln 80 mg/mL (240 mL). Prevents cleavage of protein precursors required for HIV maturation, reproduction, and infection of new cells. Serious: Greater than 200% increase in triglycerides, hepatitis, pancreatitis. Can prolong PR interval; rare cases of second/third degree AV block reported. Frequent: GI complaints, paresthesias, asthenia, taste perversion, increased CPK and uric acid. Class effects: Hyperglycemia, fat redistribution, lipid abnormalities, spontaneous bleeding in hemophiliacs.

> **Nursing Implications** Observe patients for severe allergic reactions such as hives, urticaria, shortness of breath, tightness in the chest, swelling of the mouth, face, lips, or tongue, and unusual hoarseness. Patients should also be observed for unusual signs of bleeding; mouth sores; red, blistered, peeling skin; nausea and vomiting. Patients should be advised to take this medication with food and the tab should be taken whole and not broken. Patients should be advised that hormonal birth control methods may not be as effective when on this medication, and other forms of birth control should be used. Patients need to be advised that this medication does not prevent the spread of HIV to others through blood or sexual contact.

Carbapenems

ERTAPENEM (*Invanz*) 1 g IV/IM q 24 h. Prophylaxis, colorectal surgery: 1 g IV 1 h before incision. Peds, younger than 13 yo: 15 mg/kg IV/IM q 12 h (up to 1 g/day). Infuse IV over 30 min. ▶K ♀B ▶? © $$$$$ Beta-lactam resistant to hydrolysis by most beta-lactamases, including extended-spectrum beta-lactamases. Serious: Cross-sensitivity with other beta-lactams, *C. difficile*–associated diarrhea, superinfection, seizures (0.5% of patients). Frequent: Diarrhea, N/V, infusion site reactions. Lidocaine diluent can cause allergy.

> Nursing Implications IM: Reconstitute per manufacture drug insert. Inject deep into large muscle mass. Intermittent infusion: Administer within 6 h of mixing. Rate: Over 30 min.

MEROPENEM (*Merrem IV*) Complicated skin infections: 10 mg/kg up to 500 mg IV q 8 h. Intra-abdominal infections: 20 mg/kg up to 1 g IV q 8 h. Peds meningitis: 40 mg/kg IV q 8 h for age 3 mo or older; 2 g IV q 8 h for wt greater than 50 kg. ▶K ♀B ▶? © $$$$$ Beta-lactam resistant to hydrolysis by most beta-lactamases, including extended-spectrum beta-lactamases. Serious: Cross-sensitivity with other beta-lactams, *C. difficile*–associated diarrhea, superinfection, seizures, thrombocytopenia in renal dysfunction. Frequent: Diarrhea.

> Nursing Implications Administer by IV infusion. Monitor for severe allergic reaction/anaphylaxis including seizures, weakness, bleeding/bruising, and severe diarrhea. Shake and let stand until clear when preparing soln, use immediately, and do not administer with other drugs; do not freeze reconstituted solns. Teach pt that the following may occasionally occur: flu-like symptoms, GI disturbances, rash, breathing problems, anemia, and pain. Assess pt for prior penicillin hypersensitivity which may indicate hypersensitivity to Megace; alert prescriber.

Cephalosporins—1st Generation

CEFADROXIL (*Duricef*) 1 to 2 g/day PO once daily or divided two times per day. Peds: 30 mg/kg/day divided two times per day. ▶K ♀B ▶+ © $$$ Generic only: Tabs 1 g. Caps 500 mg. Susp 125, 250, 500 mg/5 mL. Beta-lactam antibiotic that inhibits the biosynthesis of cell wall mucopeptide. (Beta-lactam fused to different ring structure from penicillins.) Serious: Cross-sensitivity with penicillins, *C. difficile*–associated diarrhea. Frequent: diarrhea.

> Nursing Implications Administer with 8 ounces of water. Do not use in patients allergic to this drug or other cephalosporin antibiotics. Use cautiously in patients with kidney disease, diabetes, or a history of intestinal problems. Promote completion of entire course of therapy. Monitor for watery diarrhea, flu-like symptoms, unusual bleeding or bruising, seizures, yellowing of skin or eyes, confusion, joint pain, rash, sore throat, increased thirst, shortness of breath, loss of appetite, and decreased urination.

CEFAZOLIN (*Ancef*) 0.5 to 1.5 g IM/IV q 6 to 8 h. Peds: 25 to 50 mg/kg/day divided q 6 to 8 h (up to 100 mg/kg/day for severe infections). ▶K ♀B ▶+ © $$ Beta-lactam antibiotic that inhibits the biosynthesis of cell wall mucopeptide. (Beta-lactam fused to different ring structure from penicillins.) Serious: Cross-sensitivity with penicillins, *C. difficile*–associated diarrhea. Frequent: Hypersensitivity.

CEPHALOSPORINS –GENERAL ANTIMICROBIAL SPECTRUM

1st generation	Gram-positive (including *Staphylococcus aureus*); basic Gram-negative coverage
2nd generation	diminished *S. aureus*, improved Gram-negative coverage compared to 1st generation; some with anaerobic coverage
3rd generation	further diminished *S. aureus*, further improved Gram-negative coverage compared to 1st and 2nd generation; some with Pseudomonal coverage and diminished Gram-positive coverage
4th generation	same as 3rd generation plus coverage against *Pseudomonas*
5th generation	Gram-negative coverage similar to 3rd generation; also active against *S. aureus* (including MRSA) and *S. pneumoniae*

> **Nursing Implications** Follow manufacturer's instructions for injection of cefazolin. Do not use in patients allergic to this drug or other cephalosporin antibiotics. Use cautiously in patients with kidney or liver disease, or a history of intestinal problems. Promote completion of entire course of therapy. Monitor for watery diarrhea, flu-like symptoms, unusual bleeding or bruising, seizures, yellowing of skin or eyes, confusion, joint pain, rash, sore throat, increased thirst, shortness of breath, loss of appetite, and decreased urination.

CEPHALEXIN (*Keflex, Panixine DisperDose*) 250 to 500 mg PO four times per day. Peds: 25 to 50 mg/kg/day. Not for otitis media, sinusitis. ▶K ♀B ▶? © $$$ Generic/Trade: Caps 250, 500 mg. Generic only: Tabs 250, 500 mg. Susp 125, 250 mg/5 mL. Panixine DisperDose 125, 250 mg scored tabs for oral susp. Trade only: Caps 333, 750 mg. Beta-lactam antibiotic that inhibits the biosynthesis of cell wall mucopeptide. (Beta-lactam fused to different ring structure from penicillins.) Serious: Cross-sensitivity with penicillins, *C. difficile*–associated diarrhea. Frequent: Eosinophilia.

> **Nursing Implications** Administer with 8 ounces of water. Do not use in patients allergic to this drug, penicillin antibiotics, or other cephalosporin antibiotics. Use cautiously in patients with kidney disease, diabetes, those who are malnourished, or a history of intestinal problems.

Cephalosporins—3rd Generation

CEFTAZIDIME (*Fortaz, Tazicef*) 1 g IM/IV or 2 g IV q 8 to 12 h. Peds: 30 to 50 mg/kg IV q 8 h. ▶K ♀B ▶+ © $$$$$ Beta-lactam antibiotic that inhibits the biosynthesis of cell wall mucopeptide. (Beta-lactam fused to different ring structure from penicillins.) Serious: Cross-sensitivity with penicillins, *C. difficile*–associated diarrhea, CNS toxicity with high levels in patients with renal dysfunction. Frequent: Coombs plus anemia, eosinophilia, increased LFTs.

> **Nursing Implications** Administer IM or IV. Caution in use for pts with impaired kidney function. IV route preferable if infection is severe (ie, bacterial septicemia, meningitis or peritonitis). Frozen sterile solns are stable for 6 mos. Thaw only at room temperature not in water bath. Do not refreeze. Monitor pt for allergic reaction ie, rash, fever, erythema, angioedema, and anaphylaxis; GI symptoms; headache and dizziness; pain at injection site and renal function.

CEFTRIAXONE (*Rocephin*) 1 to 2 g IM/IV q 24 h. Meningitis: 2 g IV q 12 h. Gonorrhea: 250 mg IM plus azithromycin 1 g PO, both single dose. Peds: 50 to 75 mg/kg/day (up to 2 g/day) divided q 12 to 24 h. Peds meningitis: 100 mg/kg/day (up to 4 g/day) IV divided q 12 to 24 h. Otitis media: 50 mg/kg up to 1 g IM single dose. May dilute in 1% lidocaine for IM. Contraindicated in neonates who require (or are expected to require) IV calcium (including calcium in TPN); fatal lung/kidney precipitation of calcium ceftriaxone has been reported in neonates. In other patients, do not give ceftriaxone and calcium-containing solns simultaneously, but sequential administration is acceptable if lines are flushed with a compatible fluid between infusions. ▶K/Bile ♀B ▶+ © $$$ Beta-lactam antibiotic that inhibits the biosynthesis of cell wall mucopeptide. (Beta-lactam fused to different ring structure from penicillins.) Serious: Cross-sensitivity with penicillins, *C. difficile*–associated diarrhea, prolonged prothrombin time due to vitamin K deficiency, biliary sludging/symptoms of gallbladder disease, hemolytic anemia. Fatal precipitation with calcium in lungs/kidneys of neonates. Frequent: Eosinophilia.

> **Nursing Implications** Do not administer to pts with allergies to cephalosporins or penicillin. Assess pt for previous gall bladder, kidney, liver or GI diseases, and pregnancy and report to prescriber before use. Monitor for allergic reactions, pounding or irregular HB, weakness, fatigue, jaundice, dark urine or change in urine amount, chest pain, breathing problems, or confusion. Alert pt that with prolonged use drug may cause vaginal yeast infection, thrush, or diarrhea. Persistent diarrhea or bloody stool should be reported immediately to prescriber. May interfere with efficacy of birth control pills or accuracy of certain lab tests.

Cephalosporins—4th Generation

CEFEPIME (*Maxipime*) 0.5 to 2 g IM/IV q 12 h. Peds: 50 mg/kg IV q 8 to 12 h. ▶K ♀B ▶? © $$$$$ Beta-lactam antibiotic that inhibits the biosynthesis of cell wall mucopeptide. (Beta-lactam fused to different ring structure from penicillins.) Serious: Cross-sensitivity with penicillins, *C. difficile*–associated diarrhea, CNS toxicity (encephalopathy, myoclonus, seizures) due to high levels of cefepime, especially in patients with renal dysfunction. An FDA safety review did not find higher mortality with cefepime than with other beta-lactams. Frequent: Coombs plus anemia.

Nursing Implications Follow manufacturer's instructions for infusion via injection or IV. Do not use in patients allergic to this drug or other penicillin antibiotics. Use cautiously in patients with kidney or liver disease, or a history of intestinal problems. Promote seeking of emergency medical help if the following symptoms occur: watery diarrhea, flu-like symptoms, unusual bleeding or bruising, seizures, yellowing of skin or eyes, confusion, joint pain, rash, sore throat, increased thirst, shortness of breath, loss of appetite, and decreased urination. Administer over 30 min.

Cephalosporins—5th Generation

NOTE: *Cephalosporins can be cross-sensitive with penicillins and can cause C. difficile–associated diarrhea.*

CEFTAROLINE (*Teflaro*) Community-acquired bacterial pneumonia, acute bacterial skin and skin structure infections: 600 mg IV q 12 h infused over 1 h. ▶K ♀B ▶? © $$$$$ Beta-lactam antibiotic that inhibits the biosynthesis of cell wall mucopeptide. (Beta-lactam fused to different ring structure from penicillins). Serious: Serious: Cross-sensitivity with penicillins, *C. difficile*–associated diarrhea. Coombs and anemia possible. Frequent: Diarrhea, nausea, rash.

Nursing Implications Must be diluted in 250 mL; stable for 6 h at room temperature; 24 h if refrigerated. No compatibility studies are known; avoid mixing with other products.

Other Antimicrobials

LINEZOLID (*Zyvox*, ✦ *Zyvoxam*) Pneumonia, complicated skin infections (including MRSA), vancomycin-resistant *E. faecium* infections: 10 mg/kg (up to 600 mg) IV/PO q 8 h for age younger than 12 yo, 600 mg IV/PO q 12 h for adults and age 12 yo or older. Myelosuppression, drug interactions due to MAO inhibition. Limit tyramine foods to less than 100 mg/meal. ▶Oxidation/K ♀C ▶? © $$$$$ Trade only: Tabs 600 mg. Susp 100 mg/ 5 mL. Oxazolidinone that inhibits bacterial protein synthesis by binding with 50S ribosome (may compete for binding with chloramphenicol). Bacteriostatic. Serious: Myelosuppression, reports of serotonin syndrome, peripheral and optic neuropathy (with long-term use; optic neuropathy sometimes progressing to vision loss), lactic acidosis (immediate evaluation if recurrent N/V, unexplained acidosis, low bicarbonate). Hypoglycemia reported in diabetics treated with insulin or oral hypoglycemics. In a study comparing linezolid with vancomycin, oxacillin, dicloxacillin for catheter-related bloodstream infections, mortality was increased in linezolid-treated patients infected only with Gram-negative bacteria. Frequent: Thrombocytopenia, N/V, diarrhea. Tooth discoloration (removable with cleaning).

Nursing Implications Any allergies should be considered before starting Zyvox. Other drugs, toabcco, and alcohol should not be used with Zyvox. Patients must be on a low-tyramine diet when on this medication and for a minimum of 2 days following discontiuation of this medication. A low-tyramine diet includes not eating foods high in preservatives, caffeine, or highly processed foods. Most cheeses must be avoided with the exception of cottage and cream cheese. Certain wines must be avoided. Nuts, bananas, figs, dried fruit must be avoided. For a complete list of foods, please consult information on low-tyramine diets. This medication needs to be taken with food. One of the most common side effects is diarrhea. This medication may also lower the blood sugar, so diabetic patients should monitor blood sugar levels closely.

NITROFURANTOIN (*Furadantin, Macrodantin, Macrobid*) 50 to 100 mg PO four times per day. Peds: 5 to 7 mg/kg/day divided four times per day. Macrobid: 100 mg PO two times per day. ▶KL ♀B ▶+? © $ Generic/Trade (Macrodantin): Caps 25, 50, 100 mg. Generic/Trade (Macrobid): Caps 100 mg. Generic/Trade (Furadantin): Susp 25 mg/5 mL. Appears to interact with ribosomal proteins and damage bacterial DNA. Serious: Pulmonary fibrosis with prolonged use, hepatotoxicity, peripheral neuropathy, hemolytic anemia in G6PD deficiency. Frequent: N/V, allergy, brown discoloration of urine.

Nursing Implications Patients should be educated to take this medication with food in order to improve drug absorption. Nursing should observe patients for signs and symptoms of pulmonary reactions, which can be fatal; hepatoxicity; neuropathy; optic neuritis; and hemolytic anemia. Patients should be advised to report any signs or symptoms of diarrhea as *C. difficile*–associated diarrhea has been associated with taking this medication. This medication should be discontinued if any of these adverse reactions occur.

RIFAXIMIN   (*Xifaxan*) Traveler's diarrhea: 200 mg PO three times per day for 3 days. Prevention of recurrent hepatic encephalopathy ($$$$$): 550 mg PO two times per day. ▶Feces, no GI absorption ♀C ▶? © $$$ Trade only: Tabs 200, 550 mg. Rifamycin structurally related to rifampin. Inhibits bacterial RNA synthesis by binding with beta-subunit of bacterial DNA-dependent RNA polymerase. Active against entero-toxigenic or -aggregative *E. coli*. Serious: None found. Frequent: None found.

> Nursing Implications Administer with or without food.

TIGECYCLINE   (*Tygacil*) Complicated skin infections, complicated intra-abdominal infections, community-acquired pneumonia: 100 mg IV first dose, then 50 mg IV q 12 h. Infuse over 30 to 60 min. Consider other antibiotics for severe infection because mortality is higher with tigecycline, especially in ventilator-associated pneumonia. ▶Bile, K ♀D ▶?+ © $$$$$ Inhibits bacterial protein synthesis by binding with ribosomal 30S subunit and blocking addition of amino acids to peptide chain. Bacteriostatic. Serious: Higher mortality than other antibiotics, especially in ventilator-associated pneumonia. Anaphylaxis/anaphylactoid reactions, acute pancreatitis, hepatic dysfunction. Other adverse effects may be similar to tetracyclines (Serious: Pseudotumor cerebri, anti-anabolic effects, photosensitivity, teeth staining in children younger than 8 yo.) Frequent: N/V.

> Nursing Implications Tygacil should not be used in women who are pregnant, nursing, or planning to become pregnant; people allergic to tetracycline, or those with a history of pancreatitis. Patients should be advised to use other forms of birth control as this medication may lower the efficacy of hormonal birth control. Common side effects are to the gastrointestinal system such as abdominal cramps and pain and diarrhea. This medication is teratogenic.

VANCOMYCIN   (*Vancocin*) Usual dose: 15 to 20 mg/kg IV q 8 to 12 h; consider loading dose of 25 to 30 mg/kg for severe infection. Infuse over 1 h; infuse over 1.5 to 2 h if dose greater than 1 g. Peds: 10 to 15 mg/kg IV q 6 h. *C. difficile* diarrhea: 40 mg/kg/day PO up to 500 mg/day divided four times per day for 10 to 14 days. IV administration ineffective for this indication. Dose depends on severity and complications, see table for management of *C. difficile* infection in adults. ▶K ♀C ▶? © $$$$$ Trade only: Caps 125, 250 mg. Bactericidal glycopeptide that inhibits synthesis of cell wall peptidoglycan polymers. May also have other mechanisms of action. Serious: Reversible neutropenia, ototoxicity (rare and reversible with monotherapy) or nephrotoxicity (rare; risk may be increased by high doses, poor renal function, old age, or nephrotoxic drug), superinfection. Can cause *C. difficile*–associated diarrhea. Frequent: "Red Neck" (or "Red Man") syndrome with rapid IV administration, vein irritation with IV extravasation.

> Nursing Implications Observe for signs and symptoms of severe allergic reactions such as hives, urticaria, shortness of breath, tightness in the chest, and swelling of the mouth, face, lips, or tongue. This medication is administered as an injection, usually intravenously in a hospital setting. Common side effects are stomach pain and cramping as well as diarrhea. This medication can cause ototoxicity and renal toxicity. Patients should have hearing acuity testing and renal function tests (BUN and creatinine) prior to starting this medication. This medication has been found in breastmilk. Vancomycin should not be used with methotrexate or aminoglycosides because of increased risk of renal and ototoxicities.

Penicillins—1st generation—Natural

PENICILLIN V   (◆ *PVF-K*) Adults: 250 to 500 mg PO four times per day. Peds: 25 to 50 mg/kg/day divided two to four times per day. AHA doses for pharyngitis: 250 mg (peds 27 kg or less) or 500 mg (adults and peds greater than 27 kg) PO two to three times per day for 10 days. ▶K ♀B ▶? © $ Generic only: Tabs 250, 500 mg, oral soln 125, 250 mg/5 mL. Beta-lactam antibiotic that inhibits the biosynthesis of cell wall mucopeptide. Serious: Anaphylaxis (rare), cross-sensitivity with cephalosporins, Coombs and hemolytic anemia. Frequent: Allergy.

> Nursing Implications Patients need to be advised that severe allergic reactions (rash, hives, itching, difficulty breathing, tightness in the chest, swelling of the mouth, face, lips, or tongue) may occur when taking this medication. If side effects occur, medication should be stopped immediately and patients should seek emergency treatment ASAP. The most common side effects of this medication affect the gastrointestinal track, such as nausea, vomiting and diarrhea. Patients need to be educated that hormonal birth control may not work while taking this medication and patients should utilize additional birth control methods.

PROPHYLAXIS FOR BACTERIAL ENDOCARDITIS*

Limited to dental or respiratory tract procedures in patients at highest risk. All regimens are single doses administered 30–60 minutes prior to procedure.	
Standard regimen	Amoxicillin 2 g PO
Unable to take oral meds	Ampicillin 2 g IM/IV; or cefazolin† or ceftriaxone† 1 g IM/IV
Allergic to penicillin	Clindamycin 600 mg PO; or cephalexin† 2 g PO; or azithromycin or clarithromycin 500 mg PO
Allergic to penicillin and unable to take oral meds	Clindamycin 600 mg IM/IV; or cefazolin† or ceftriaxone† 1 g IM/IV
Pediatric drug doses	Pediatric dose should not exceed adult dose. Amoxicillin 50 mg/kg, ampicillin 50 mg/kg, azithromycin 15 mg/kg, cephalexin† 50 mg/kg, cefazolin† 50 mg/kg, ceftriaxone† 50 mg/kg, clarithromycin 15 mg/kg, clindamycin 20 mg/kg.

*For additional details of the 2007 AHA guidelines, see http://www.americanheart.org.
†Avoid cephalosporins if prior penicillin-associated anaphylaxis, angioedema, or urticaria.

PENICILLINS—GENERAL ANTIMICROBIAL SPECTRUM

1st generation	Most streptococci; oral anaerobic coverage
2nd generation	Most streptococci; *S.aureus* (but not MRSA)
3rd generation	Most streptococci; basic Gram-negative coverage
4th generation	*Pseudomonas*

Penicillins—3rd generation—Aminopenicillins

AMOXICILLIN (*DisperMox, Moxatag*) 250 to 500 mg PO three times per day, or 500 to 875 mg PO two times per day. High-dose for community-acquired pneumonia, acute sinusitis: 1 g PO three times per day. Lyme disease: 500 mg PO three times per day for 14 days for early disease, 28 days for Lyme arthritis. Chlamydia in pregnancy: 500 mg PO three times per day for 7 days. AHA dosing for group A streptococcal pharyngitis: 50 mg/kg (max 1 g) PO once daily for 10 days. Group A streptococcal pharyngitis/ tonsillitis: 775 mg ER tab (Moxatag) PO for 10 days for age 12 yo or older. Peds AAP otitis media: 90 mg/kg/day divided two times per day. AAP recommends 5 to 7 days of therapy for age 6 yo or older with non severe otitis media, and 10 days for younger children and those with severe disease. Peds infections other than otitis media: 40 mg/kg/day PO divided three times per day or 45 mg/kg/day divided two times per day. ▶K ♀B ▶+ © $ Generic only: Caps 250, 500 mg, Tabs 500, 875 mg, Chewable tabs 125, 200, 250, 400 mg. Susp 125, 250 mg/5 mL. Susp 200, 400 mg/5 mL. Infant gtts 50 mg/mL. DisperMox 200, 400, 600 mg tabs for oral susp, Moxatag 775 mg extended-release tab. Beta-lactam antibiotic that inhibits the biosynthesis of cell wall mucopeptide. Aminopenicillins are more active than natural penicillins against Gram-negative cocci and Enterobacteriaceae. Serious: Anaphylaxis (rare), cross-sensitivity with cephalosporins. Frequent: Rash (nonallergic in patients with mononucleosis, chronic myelogenous leukemia, or allopurinol therapy), diarrhea.

> Nursing Implications   Follow directions for dosage as prescribed by healthcare provider. Can be taken with or without food. Do not use in patients allergic to amoxicillin or penicillin drugs. Use cautiously in patients allergic to cephalosporin antibiotics. Use cautiously in patients with renal or liver dysfunction, asthma, history of diarrhea while taking antibiotics, history of allergies, or mononucleosis.

AMOXICILLIN-CLAVULANATE (*Augmentin, Augmentin ES-600, Augmentin XR, ◆ Clavulin*) Adults, usual dose: 500 to 875 mg PO two times per day or 250 to 500 mg three times per day. Augmentin XR: 2 tabs PO q 12 h with meals. See table for management of acute sinusitis in adults and children. Peds, usual dose: 45 mg/kg/day PO divided two times per day or 40 mg/kg/day divided three times per day. High-dose for community-acquired pneumonia, otitis media, sinusitis: 90 mg/kg/day PO divided two times per day (max dose of 2 g PO two times per day for age 5 yo and older). Treat pneumonia for up to 10 days; otitis media for 5 to 7 days in age 6 yo or older with non severe infection or 10 days for younger children or those with severe infection; sinusitis for 10 to 14 days. ▶K ♀B ▶? © $$$$ Generic/Trade: (amoxicillin-clavulanate) Tabs 250/125, 500/125, 875/125 mg. Chewables, Susp 200/28.5, 400/57 mg per tab or 5 mL, 250/62.5 mg per 5 mL. (ES) Susp 600/42.9 mg per 5 mL. Trade only: Chewables, Susp 125/31.25 per tab or 5 mL, 250/62.5 per tab. Extended-release tabs (Augmentin XR) 1000/62.5 mg. Beta-lactam antibiotic that inhibits the biosynthesis of cell wall mucopeptide. Aminopenicillins are more active than natural penicillins against Gram-negative cocci and Enterobacteriaceae. Clavulanate is a beta-lactamase inhibitor. Serious: Anaphylaxis (rare), cross-sensitivity with cephalosporins, clavulanate-induced cholestatic hepatitis (esp. in elderly men treated for more than 2 weeks). Frequent: Diarrhea (less with twice daily dosing, incidence related to clavulanate dose), rash (nonallergic in patients with mononucleosis, chronic myelogenous leukemia, or allopurinol therapy).

> Nursing Implications Follow directions for dosage as prescribed by healthcare provider. Administer dosage with 8 ounces of water and with food to reduce stomach upset. Do not use in patients allergic to amoxicillin or clavulanate potassium. Do not use in patients with penicillin allergies. Use cautiously in patients with renal or liver dysfunction, mononucleosis, or patients allergic to cephalosporin antibiotics. Promote completion of entire course of therapy.

AMPICILLIN (✦ *Penbritin*) Usual dose: 1 to 2 g IV q 4 to 6 h. Sepsis, meningitis: 150 to 200 mg/kg/ day IV divided q 3 to 4 h. Peds: 100 to 400 mg/kg/day IM/IV divided q 4 to 6 h. ▶K ♀B ▶? © $ PO $$$$$ IV Generic only: Caps 250, 500 mg. Susp 125, 250 mg/5 mL. Beta-lactam antibiotic that inhibits the biosynthesis of cell wall mucopeptide. Aminopenicillins are more active than natural penicillins against Gram-negative cocci and Enterobacteriaceae. Serious: Anaphylaxis (rare), cross-sensitivity with cephalosporins, *C. difficile*–associated diarrhea. Frequent: Nonallergic rash in patients with mononucleosis, chronic myelogenous leukemia, or allopurinol therapy; eosinophilia; diarrhea (especially with PO).

> Nursing Implications Follow directions for dosage as prescribed by healthcare provider. Administer dosage with 8 ounces of water and on an empty stomach at least 1 to 2 h before a meal. Do not use in patients allergic to ampicillin or other penicillin drugs. Use cautiously in patients allergic to cephalosporin antibiotics. Use cautiously in patients with renal dysfunction, asthma, bleeding or clotting disorders, history of diarrhea while taking antibiotics, history of allergies, or mononucleosis. Promote regular follow-up with provider for blood testing.

Penicillins—4th Generation—Extended Spectrum

PIPERACILLIN-TAZOBACTAM (*Zosyn*, ✦ *Tazocin*) 3.375 to 4.5 g IV q 6 h. Peds appendicitis or peritonitis: 80 mg/kg IV q 8 h for age 2 to 9 mo, 100 mg/kg piperacillin IV q 8 h for age older than 9 mo, use adult dose for wt greater than 40 kg. ▶K ♀B ▶? © $$$$$ Beta-lactam antibiotic that inhibits the biosynthesis of cell wall mucopeptide. Tazobactam is beta-lactamase inhibitor. Serious: Anaphylaxis (rare), cross-sensitivity with cephalosporins, hypokalemia, bleeding, and coagulation abnormalities (especially with renal impairment). Frequent: N/V, diarrhea, headache.

> Nursing Implications Zosyn should not be used by patients with a history of allergic reactions to any penicillin, cephalosporin, beta-lactam antibiotic, or beta-lactamase inhibitor. People with cystic fibrosis, bleeding problems, congestive heart failure, bowel inflammation, kidney problems, low blood potassium, or salt-restrictive diet should not use Zosyn. Patients should be advised to avoid activities that may result in bruising or injuries as this medication can decrease the platelet count. Diabetic patients should check their blood sugar more frequently. The most common side effects are gastrointestinal in nature, such as stomach cramping or pain and diarrhea.

Quinolones—2nd Generation

CIPROFLOXACIN (*Cipro, Cipro XR, ProQuin XR*) 200 to 400 mg IV q 8 to 12 h. 250 to 750 mg PO two times per day. Simple UTI: 250 mg two times per day for 3 days or Cipro XR/ProQuin XR 500 mg PO daily for 3 days. Give ProQuin XR with main meal of day. Cipro XR for pyelonephritis or complicated UTI: 1000 mg PO daily for 7 to 14 days. ▶LK ♀C but teratogenicity unlikely ▶?+ © $ Generic/Trade: Tabs 100, 250, 500, 750 mg. Extended-release tabs 500, 1000 mg. Trade only (ProQuin XR): Extended-release tabs 500 mg, blister pack 500 mg (#3 tabs). Inhibits bacterial DNA synthesis by binding with DNA gyrase and topoisomerase IV. Serious: Tendon rupture (rare), phototoxicity, CNS toxicity, crystalluria

QUINOLONES—GENERAL ANTIMICROBIAL SPECTRUM

1st generation	1st generation quinolones are no longer available
2nd generation	Gram-negative (including *Pseudomonas*); *S. aureus* (but not MRSA or *pneumococcus*); some atypicals
3rd generation	Gram-negative (including *Pseudomonas*); Gram-positive, including *Pneumococcus* and *S aureus* (but not MRSA); expanded atypical coverage
4th generation	same as 3rd generation plus enhanced coverage of *Pneumococcus*, decreased *Pseudomonas activity*

if alkaline urine, peripheral neuropathy (rare), hypersensitivity. Theoretical risk of cartilage toxicity in children, but no clinical evidence of harm other than transient large-joint arthralgias. Musculoskeletal adverse events reported with ciprofloxacin treatment of complicated UTI in peds patients were mild to moderate in severity and resolved within 1 month after treatment. Frequent: N/V. More GI, neurologic, and musculoskeletal adverse reactions reported during postexposure prophylaxis of bioterrorism anthrax.

> Nursing Implications Administer with 8 ounces of water. Do not crush, chew, or break tablet. May be taken with or without food, and must be taken at same time each day. Do not administer with dairy or milk products, or with calcium-enriched juices. Do not use in patients currently taking tizanidine, or in those allergic to ciprofloxacin or similar medications such as levofloxacin, lomefloxacin, moxifloxacin, ofloxacin, and norfloxacin. Use cautiously in patients with heart rhythm disorders, or in those being treated with quinidine, disopyramide, procainamide, amiodarone, or sotalol. Use cautiously in patients with a history of renal or liver dysfunction, epilepsy or seizures, diabetes, joint problems, a history of long QT syndrome, low levels of potassium, or a history of allergy to antibiotics. Promote increased hydration during entire course of therapy.

Quinolones—3rd Generation

LEVOFLOXACIN (***Levaquin***) 250 to 750 mg PO/IV daily. See table for management of acute sinusitis in adults and children. ▶KL ♀C ▶? © $ Generic/Trade: Tabs 250, 500, 750 mg, Oral soln 25 mg/mL. Trade only: Leva-Pak: #5, 750 mg tabs. Inhibits bacterial DNA synthesis by binding with DNA gyrase and topoisomerase IV. Serious: QT interval prolongation, tendon rupture (rare), phototoxicity (rare), peripheral neuropathy (rare), CNS toxicity, hepatotoxicity, and hypersensitivity. Frequent: Headache. Musculoskeletal disorders (arthralgia, arthritis, tendinopathy, gait abnormality) reported in children; safety for treatment duration more than 14 days not established.

> Nursing Implications PO or IV injection. Increases risk of tendonitis, tendon rupture thus vigorous exercise should be avoided during treatment. Elderly pts and those on steroids are especially prone to tendonitis as well as those who have had organ transplants. Avoid use in pts with myasthenia gravis. Pt should call prescriber if allergic reaction occurs: fainting or rapid, pounding HR; joint swelling in arm or ankles; watery, bloody diarrhea; urine problems; skin rash (even mild); bruising/bleeding; seizures; or mental confusion. Numbness, burning or pains in hands and feet and symptoms of hypo- or hyperglycemia should be reported to prescriber. Teach pt that other side effects may occur including GI disturbances, restlessness, headache, problems sleeping, and skin and vaginal itching. Pt should avoid antacids and exposure to strong sun and light.

Tetracyclines

NOTE: *Tetracyclines can cause photosensitivity and pseudotumor cerebri (avoid with isotretinoin which is also linked to pseudotumor cerebri). May decrease efficacy of oral contraceptives. Increased INR with warfarin. May increase risk of ergotism with ergot alkaloids.*

MINOCYCLINE (***Minocin, Dynacin, Solodyn***, ✦ ***Enca***) 200 mg IV/PO initially, then 100 mg q 12 h. Community-acquired MRSA skin infections: 200 mg PO first dose, then 100 mg PO two times per day for 5 to 10 days. Acne (traditional dosing, not Solodyn): 50 mg PO two times per day. Solodyn ($$$$$)

for inflammatory acne in adults and children 12 yo and older: Give PO once daily at dose of 45 mg for wt 45 to 54 kg, 65 mg for wt 55 to 77 kg, 90 mg for wt 78 to 102 kg, 115 mg for wt 103 to 125 kg, 135 mg for wt 126 to 136 kg. ▶LK ♀D ▶?+ © $$ Generic/Trade: Caps, Tabs 50, 75, 100 mg. Tabs, extended-release (Solodyn) 45, 90, 135 mg. Trade only: Tabs, extended-release (Solodyn) 65, 115 mg. Inhibits bacterial protein synthesis by binding with ribosomal 30S subunit and blocking addition of amino acids to peptide chain. Active against intracellular bacteria. Bacteriostatic. Subantimicrobial doses have anti-inflammatory effects. Serious: Pseudotumor cerebri, serum sickness, Stevens-Johnson syndrome, drug rash with eosinophilia and systemic symptoms (DRESS), increased BUN, photosensitivity, hepatotoxicity, lupus, hypersensitivity pneumonitis, hyperpigmentation, teeth staining in children younger than 8 yo. Frequent: Dizziness/vestibular toxicity.

> Nursing Implications   Observe patients for severe allergic reactions such as hives, urticaria, shortness of breath, tightness in the chest, and swelling of the mouth, face, lips, or tongue. This medication should be used cautiously in children when bones and teeth are developing. Patients should be advised to avoid sun exposure and tanning beds; secondary to photosensitivity from this medication. This medication may cause permanent discoloration of teeth. Iron supplements, multivitamins, calcium supplements, laxatives, and antacids make minocycline less effective.

CARDIOVASCULAR

ACE Inhibitors

NOTE: *See also Antihypertensive Combinations. Hyperkalemia possible, especially if used concomitantly with other drugs that increase K+ (including K+ containing salt substitutes) and in patients with heart failure, diabetes mellitus, or renal impairment. Monitor closely for hypoglycemia, especially during first month of treatment when combined with insulin or oral antidiabetic agents. ACE inhibitors are contra-indicated during pregnancy. Contraindicated with a history of angioedema. Renoprotection and decreased cardiovascular morbidity/mortality seen with some ACE inhibitors are most likely a class effect.*

ENALAPRIL (enalaprilat, *Vasotec*) HTN: Start 5 mg PO daily, usual maintenance dose 10 to 40 mg PO daily or divided two times per day, max 40 mg/day. If oral therapy not possible, can use enalaprilat 1.25 mg IV q 6 h over 5 min, and increase up to 5 mg IV q 6 h if needed. Renal impairment or concomitant diuretic therapy: Start 2.5 mg PO daily. Heart failure: Start 2.5 mg PO two times per day, usual dose 10 to 20 mg PO two times per day, max 40 mg/day. ▶LK ♀D ▶+ © $$ Generic/Trade: Tabs, scored 2.5, 5 mg, unscored 10, 20 mg. Inhibits angiotensin-converting enzyme which converts angiotensin I to angiotensin II. Serious: Angioedema, hyperkalemia, renal impairment. Frequent: Cough.

> Nursing Implications   Do not use in pregnancy. Use cautiously in patients with liver and heart disease, or taking diuretics; in elderly, breastfeeding women, and children. Give with food or beverage. Monitor for CNS symptoms including mood changes and neuropathy, gastric symptoms, cough, skin rash, enlarged lymph nodes, flu-like symptoms, infections such as herpes. Drug must be weaned; teach patient to immediately report rash, fever, chills, N/V, and injection site reaction.

LISINOPRIL (*Prinivil, Zestril*) HTN: Start 10 mg PO daily, usual maintenance dose 20 to 40 mg PO daily, max 80 mg/day. Heart failure, acute MI: Start 2.5 to 5 mg PO daily, usual dose 5 to 20 mg PO daily, max dose 40 mg. ▶K ♀D ▶? © $ Generic/Trade: Tabs unscored (Zestril) 2.5, 5, 10, 20, 30, 40 mg. Tabs scored (Prinivil) 10, 20, 40 mg. Serious: Angioedema, hyperkalemia, renal impairment. Frequent: Cough.

> Nursing Implications   The most common side effect is a dry cough. This medication can also affect libido. This medication is teratogenic and patients contemplating pregnancy should not be prescribed this medication.

QUINAPRIL (*Accupril*) HTN: Start 10 to 20 mg PO daily (start 10 mg/day if elderly), usual maintenance dose 20 to 80 mg PO daily or divided two times per day, max 80 mg/day. Heart failure: Start 5 mg PO two times per day, usual maintenance dose 10 to 20 mg two times per day. ▶LK ♀D ▶? © $$ Generic/Trade: Tabs scored 5, unscored 10, 20, 40 mg. Inhibits angiotensin-converting enzyme which converts angiotensin I to angiotensin II. Serious: Angioedema, hyperkalemia, renal impairment. Frequent: Cough.

ACE INHIBITOR DOSING	HTN		Heart Failure	
	Initial	Max/day	Initial	Max/day
benazepril (*Lotensin*)	10 mg daily*	80 mg	-	-
captopril (*Capoten*)	25 mg two to three times per day	450 mg	6.25 mg three times per day	450 mg
enalapril (*Vasotec*)	5 mg daily*	40 mg	2.5 mg bid twice daily	40 mg
fosinopril (*Monopril*)	10 mg daily*	80 mg	5–10 mg daily	40 mg
lisinopril (*Zestril/ Prinivil*)	10 mg daily	80 mg	2.5–5 mg daily	40 mg
moexipril (*Univasc*)	7.5 mg daily*	30 mg	-	-
perindopril (*Aceon*)	4 mg daily*	16 mg	2 mg daily	16 mg
quinapril (*Accupril*)	10–20 mg daily*	80 mg	5 mg bid	40 mg
ramipril (*Altace*)	2.5 mg daily*	20 mg	1.25–2.5 mg bid twice daily	10 mg
trandolapril (*Mavik*)	1–2 mg daily*	8 mg	1 mg daily	4 mg

bid = two times per day; tid = three times per day.
Data taken from prescribing information and *Circulation* 2009;119:e391–e479.
* May require twice daily dosing for 24-h BP control.

Nursing Implications This medication should be taken 1 h prior to eating or 2 h prior to bedtime after eating. Tetracyclines and the fluoroquiniolones should be taken 3 h prior to bedtime apart from this medication. Patients should be advised to avoid the use of alcohol when taking this medication. Patients should not take diet pills, cold medicines, or other stimulant types of medications. May cause depression in patients. Discontinue if angioedema occurs to the face, including tongue and lips. Also watch for hypotensive effects within 1 to 3 h of taking initial dose or increased dosage. Diabetic patients need to have frequent blood sugar assessments. This medication is teratogenic. Blood pressure, heart rate, electrolytes, renal and hepatic function need to be assessed on a periodic basis.

RAMIPRIL (*Altace*) HTN: 2.5 mg PO daily, usual maintenance dose 2.5 to 20 mg PO daily or divided two times per day, max 20 mg/day. Heart failure post-MI: Start 2.5 mg PO two times per day, usual maintenance dose 5 mg PO two times per day. Reduce risk of MI, CVA, death from cardiovascular causes: 2.5 mg PO daily for 1 week, then 5 mg daily for 3 weeks, increase as tolerated to max 10 mg/day. ▶LK ♀D ▶? © $$$ Generic/Trade: Caps 1.25, 2.5, 5, 10 mg. Inhibits angiotensin-converting enzyme which converts angiotensin I to angiotensin II. Serious: Angioedema, hepatotoxicity, hyperkalemia, pancreatitis, renal impairment. Frequent: Cough.

Nursing Implications Monitor creatine, wt, pulse, BP, edema, WBC, and BUN. Renal and hepatic function need to be periodically assessed. The blood pressure should be checked frequently. Alcohol should be avoided when on this medication. It is not recommended that this medication be administered to pregnant patients. Coomon side effects include dizziness, vertigo and a feeling of tiredness.

Aldosterone Antagonists

NOTE: *Hyperkalemia possible, especially if used concomitantly with other drugs that increase K+ (including K+ containing salt substitutes) and in patients with heart failure, diabetes mellitus, or renal impairment.*

SPIRONOLACTONE (*Aldactone*) HTN: 50 to 100 mg PO daily or divided two times per day. Edema: 25 to 200 mg/day. Hypokalemia: 25 to 100 mg PO daily. Primary hyperaldosteronism, maintenance: 100 to 400 mg/day PO. Heart failure, NYHA III or IV: 25 to 50 mg PO daily. ▶LK ♀D ▶+ © $ Generic/Trade: Tabs unscored 25 mg, scored 50, 100 mg. Blocks the binding of aldosterone to mineralocorticoid receptors. Serious: Agranulocytosis, hyperkalemia (rare), hypersensitivity, Stevens-Johnson syndrome. Frequent: Gynecomastia, headache, impotence, irregular menses.

> Nursing Implications PO with or without food. Patients should be educated that this medication will cause the patient to urinate more frequently. This medication is a potassium-sparing diuretic and the serum potassium level may rise when one is taking this medication. This medication should be used cautiously in the elderly and with individuals who have renal or hepatic problems. A side effect in men may be breast enlargement, which usually resolves after discontinuation of this medication. Patients need to have renal function, serum electrolytes, and blood pressure monitored periodically.

Angiotensin Receptor Blockers (ARBs)

NOTE: *See also Antihypertensive Combinations. An increase in serum creatinine up to 35% above baseline is acceptable and is not reason to withhold therapy unless hyperkalemia occurs. Do not use during pregnancy. Dual blockade of the renin-angiotensin-aldosterone system has been associated with non-fatal stroke (when used with aliskiren), hypotension, syncope, hyperkalemia, and renal complications. Coadministration with NSAIDs, including selective COX-2 inhibitors, may further deteriorate renal function (usually reversible) and decrease antihypertensive effects.*

LOSARTAN   (***Cozaar***) *HTN: Start 50 mg PO daily, max 100 mg/day given once daily or divided two times per day. Volume-depleted patients or history of hepatic impairment: Start 25 mg PO daily. CVA risk reduction in patients with HTN and LV hypertrophy (may not be effective in black patients): Start 50 mg PO daily. If need more BP reduction add HCTZ 12.5 mg PO daily, then increase losartan to 100 mg/day, then increase HCTZ to 25 mg/day. Type 2 diabetic nephropathy: Start 50 mg PO daily, target dose 100 mg daily.* ▶L ♀D ▶? © $$$ *Generic/Trade: Tabs unscored 25, 50, 100 mg. Blocks binding of angiotensin II to the angiotensin subtype 1 receptor. Serious: Hyperkalemia, renal impairment, thrombocytopenia (rare).*

> Nursing Implications May take 3 to 6 weeks for therapeutic effect; patients should avoid potassium salts/supplements. Pt should contact prescriber immediately if pregnancy is suspected. Monitor for hypersensitivity, BP, liver and kidney function. Teach pt to avoid alcohol and to call prescriber if faintness, urinary problems, pain in chest, bruising or bleeding, slow HR, or swelling in hands or feet occur.

Anti-Dysrhythmics/Cardiac Arrest

ADENOSINE   (***Adenocard***) *PSVT conversion (not A-fib): Adult and peds wt 50 kg or greater: 6 mg rapid IV and flush, preferably through a central line. If no response after 1 to 2 min, then 12 mg. A 3rd dose of 12 mg may be given prn. Peds wt less than 50 kg: Initial dose 50 to 100 mcg/kg, subsequent doses 100 to 200 mcg/kg q 1 to 2 min prn up to a max single dose of 300 mcg/kg or 12 mg, whichever is less. Half-life is less than 10 sec. Give doses by rapid IV push followed by NS flush. Need higher dose if on theophylline or caffeine, lower dose if on dipyridamole or carbamazepine.* ▶Plasma ♀C ▶? © $$$ *Blocks cardiac conduction through the AV node. Serious: Arrhythmias, heart block, bronchoconstriction, seizures. Frequent: Flushing, chest tightness.*

> Nursing Implications This medication is utilized primarily for the treatment of supraventricular tachycardia and other atrial tachycardias. It can also be utilized initially to differentiate monomorphic ventricular tachycardia from supraventricular tachycardia with aberrancy. This medication has an extremely short half-life (approximately 9 seconds), so this medication must be administered by rapid intravenous push in less than 3 seconds followed immediately by a 20 milliliter to 30 milliliter saline bolus. It is common for the patient to experience a short run (5 to 8 seconds) of asystole after the dose is administered. Denervated hearts in heart transplant patients are very sensitive to Adenosine.

AMIODARONE   (***Cordarone, Pacerone***) *Proarrhythmic. Life-threatening ventricular arrhythmia without cardiac arrest: Load 150 mg IV over 10 min, then 1 mg/min for 6 h, then 0.5 mg/min for 18 h. Mix in D5W. Oral loading dose 800 to 1600 mg PO daily for 1 to 3 weeks, reduce to 400 to 800 mg PO daily for 1 month when arrhythmia is controlled, reduce to lowest effective dose thereafter, usually 200 to 400 mg PO daily. Photosensitivity with oral therapy. Pulmonary and hepatic toxicity. Hypo- or hyperthyroidism possible. Coadministration of fluoroquinolones, macrolides, loratadine, trazodone, azoles, or Class IA and*

III antiarrhythmic drugs may prolong QTc. May increase digoxin levels; discontinue digoxin or decrease dose by 50%. May increase INR with warfarin; decrease warfarin dose by 33 to 50%. Do not use with grapefruit juice. Do not use with simvastatin dose greater than 20 mg/day, lovastatin dose greater than 40 mg/day; may increase atorvastatin level; increases risk of myopathy and rhabdomyolysis. Caution with beta-blockers and calcium channel blockers. IV therapy may cause hypotension. Contraindicated with marked sinus bradycardia and 2nd or 3rd degree heart block in the absence of a functioning pacemaker. ▶L ♀D ▶– © $$$$ Trade only (Pacerone): tabs unscored 100 mg. Generic/Trade: Tabs scored 200, 400 mg. Prolongs cardiac repolarization (Class III antiarrhythmic properties). Also has sodium channel blockade, beta adrenergic blockade, and calcium channel blockade effects (Class I, II, IV effects). Serious: Pulmonary toxicity, thyroid toxicity, bradycardia/heart block, arrhythmias, rhabdomyolysis, blindness, visual impairment, SIADH, hepatotoxicity, acute renal failure, agranulocytosis. Frequent: Hypotension, elevated LFTs, photosensitivity, GI intolerance, corneal microdeposits.

> Nursing Implications Teach patient to immediately report irregular, rapid, slow, or pounding heartbeats; chest pain; faintness; wheezing cough; or breathing problems. Advise against driving, operating machinery, or other complex activity until used to drug. Advise patient to wear sunscreen and avoid alcoholic beverages. Closely monitor patient when initial loading dose is given. Neurologic side effects are common. Worsening of arrhythmias may occur and can be fatal. Teach patient or family member to monitor blood pressure regularly.

DIGOXIN (*Lanoxin, Lanoxicaps, Digitek*) Proarrhythmic. Systolic heart failure/rate control of chronic A-fib: younger than 70 yo: 0.25 mg PO daily; age 70 yo or older: 0.125 mg PO daily; impaired renal function: 0.0625 to 0.125 mg PO daily. Rapid A-fib: Total loading dose (TLD), 10 to 15 mcg/kg IV/PO, give in 3 divided doses every 6 to 8 h; give ~50% TLD for 1 dose, then ~25% TLD for 2 doses (eg, 70 kg with normal renal function: 0.5 mg, then 0.25 mg q 6 to 8 h for 2 doses). Impaired renal function, 6 to 10 mcg/kg IV/PO TLD, given in 3 divided 0.125 to 0.375 mg IV/PO daily. ▶KL ♀C ▶+ © $ Generic/Trade: Tabs, scored (Lanoxin, Digitek) 0.125, 0.25 mg; elixir 0.05 mg/mL. Trade only: Caps (Lanoxicaps), 0.1, 0.2 mg. Slows cardiac conduction through the AV node, increases force of myocardial contraction. Serious: Arrhythmias, heart block. Frequent: More frequent with higher doses. Dizziness, N/V, diarrhea.

> Nursing Implications Cautionary use with kidney disease. Monitor for visual disturbances, abdominal pain, heart block, skin rash, nausea and vomiting; low potassium or magnesium: high calcium can potentiate digoxin toxicity resulting in serious heart arrhythmias; take pulse before administering. Take 2 h before or after eating high-fiber foods such as oat bran; instruct pt to store in dry, cool place.

HTN Therapy[1]

Area of Concern	BP Target	Preferred Therapy[2]	Comments
General CAD prevention	<140/90 mm Hg	ACEI, ARB, CCB, thiazide, or combination	Start 2 drugs if systolic BP ≥ 160 or diastolic BP ≥ 100
High CAD risk[3]	<130/80 mm Hg		
Stable angina, unstable angina, MI	<130/80 mm Hg	Beta-blocker[4] + (ACEI or ARB)[5]	May add dihydropyridine CCB or thiazide
Left heart failure[6,7]	<120/80 mm Hg	Beta-blocker + (ACEI or ARB) + diuretic[8] + aldosterone antagonist[9]	

[1]ACEI = angiotensin-converting enzyme inhibitor; ARB = angiotensin-receptor blocker; CCB = calcium-channel blocker; MI = myocardial infarction. Adapted from *Circulation* 2007;115:2761–2788.
[2]All patients should attempt lifestyle modifications: optimize wt, healthy diet, sodium restriction, exercise, smoking cessation, alcohol moderation.
[3]DM, chronic kidney disease, known CAD or risk equivalent (eg, peripheral artery disease, abdominal aortic aneurysm, carotid artery disease, and prior ischemic CVA/TIA), 10-year Framingham risk score ≥ 10%.
[4]Use only if hemodynamically stable. If beta-blocker contraindications or intolerable side effects (and no bradycardia or heart failure), may substitute verapamil or diltiazem.
[5]Preferred if anterior wall MI, persistent HTN, heart failure, or DM.
[6]Avoid verapamil, diltiazem, clonidine, alpha-blockers.
[7]For blacks with NYHA class III or IV HF, consider adding hydralazine/isosorbide dinitrate.
[8]Loop or thiazide.
[9]Use if NYHA class III or IV, or if clinical heart failure + LVEF < 40%.

DIGOXIN IMMUNE FAB (*Digibind, DigiFab*) Digoxin toxicity: Acute ingestion of known amount: 1 vial binds approximately 0.5 mg digoxin. Acute ingestion of unknown amount: 10 vials IV, may repeat once. Toxicity during chronic therapy: 6 vials usually adequate; one formula is: Number vials = (serum dig level in ng/mL) × (kg)/100. ▶K ♀C ▶? © $$$$$ Binds digoxin, preventing interaction with sodium pump receptor. Serious: Hypersensitivity (rare), hypokalemia.

> Nursing Implications Cautionary use with kidney disease; monitor for visual disturbances, abdominal pain, heart block, skin rash, nausea and vomiting. Low potassium or magnesium, high calcium can potentiate digoxin toxicity resulting in serious heart arrhythmias; take pulse before administering. Wait 2 h before or after eating high fiber foods such as oat bran; instruct patient to store in dry, cool place.

DRONEDARONE (*Multaq*) Proarrhythmic. Reduce hospitalization risk for patients with atrial fib who are in sinus rhythm and have a history of paroxysmal or persistent atrial fib: 400 mg PO two times per day with morning and evening meals. Do not use with permanent atrial fibrillation; NYHA Class IV heart failure or NYHA Class II–III heart failure with recent decompensation requiring hospitalization or

SELECTED DRUGS THAT MAY PROLONG THE QT INTERVAL			
alfuzosin	erythromycin*†	levofloxacin	quetiapine‡
amantadine	escitalopram	lithium	quinidine*†
amiodarone*†	famotidine	methadone*†	ranolazine
arsenic trioxide*	felbamate	moexipril/HCTZ	risperidone‡
atazanavir	fingolimod	moxifloxacin*	sertindole
azithromycin*	flecainide*	nicardipine	sotalol*†
chloroquine*	foscarnet	nilotinib	sunitinib
chlorpromazine*	fosphenytoin	octreotide	tacrolimus
cisapride*	gatifloxacin	ofloxacin	tamoxifen
citalopram*	gemifloxacin	ondansetron	telithromycin
clarithromycin*	granisetron	oxytocin	thioridazine*
clozapine	halofantrine*†	paliperidone	tizanidine
disopyramide*†	haloperidol*‡	pentamidine*†	tolterodine
dofetilide*†	ibutilide*†	perflutren lipid	vandetanib*
dolasetron	iloperidone	microspheres	vardenafil
dronedarone	indapamide	phenothiazines‡	venlafaxine
droperidol*	isradipine	pimozide*†	voriconazole
eribulin	lapatinib	procainamide*	ziprasidone‡

NOTE: This table may not include all drugs that prolong the QT interval or cause torsades. Risk of drug-induced QT prolongation may be increased in women, elderly, hypokalemia, hypomagnesemia, bradycardia, starvation, CHF, & CNS injuries. Hepa-torenal dysfunction & drug interactions can the concentration of QT interval-prolonging drugs. Coadministration of QT interval-prolonging drugs can have additive effects. Avoid these (and other) drugs in congenital prolonged QT syndrome (www.qtdrugs.org).

*Torsades reported in product labeling/case reports.

†Increased in women.

‡QT prolongation: thioridazine > ziprasidone > risperidone, quetiapine, haloperidol.

referral to heart failure clinic; 2nd or 3rd degree AV block or sick sinus syndrome without functioning pacemaker; bradycardia less than 50 bpm; QTc Bazett interval greater than 500 ms; liver toxicity related to previous amiodarone use; severe hepatic impairment; pregnancy; lactation; grapefruit juice; drugs or herbals that increase QT interval; antiarrhythmic agents; potent inhibitors of CYP3A4 enzyme system (clarithromycin, itraconazole, ketoconazole, nefazodone, ritonavir, voriconazole); or inducers of CYP3A4 enzyme system (carbamazepine, phenytoin, phenobarbital, rifampin, St. John's wort). Correct hypo/hyperkalemia and hypomagnesium before giving. Monitor EKG every 3 months; if in atrial fib, then either discontinue dronedarone or cardiovert. May initiate or worsen heart failure symptoms. May be associated with hepatic injury; discontinue if hepatic injury is suspected. Serum creatinine and/or BUN may increase during first weeks, but does not reflect change in renal function; reversible when discontinued. Give with appropriate antithrombotic therapy. May increase INR when used with warfarin. May increase dabigatran level. May increase digoxin level; discontinue digoxin or decrease dose by 50%. Use cautiously with beta-blockers (BB) and calcium channel blockers (CCB); initiate lower doses of BB or CCB; initiate at low dose and monitor EKG. Do not use with more than 10 mg of simvastatin. May increase level of sirolimus, tacrolimus, or CYP3A4 substrates with narrow therapeutic index. ▶L ♀X ▶ © $$$$ Trade: Tabs unscored 400 mg. Has sodium channel blockade, beta adrenergic blockade, cardiac repolarization, and calcium channel blockade effects (Class I, II, III, IV effects). Serious: New/worsening heart failure, bradycardia/heart block, arrhythmias, hepatotoxicity, pulmonary toxicity. Frequent: Abdominal pain, asthenia, diarrhea, nausea.

> **Nursing Implications** Give with food. Teach patients to report symptoms of new or worsening heart failure (eg, wt gain, edema, SOB). Teach patients to report symptoms of hepatic injury (eg, anorexia, nausea, vomiting, fatigue, malaise, right upper quadrant discomfort, jaundice, dark urine).

FLECAINIDE (*Tambocor*) Proarrhythmic. Prevention of paroxysmal atrial fib/flutter or PSVT, with symptoms and no structural heart disease: Start 50 mg PO q 12 h, may increase by 50 mg two times per day q 4 days, max 300 mg/day. Use with AV nodal slowing agent (beta-blocker, verapamil, diltiazem) to minimize risk of 1:1 atrial flutter. Life-threatening ventricular arrhythmias without structural heart disease: Start 100 mg PO q 12 h, may increase by 50 mg two times per day q 4 days, max 400 mg/day. With CrCl less than 35 mL/min: Start 50 mg PO two times per day. ▶K ♀C ▶– © $$$$ Generic/Trade: Tabs unscored 50 mg, scored 100, 150 mg. Depresses phase 0 depolarization significantly, slows cardiac conduction significantly (Class 1C). Serious: Arrhythmias, depressed conduction/widened QRS at higher heart rates. Frequent: Dizziness, headache, nausea, dyspnea, fatigue, visual disturbances.

> **Nursing Implications** Do not give to pts prone to ventricular or atrial fibrillation. Caution in pts with heart and renal disease, pregnant or breastfeeding women, children, or pts taking beta-blockers. Monitor for dizziness, anxiety, depression, tremors, chest pain, signs of heart failure, visual disturbances, GI symptoms, hepatitis, shortness of breath, skin rash, or edema. Carefully monitor potassium levels and liver tests. Teach pt to immediately report cardiac symptoms including fatigue, skin or eye jaundice. Avoid driving until effect of drug is known. Advise pt to eat small, frequent meals and intake adequate fluids. Regular blood testing during therapy is required.

LIDOCAINE (*Xylocaine, Xylocard*) Ventricular arrhythmia: Load 1 mg/kg IV, then 0.5 mg/kg q 8 to 10 min prn to max 3 mg/kg. IV infusion: 4 g in 500 mL D5W (8 mg/mL) run at rate of 7.5 to 30 mL/h to deliver 1 to 4 mg/min. Peds: 20 to 50 mcg/kg/min. ▶LK ♀B ▶? © $ Depresses phase 0 depolarization slightly, shortens cardiac action potential duration (Class 1B). Serious: Arrhythmias, hypersensitivity (rare), seizures (rare). Frequent: Hypotension, dizziness, drowsiness.

> **Nursing Implications** Throat spray: This medication has various uses: an agent to anesthetize soft tissues prior to suturing a wound, and as a cardiac antidysrhythmic medication for ventricular dysrhythmias. The product literature on this medication should be reviewed carefully prior to use of this medication. This medication can be administered at half the initial calculated dosage every 3 to 5 minutes not to exceed a total dosage of 3 milligrams per kilogram of body weight. A maintenance drip usually follows IV bolus dose administration. Each hospital's pharmacy and therapeutics committee should have established guidelines for maintenance drips. Overdose situations can result in seizures, coma and death.

QUINIDINE (◆ *Biquin Durules*) Proarrhythmic. Arrhythmia: Gluconate, extended-release: 324 to 648 mg PO q 8 to 12 h; sulfate, immediate-release: 200 to 400 mg PO q 6 to 8 h; sulfate, extended-release: 300 to 600 mg PO q 8 to 12 h. ▶LK ♀C ▶+ © $$$-gluconate, $-sulfate. Generic gluconate: Tabs, extended-release unscored 324 mg. Generic sulfate: Tabs, scored immediate-release 200, 300 mg, Tabs, extended-release 300 mg. Depresses phase 0 depolarization, prolongs cardiac action potential duration (Class 1A). Unknown antimalarial mechanism. Serious: Arrhythmias, syncope (rare), hypersensitivity (rare). Frequent: Diarrhea, hypotension, N/V, cinchonism (disturbed hearing, headaches, visual changes, confusion).

> Nursing Implications Monitor cardiac functions and report to physician immediately should serious signs develop such as a significant change in heart rate, changes in refractory or QT interval, QRS complex widening in excess of 25%, P wave disappearance, an increase in ectopic ventricular beats, any other minor side effects that worsen. Continue BP and ECG monitoring. Observe patients following each parenteral dose. Monitor patient's vital signs more often for acute treatment duration. Report any sudden changes in heart rate or blood pressure. Patients receiving high oral doses are more than likely to develop hypotension. Can cause rhythm abnormalities in the heart. Lab work should be done for renal and hepatic functions. Assess periodic blood counts and serum electrolytes.

SOTALOL (*Betapace*, *Betapace AF*, ◆ *Rylosol*) Proarrhythmic. Ventricular arrhythmia (Betapace), A-fib/A-flutter (Betapace AF): Start 80 mg PO two times per day, max 640 mg/ day. Initiate or re-initiate this product in a facility with cardiac resuscitation capacity, continuous EKG and CrCl monitoring. Do not substitute Betapace for Betapace AF. ▶K ♀B ▶– © $$$$ Generic/Trade: Tabs, scored 80, 120, 160, 240 mg, Tabs, scored (Betapace AF) 80, 120, 160 mg. Prolongs cardiac repolarization (Class III antiarrhythmic properties). Serious: Arrhythmias, bradycardia, exacerbation of heart failure.

> Nursing Implications Peform baseline EKG prior to starting the medication. Monitor vital signs (blood pressure and pulse rate) especially during medication dosing adjustments. Perform baseline serum electrolyte levels and correct hypomagnesemia imbalances prior to therapy. Monitor cardiac status throughout treatment. Special caution is highly exercised while medication is concurrently used with calcium channel blockers, digoxin, and antiarrhythmics. Monitor diabetics and bronchospastic disease patients. This medication should not be withdrawn abruptly as patients may experience an exacerbation of angina pectoris, cardiac dysrhythmias, and myocardial infarction.

Anti-Hyperlipidemic Agents—Bile Acid Sequestrants

COLESEVELAM (*Welchol*) LDL-C reduction or glycemic control of type 2 diabetes: 3.75 g once daily or 1.875 g PO two times per day, max 3.75 g/day. Give with meal and 4 to 8 ounces of water, fruit juice, or diet soft drink. 3.75 g is equivalent to 6 tabs; 1.875 g is equivalent to 3 tabs. ▶Not absorbed ♀B ▶+ © $$$$$ Trade only: Tabs unscored 625 mg. Powder single-dose packets 1.875, 3.75 g. Binds bile acid in the intestine preventing absorption. Serious: Fecal impaction (rare). Frequent: Constipation, dyspepsia, nausea.

> Nursing Implications Administer PO once or twice daily with a full glass of water. Administer other drugs at least 4 h or more before colesevelam to avoid decreased absorption of the other drug.

Anti-Hyperlipidemic Agents—HMG-CoA Reductase Inhibitors ("Statins") and Combinations

NOTE: *Each statin has restricted maximum doses that are lower than typical maximum doses when used with certain interacting medications; see prescribing information for complete information. Muscle issues: Measure creatine kinase before starting therapy. Evaluate muscle symptoms before starting therapy, 6 to 12 weeks after starting/increasing therapy and at each follow-up visit. Risk of muscle issues increases with advanced age (65 yo or older), female gender, uncontrolled hypothyroidism, renal impairment, higher statin doses, and concomitant use of certain medicines (eg, fibrates, niacin 1 g or more, colchicine, or ranolazine). Teach patients to report promptly unexplained muscle pain, tenderness, or weakness; rule out common causes; discontinue if myopathy diagnosed or suspected. Obtain creatine kinase, TSH, vitamin D level when patient complains of muscle soreness, tenderness, weakness, or pain. Hepatotoxicity: Rare. Monitor LFTs before initiating statin therapy and as clinically indicated thereafter. Statins may increase the risk of hyperglycemia (and type 2 diabetes) or transient memory problems; benefits usually outweigh risks.*

ATORVASTATIN   (*Lipitor*) Hyperlipidemia/prevention of cardiovascular events, including type 2 diabetes mellitus: Start 10 to 40 mg PO daily, max 80 mg/day. Do not give with cyclosporine; tipranavir + ritonavir; or telaprevir. Use with caution and lowest dose necessary with lopinavir + ritonavir. Do not exceed 20 mg/day when given with clarithromycin, itraconazole, other protease inhibitors (saquinavir + ritonavir, darunavir + ritonavir, fosamprenavir, or fosamprenavir + ritonavir). Do not exceed 40 mg/day when given with nelfinavir. ▶L ♀X ▶– © $$$$ Generic/Trade Tabs unscored 10, 20, 40, 80 mg. Inhibits 3-hydroxy-3-methyl-glutaryl-coenzyme A (HMG-CoA) reductase which converts HMG-CoA to mevalonate in cholesterol biosynthesis. Serious: Hepatotoxicity (rare), myopathy/rhabdomyolysis (rare). Frequent: Headache, dyspepsia.

> Nursing Implications   Monitor for signs of allergic reaction and for muscle pain or tenderness, flu-like symptoms, nausea, GI pain, appetite loss, jaundice, clay stools or dark urine. If patient has HIV, check precautions or avoidance of use criteria such as with protease inhibitors. Skeletal muscle effects may occur if patient is also taking niacin. Teach patient to avoid alcohol and to always disclose the use of Lipitor to health providers. Should not be used if patient is pregnant.

PRAVASTATIN   (*Pravachol*) Hyperlipidemia/prevention of cardiovascular events: Start 40 mg PO daily, max 80 mg/day. Do not exceed 20 mg/day when given with cyclosporine. Do not exceed 40 mg/day when given with clarithromycin. ▶L ♀X ▶– © $ Generic/Trade: Tabs unscored 10, 20, 40, 80 mg. Inhibits 3-hydroxy-3-methyl-glutaryl-coenzyme A (HMG-CoA) reductase, which converts HMG-CoA to mevalonate in cholesterol biosynthesis. Serious: Hepatotoxicity (rare), myopathy/rhabdomyolysis (rare). Frequent: Headache, dyspepsia.

> Nursing Implications   This medication can cause myalgias and a rhabdomyolysis.

ROSUVASTATIN   (*Crestor*) Hyperlipidemia/slow progression of atherosclerosis/primary prevention of cardiovascular disease: Start 10 to 20 mg PO daily, max 40 mg/day. Renal impairment (CrCl less than 30 mL/min and not on hemodialysis): Start 5 mg PO daily, max 10 mg/day. Asians: Start 5 mg PO daily. When given with atazanavir with or without ritonavir or lopinavir with ritonavir, do not exceed 10 mg/day. When given with cyclosporine, do not exceed 5 mg/day. Avoid using with gemfibrozil; if used concomitantly, do not exceed 10 mg/day. ▶L ♀X ▶– © $$$$ Trade only: Tabs unscored 5, 10, 20, 40 mg. Inhibits 3-hydroxy-3-methyl-glutaryl-coenzyme A (HMG-CoA) reductase which converts HMG-CoA to mevalonate in cholesterol biosynthesis. Serious: Hepatotoxicity (rare), myopathy/rhabdomyolysis (rare). Frequent: Myalgia, constipation, nausea, asthenia, abdominal pain, proteinuria (transient), hematuria (transient).

LIPID REDUCTION BY CLASS/AGENT[1]

Drug class/agent	LDL	HDL	TG
Bile acid sequestrants[2]	↓ 15–30%	↑ 3–5%	No change or ↑
Cholesterol absorption inhibitor[3]	↓ 18%	↑ 1%	↓ 8%
Fibrates[4]	↓ 5–20%	↑ 10–20%	↓ 20–50%
Lovastatin+ext'd release niacin[5]*	↓ 30–42%	↑ 20–30%	↓ 32–44%
Niacin[6]*	↓ 5–25%	↑ 15–35%	↓ 20–50%
Omega 3 fatty acids[7]	↓ 5% or ↑ 44%	↓ 4% or ↑ 9%	↓ 27-45
Statins[8]	↓ 18–63%	↑ 5–15%	↓ 7–35%
Simvastatin+ezetimibe[9]	↓ 45–59%	↑ 6–10%	↓ 23–31%

[1] LDL = low density lipoprotein. HDL = high density lipoprotein. TG = triglycerides. Adapted from NCEP: *JAMA* 2001; 285:2486 and prescribing information.
[2] Cholestyramine (4–16 g), colestipol (5–20 g), colesevelam (2.6–3.8 g).
[3] Ezetimibe (10 mg). When added to statin therapy, will ↓ LDL 25%, ↑ HDL 3%, ↓ TG 14% in addition to statin effects.
[4] Fenofibrate (145–200 mg), gemfibrozil (600 mg two times per day).
[5] Advicor® (20/1000–40/2000 mg).
[6] Extended release nicotinic acid (Niaspan® 1–2 g), immediate release (crystalline) nicotinic acid (1.5–3 g), sustained release nicotinic acid (Slo-Niacin® 1–2 g).
[7] Lovaza (4 g), Vascepa (4 g)
[8] Atorvastatin (10–80 mg), fluvastatin (20–80 mg), lovastatin (20–80 mg), pravastatin (20–80 mg), rosuvastatin (5–40 mg), simvastatin (20–40 mg).
[9] Vytorin® (10/10–10/40 mg).
*Lowers lipoprotein a.

> Nursing Implications Should be used in concert with dietary changes; liver function must be monitored along with signs of rhabdomyolysis; cautionary use with Japanese and Chinese patients. Patient should avoid alcohol, caffeine, ephedra, oat bran. Antacids should be taken 2 h after drug. Patient should immediately report muscle pain, tenderness, or weakness. Discontinue if pregnant.

SIMVASTATIN   (*Zocor*) Do not initiate therapy with or titrate to 80 mg/day; only use 80 mg/day in patients who have taken this dose for more than 12 months without evidence of muscle toxicity. Hyperlipidemia: Start 10 to 20 mg PO q pm, max 40 mg/day. Reduce cardiovascular mortality/events in high risk for coronary heart disease event: Start 40 mg PO q pm, max 40 mg/day. Severe renal impairment: Start 5 mg/day, closely monitor. Chinese patients: Do not exceed 20 mg/day with niacin 1 g or more daily. Do not use with boceprevir, clarithromycin, cyclosporine, danazol, erythromycin, gemfibrozil, grapefruit juice more than 1 quart/day, HIV protease inhibitors, itraconazole, ketoconazole, nefazodone, posaconazole, telaprevir, telithromycin; increases risk of myopathy. Do not exceed 10 mg/day when used with diltiazem, dronedarone, or verapamil. Do not exceed 20 mg/day when used with amiodarone, amlodipine, or ranolazine. ▶L ♀X ▶– © $$$$ Generic/Trade: Tabs unscored 5, 10, 20, 40, 80 mg. Inhibits 3-hydroxy-3-methyl-glutaryl-coenzyme A (HMG-CoA) reductase which converts HMG-CoA to mevalonate in cholesterol biosynthesis. Serious: Hepatotoxicity, myopathy/rhabdomyolysis (rare). Frequent: Headache, dyspepsia.

> Nursing Implications Observe for signs and symptoms of severe allergic reactions (rash; hives; itching; difficulty breathing; tightness in the chest; swelling of the mouth, face, lips, or tongue). Do not prescribe if a patient is currently using nitrate medications for chest pain and heart problems/conditions. Taking Revatio with a nitrate medication can cause a severe and sudden decrease in blood pressure. Patients should avoid alcohol when taking this medication. May increase the risk of heart-related and other side effects such as chest, shoulder, neck, and jaw pain; paresthesia; dizziness; fainting, and vision changes.

VYTORIN   (ezetimibe + simvastatin) Hyperlipidemia: Start 10/10 or 10/20 mg PO q pm, max 10/40 mg/day. Restrict the use of the 10/80 mg dose to patients who have taken it at least 12 months without muscle toxicity. See simvastatin monograph for other dose restrictions. ▶L ♀X ▶– © $$$$ Trade only: Tabs, unscored ezetimibe/simvastatin 10/10, 10/20, 10/40, 10/80 mg. See component drugs.

> Nursing Implications This medication works both on the genetic component of cholesterol as well as the dietary etiology to increased cholesterol levels. This medication can also cause myalgias and rhabdomyolysis.

Anti-Hyperlipidemic Agents—Other

EZETIMIBE   (*Zetia*, ✦ *Ezetrol*) Hyperlipidemia: 10 mg PO daily. ▶L ♀C ▶? © $$$$ Trade only: Tabs, unscored 10 mg. Selectively inhibits small intestine cholesterol absorption. Decreases lipoproteins associated with high total cholesterol, LDL-C, APO B, and triglycerides. Serious: Anaphylaxis, angioedema, cholelithiasis, cholecystitis, myopathy/rhabdomyolysis (rare), pancreatitis, thrombocytopenia. Frequent: Arthralgia, back pain, diarrhea, rash.

> Nursing Implications Observe for severe allergic reactions such as hives, urticaria, urticaria, shortness of breath, tightness in the chest, unusual hoarseness, and swelling of the mouth, face, lips, or tongue. Zetia should not be taken with fibrates, cholestyramine, anticoagulants, or if the patient has kidney problems or thyroid problems; a history of liver problems; unexplained muscle pain, tenderness, or weakness; or moderate to severe liver problems. Patients should be instructed to avoid alcohol while on this medication. This medication should be utilized in combination with exercise, a low-cholesterol and low-fat diet and a wt loss program. Liver function and cholesterol levels should be done prior to starting this medication and periodically thereafter. Muscle pain and tenderness should be reported promptly as the medication may need to be discontinued.

FENOFIBRATE   (*TriCor, Antara, Fenoglide, Lipofen, Triglide*, ✦ *Lipidil Micro, Lipidil Supra, Lipidil EZ*) Hypertriglyceridemia: TriCor tabs: 48 to 145 mg PO daily, max 145 mg daily. Antara: 43 to 130 mg PO daily, max 130 mg daily. Fenoglide: 40 to 120 mg PO daily, max 120 mg daily. Lipofen: 50 to 150 mg PO daily, max 150 mg daily. Triglide: 50 to 160 mg PO daily, max 160 mg daily. Generic tabs: 54 to 160 mg, max 160 mg daily. Generic caps: 67 to 200 mg PO daily; max 200 mg daily. Hypercholesterolemia/mixed dyslipidemia: TriCor tabs: 145 mg PO daily. Antara: 130 mg PO daily. Fenoglide: 120 mg daily. Lipofen: 150 mg daily. Triglide: 160 mg daily. Generic tabs: 160 mg daily. Generic caps 200 mg PO daily. All formulations, except Antara, TriCor, and Triglide, should be taken with food. ▶LK ♀C ▶– © $$$ Generic only: Tabs unscored 54, 160 mg. Generic caps 67, 134, 200 mg. Trade only: Tabs (TriCor) unscored 48, 145 mg. Caps (Antara) 43, 130 mg. Tabs (Fenoglide) unscored 40, 120 mg. Tabs (Lipofen) unscored 50, 100, 150 mg. Tabs (Triglide) unscored 50, 160 mg. Activates lipoprotein lipase and reduces apoprotein C-III leading to elimination of triglycerides. Serious: Tumor (rare), hepatotoxicity (rare), myopathy/rhabdomyolysis (rare), cholelithiasis (rare).

| Nursing Implications | Should be taken with meals. |

Antiadrenergic Agents

CLONIDINE (*Catapres, Catapres-TTS, Jenloga, Kapvay, ✦ Dixarit*) Immediate-release, HTN: Start 0.1 mg PO two times per day, usual maintenance dose 0.2 to 0.6 mg/day in 2 to 3 divided doses, max 2.4 mg daily. Extended-release (Jenloga), HTN: Start 0.1 mg daily at bedtime, max 0.6 mg daily. Rebound HTN with abrupt discontinuation, taper dose slowly. Transdermal (Catapres-TTS), HTN: Start 0.1 mg/24 h patch once a week, titrate to desired effect, max effective dose 0.6 mg/24 h (two 0.3 mg/24 h patches). Transdermal Therapeutic System (TTS) is designed for 7-day use so that a TTS-1 delivers 0.1 mg/day for 7 days. May supplement 1st dose of TTS with oral for 2 to 3 days while therapeutic level is achieved. Extended-release (Kapvay), ADHD (6 to 17 yo): Start 0.1 mg PO at bedtime; may increase by 0.1 mg/day each week; give twice daily with equal or higher dose at bedtime, max 0.4 mg daily. Immediate-release, ADHD (unapproved peds): Start 0.05 mg PO at bedtime, titrate based on response over 8 weeks to max 0.2 mg/day (for wt less than 45 kg) or to max 0.4 mg/day (for wt 45 kg or greater) in 2 to 4 divided doses. Tourette syndrome (unapproved peds and adult): 3 to 5 mcg/kg/day PO divided two to four times per day. Opioid withdrawal, adjunct: 0.1 to 0.3 mg PO three to four times per day or 0.1 to 0.2 mg PO q 4 h for 3 days tapering off over 4 to 10 days. Alcohol withdrawal, adjunct: 0.1 to 0.2 mg PO q 4 h prn. Smoking cessation: Start 0.1 mg PO two times per day, increase 0.1 mg/day at weekly intervals to 0.75 mg/day as tolerated; transdermal (Catapres TTS): 0.1 to 0.2 mg/24 h patch once a week for 2 to 3 weeks after cessation. Menopausal flushing: 0.1 to 0.4 mg/day PO divided two to three times per day. Transdermal system applied weekly: 0.1 mg/day. May cause dizziness, drowsiness, or lightheadedness. Monitor for bradycardia when taking concomitant digitalis, nondihydropyridine calcium channel blockers, or beta blockers. ▶LK ♀C ▶? © $$ Generic/Trade: Tabs immediate-release unscored (Catapres) 0.1, 0.2, 0.3 mg. Transdermal weekly patch 0.1 mg/day (TTS-1), 0.2 mg/day (TTS-2), 0.3 mg/day (TTS-3). Generic only: Oral Susp, Extended-release, 0.09 mg/mL (118 mL). Tabs extended-release unscored (Jenloga, Kapvay) 0.1, 0.2 mg. Centrally acting alpha-2 agonist. Serious: Rebound hypertension, orthostatic hypotension, depression, bradycardia, syncope. Frequent: Dry mouth, constipation, drowsiness, dizziness, sedation, sexual dysfunction, rash.

| Nursing Implications | Frequent monitoring of BP and heart rate, delayed effect—2 to 3 days administration; do not withdraw abruptly, expect increased BP to return with discontinuation. Best taken at bedtime. Rotate transdermal patch. |

DOXAZOSIN (*Cardura, Cardura XL*) BPH: Immediate-release: Start 1 mg PO at bedtime, max 8 mg/day. Extended-release (not approved for HTN): 4 mg PO q am with breakfast, max 8 mg/day. HTN: Start 1 mg PO at bedtime, max 16 mg/day. Take first dose at bedtime to minimize orthostatic hypotension. ▶L ♀C ▶? © $$ Generic/Trade: Tabs scored 1, 2, 4, 8 mg. Trade only (Cardura XL): Tabs extended-release 4, 8 mg. Blocks binding of catecholamines to postsynaptic alpha-1 receptors; decreases urethral resistance. Serious: Postural hypotension, heart failure. Frequent: Headache, dizziness, fatigue, nausea, constipation.

| Nursing Implications | Take first dose at bedtime to avoid dizziness. Monitor for dizziness, drowsiness, sleep problems, weight gain, joint/muscle pain, sexual dysfunction, vision changes, shortness of breath, or jaw or chest pain. Avoid driving and sudden movements. Elderly and pregnant women may be more prone to side effects. Check BP regularly. |

METHYLDOPA (*Aldomet*) HTN: Start 250 mg PO 2 to 3 times daily, maximum 3000 mg/day. May be used to manage BP during pregnancy. ▶LK ♀B ▶+ © $ Generic only: Tabs unscored 125, 250, 500 mg. Stimulates central alpha-adrenergic receptors reducing sympathetic outflow. Serious: Hemolytic anemia (rare), LFT abnormalities. Frequent: Sedation, dizziness, dry mouth, constipation, impotence.

> **Nursing Implications** This medication is contraindicated in those patients with active hepatic disease and impaired liver function. This medication must be utilized cautiously in patients with previous liver disease, renal failure, dialysis patients, cerebrovascular disease, pregnancy and lactation. Patients need to have a CBC, chemistry profile and LFTs prior to initiation of therapy and periodically during therapy. The patient's blood pressure needs to be monitored during therapy. Patients need to be advised to report jaundice, skin bruising and fever.

Antihypertensive Combinations

NOTE: *Dosage should first be adjusted by using each drug separately. See component drugs for metabolism, pregnancy, and lactation.*

Diovan HCT **(valsartan + hydrochlorothiazide)** ▶See component drugs ♀See component drugs ▶See component drugs © $$$ Trade only: Tabs, unscored 80/12.5, 160/12.5, 320/12.5, 160/25, 320/25 mg. See component drugs.

> **Nursing Implications** Cautionary use with potassium-sparing diuretics or with potassium supplements; monitor for headache, dizziness, abdominal pain, diarrhea, or nausea; problems with renal function; sexual dysfunction; swelling of soft tissue. Instruct patient to report muscle pain immediately, which may be indicative of rhabdomyolysis. May take 4 weeks for drug to take full effect. Instruct patient to limit alcohol, avoid sudden movement. Cautionary use in pregnant women; may cause fetal death in 2nd and 3rd trimesters.

DYAZIDE **(triamterene + hydrochlorothiazide)** ▶See component drugs ♀See component drugs ▶See component drugs © $ Generic/Trade: Caps, (Dyazide) 37.5/25 mg. Generic only: Caps, 50/25 mg. See component drugs.

> **Nursing Implications** Triamterene and hydrochlorothiazide can be used with other antihypertensive drugs, although dosage adjustments may be necessary. Neither triamterene nor hydrochlorothiazide should be used in patients on potassium or potassium-sparing agents. Renal function should be monitored while on drug. This medication may cause increased potassium levels, especially in diabetic patients. The patient's serum potassium level, BUN and creatinine levels need to be monitored periodically. An idiosyncratic reaction can occur with resultant acute transient myopia and acute angle-closure glaucoma. This condition can lead to a permanent vision loss. Patients should be advised that any erythema of the eye, acute eye pain and a fixed pupil are an ocular emergency and prompt emergency treatment must be sought.

LOTREL **(amlodipine + benazepril)** ▶See component drugs ♀See component drugs ▶See component drugs © $$$ Generic/Trade: Caps, 2.5/10, 5/10, 5/20, 10/20 mg. Trade only: Caps, 5/40, 10/40 mg. See component drugs.

> **Nursing Implications** Administer with or without food.

STATINS

Minimum Dose for 30-40% LDL	LDL*
atorvastatin 10 mg	−39%
fluvastatin 40 mg two times per day	−36%
fluvastatin XL 80 mg	−35%
lovastatin 40 mg	−31%
pitavastatin 2 mg	−36%
pravastatin 40 mg	−34%
rosuvastatin 5 mg	−45%
simvastatin 20 mg	−38%

LDL = low-density lipoprotein. Will get ~6% decrease in LDL with every doubling of dose.
*Adapted from *Circulation* 2004;110:227-239.

MODURETIC (amiloride + hydrochlorothiazide, ✦ *Moduret*) ▶See component drugs ♀See component drugs ▶See component drugs © $ Generic only: Tabs, scored 5/50 mg. See component drugs.

> Nursing Implications Administer with 8 ounces of water, and food. Monitor blood test results for increase in potassium. Do not use in patients with renal dysfunction, urination problems, or high levels of potassium. Notify provider if patient experiences numbness or tingling, muscle pain, weakness, uneven heartbeat, changes in sleep patterns, changes in urination, increased thirst, nausea, vomiting, confusion, or yellowing of the skin or eyes. Promote avoidance of alcohol, excess potassium, and becoming overheated or dehydrated. Promote a low-salt diet.

Antihypertensives—Other

HYDRALAZINE (*Apresoline*) Hypertensive emergency: 10 to 20 mg IV or 10 to 50 mg IM, repeat prn. HTN: Start 10 mg PO two to four times per day, max 300 mg/day. Headaches, peripheral edema, systemic lupus erythematosus-like syndrome. ▶LK ♀C ▶+ © $ Generic only: Tabs unscored 10, 25, 50, 100 mg. Relaxes peripheral arterial smooth muscle (vasodilation). Serious: SLE, angina exacerbation, rash. Frequent: Tachycardia, headache, edema.

> Nursing Implications PO by tab. Assess pt for previous heart disease, valve problems, kidney disease or stroke. Teach pt self-monitoring for most common side effects: headache, upper and lower GI symptoms, appetite loss, rapid HR, tightness in chest. Caution pt not to take with MAO inhibitors. Monitor pt carefully for hypotension if prescribed with another antihypertensive. Teach pt to comply with periodic blood tests.

Antiplatelet Drugs

ABCIXIMAB (*ReoPro*) Platelet aggregation inhibition, percutaneous coronary intervention: 0.25 mg/kg IV bolus via separate infusion line before procedure, then 0.125 mcg/kg/min (max 10 mcg/min) IV infusion for 12 h. ▶Plasma ♀C ▶? © $$$$$ Inhibits platelet aggregation by blocking the effects of fibrinogen and other substances at platelet glycoprotein IIb/IIIa receptors. Serious: Bleeding, hypersensitivity (rare), thrombocytopenia (rare). Frequent: Pain.

> Nursing Implications Administer by IV infusion. Do not mix with other medication in IV lines. Risk of bleeding increases if used with heparin. Bleeding during first 36 h can occur particularly at arterial access in groin. Pt may experience low BP and low HR, GI disturbances, chest and back pain, and headache. Used concommitantly with a wide range of cardiac medications including heparin and aspirin.

CLOPIDOGREL (*Plavix*) Reduction of thrombotic events, recent acute MI/CVA, established peripheral arterial disease: 75 mg PO daily; non-ST segment elevation acute coronary syndrome: 300 to 600 mg loading dose, then 75 mg PO daily in combination with aspirin. ST segment elevation MI: Start with/without 300 mg loading dose, then 75 mg PO daily in combination with aspirin, with/without thrombolytic. Avoid drugs that are strong or moderate CYP2C19 inhibitors (eg, omeprazole, esomeprazole, cimetidine, etravirine, felbamate, fluconazole, fluoxetine, fluvoxamine, ketoconazole, voriconazole). ▶LK ♀B ▶? © $$$$ Generic/Trade Tabs unscored 75, 300 mg. Inhibits platelet aggregation by blocking the effects of adenosine diphosphate at its platelet receptor. Serious: Acute liver failure, anaphylaxis, angioedema, aplastic anemia, agranulocytosis, bleeding, pancreatitis, Stevens-Johnson syndrome, thrombotic thrombocytopenia purpura. Frequent: Pruritus, purpura, diarrhea, rash.

> Nursing Implications Administer once daily with or without food.

EPTIFIBATIDE (*Integrilin*) Acute coronary syndrome: Load 180 mcg/kg IV bolus, then infusion 2 mcg/kg/min for up to 72 h. Discontinue infusion prior to CABG. Percutaneous coronary intervention: Load 180 mcg/kg IV bolus just before procedure, followed by infusion 2 mcg/kg/min and a 2nd 180 mcg/kg IV bolus 10 min after the first bolus. Continue infusion for up to 18 to 24 h (minimum 12 h) after procedure. CrCl less than 50 mL/min not on dialysis: Reduce infusion rate to 1 mcg/kg/min; Dialysis: contraindicated. Thrombocytopenia possible; monitor platelets. ▶K ♀B ▶? © $$$$ Inhibits platelet aggregation by blocking the effects of fibrinogen and other substances at platelet glycoprotein IIb/IIIa receptors. Serious: Bleeding, thrombocytopenia (rare). Frequent: Pain.

LDL CHOLESTEROL GOALS[1]

Risk Category	LDL Goal	Lifestyle Changes[2]	Also Consider Meds at LDL (mg/dL)[9]
High risk: CHD or equivalent risk,[4,5,6] 10-year risk > 20%	<100 (optional <70)[7]	LDL ≥100[8]	≥100 (<100: consider Rx options)[9]
Moderately high risk: 2+ risk factors,[10] 10-year risk 10–20%	<130 (optional <100)	LDL ≥130[8]	≥130 (100–129: consider Rx options)[11]
Moderate risk: 2+ risk factors,[10] 10-year risk <10%	<130 mg/dL	LDL ≥130	≥160
Lower risk: 0 to 1 risk factor[5]	<160 mg/dL	LDL ≥160	≥190 (160–189: Rx optional)

[1]CHD = coronary heart disease. LDL = low density lipoprotein. Adapted from NCEP: *JAMA* 2001; 285:2486; NCEP Report: *Circulation* 2004;110:227–239. All 10-year risks based upon Framingham stratification; calculator available at: http://hin.nhlbi.nih.gov/atpiii/calculator.asp?usertype = prof.
[2]Dietary modification, wt reduction, exercise.
[3]When using LDL-lowering therapy, achieve at least 30 to 40% LDL reduction.
[4]Equivalent risk defined as DM other atherosclerotic disease (peripheral artery disease, abdominal aortic aneurysm, symptomatic carotid artery disease, CKD, or prior ischemic CVA/TIA), or ≥ 2 risk factors such that 10-year risk >20%.
[5]History of ischemic CVA or transient ischemic attack = CHD risk equivalents (*Stroke* 2006;37:577-617).
[6]Chronic kidney disease = CHD risk equivalent [*Am J Kidney Dis* 2003 Apr;41(4 suppl 3):I-IV,S1-91].
[7]For any patient with atherosclerotic disease, may treat to LDL < 70 mg/dL (*Circulation* 2011;124:2458-73).
[8]Regardless of LDL, lifestyle changes are indicated when lifestyle-related risk factors (obesity, physical inactivity, ↑ TG, ↓ HDL, or metabolic syndrome) are present.
[9]If baseline LDL < 100, starting LDL-lowering therapy is an option based on clinical trials. With ↑ TG or ↓ HDL, consider combining fibrate or nicotinic acid with LDL-lowering drug.
[10]Risk factors: Cigarette smoking, HTN (BP ≥140/90 mmHg or on antihypertensive meds), low HDL (< 40 mg/dL), family history of CHD (1° relative: ♂ < 55 yo, ♀ < 65 yo), age (♂ ≥45 yo, ♀ ≥55 yo).
[11]At baseline or after lifestyle changes, initiating therapy to achieve LDL < 100 is an option based on clinical trials.

Nursing Implications IV administration. Prescriber must be called immediately if pt has nose or other bleeding, bloody stools, coffee ground vomit, faintness, or sudden weakness. Check soln for clarity and particulate matter. Can be given in same IV line with many drugs except furosemide. Refrigerate and store in dark place. Check pt for major bleeding at vascular access/femoral artery site, in GI or GU tracks and in pts weighing less than 155 lbs. Monitor for signs of anaphylaxis, stroke, or blood disorders such as thrombocytopenia. Hematocrit, Hg, and clotting time should be monitored through course of therapy.

Beta-Blockers

NOTE: *See also Antihypertensive Combinations. Not first line for HTN (unless to treat angina, post-MI, LV dysfunction, or heart failure). Abrupt discontinuation may precipitate angina, MI, arrhythmias, or rebound HTN; discontinue by tapering over 1 to 2 weeks. Avoid use of nonselective beta-blockers in patients with asthma/COPD. For patients with asthma/COPD, use agents with beta-1 selectivity and monitor cautiously. Beta-1 selectivity diminishes at high doses. Avoid initiating beta-blocker therapy in acute decompensated heart failure, sick sinus syndrome without pacer, and severe peripheral artery disease.*

BISOPROLOL (*Zebeta*, ✚ *Monocor*) HTN: Start 2.5 to 5 mg PO daily, max 20 mg/day. Highly beta-1 receptor selective. ▶LK ♀C ▶? © $$ Generic/Trade: Tabs unscored 5 mg, unscored 10 mg. Blocks binding of catecholamines to beta-1 receptors. Serious: Bronchoconstriction (high doses), masks hypoglycemic response and slow recovery, rebound hypertension/angina. Frequent: Bradycardia, fatigue, impotence.

Nursing Implications Administer with 8 ounces of water and take at same time every day. See manufacturer's extensive list of drug interactions. Promote regular visits to provider for blood pressure monitoring. Promote gradual stoppage of use over time as prescribed by healthcare provider. Notify provider and seek immediate medical attention if patient experiences any of the following symptoms: hives; difficulty breathing; swelling of face, tongue, lips, or throat; chest pain; irregular heartbeat; confusion; hallucinations; pain or burning during urination; numbness or tingling in extremities.

CARVEDILOL (*Coreg, Coreg CR*) Heart failure, immediate-release: Start 3.125 mg PO two times per day, double dose q 2 weeks as tolerated up to max of 25 mg two times per day (for wt 85 kg or less) or 50 mg two times per day (for wt greater than 85 kg). Heart failure, sustained-release: Start 10 mg PO daily, double dose q 2 weeks as tolerated up to max of 80 mg/day. LV dysfunction following acute MI, immediate-release: Start 3.125 to 6.25 mg PO two times per day, double dose q 3 to 10 days as tolerated to max of 25 mg two times per day. LV dysfunction following acute MI, sustained-release: Start 10 to 20 mg PO daily, double dose q 3 to 10 days as tolerated to max of 80 mg/day. HTN, immediate-release: Start 6.25 mg PO two times per day, double dose q 7 to 14 days as tolerated to max 50 mg/day. HTN, sustained-release: Start 20 mg PO daily, double dose q 7 to 14 days as tolerated to max 80 mg/day. Take with food to decrease orthostatic hypotension. Give Coreg CR in the morning. Alpha-1, beta-1, and beta-2 receptor blocker. ▶L ♀C ▶? © $$$$ Generic/Trade: Tabs immediate-release unscored 3.125, 6.25, 12.5, 25 mg. Trade only: Caps extended-release 10, 20, 40, 80 mg. Blocks binding of catecholamines to postsynaptic alpha-1, beta-1, and beta-2 receptors. Serious: Anaphylaxis, angioedema, bronchoconstriction, masks hypoglycemic response and slow recovery, rebound hypertension/angina. Frequent: Bradycardia, fatigue, impotence, hypotension.

> Nursing Implications Administer with 8 ounces of water at the same time every day. Do not use in patients with a history of breathing disorders, severe liver disease, or serious heart conditions. Use cautiously in patients with diabetes, low blood pressure, depression, congestive heart failure, kidney disease, thyroid disorders, myasthenia gravis, pheochromocytoma, or circulation problems. Promote avoidance of alcohol. Promote caution while driving or using heavy machinery. Promote adherence to provider's nutrition and exercise instructions exactly. Gradually reduce dosage over time; do not stop suddenly.

ESMOLOL (*Brevibloc*) SVT/HTN emergency: Load 500 mcg/kg over 1 min (dilute 5 g in 500 mL to make a soln of 10 mg/mL and give 3.5 mL to deliver 35 mg bolus for 70 kg patient) then start infusion 50 to 200 mcg/kg/min (40 mL/h delivers 100 mcg/kg/min for 70 kg patient). Half-life is 9 min. Beta-1 receptor selective. ▶K ♀C ▶? © $ Blocks binding of catecholamines to beta-1 receptors. Serious: Bronchoconstriction (high doses), masks hypoglycemic response and slow recovery, rebound hypertension/angina. Frequent: Bradycardia, fatigue.

> Nursing Implications Administer by IV infusion. Instruct patient that drug is for emergency use only; check IV site regularly. Observe pts for severe allergic reactions such as hives, urticaria, and SOB; swelling of mouth, face, lips or tongue, and provide emergency intervention. Cautionary use in patients with kidney and cardiac disease, diabetes, hyperthyroidism, vascular diseases. Monitor during administration for hypotension, I&O, CNS symptoms, chest pain, unusually slow or irregular pulse, low BP, GI symptoms, urine retention, difficulties breathing, flushing, or pallor.

LABETALOL (*Trandate*) HTN: Start 100 mg PO two times per day, max 2400 mg/day. HTN emergency: Start 20 mg IV slow injection, then 40 to 80 mg IV q 10 min prn up to 300 mg or IV infusion 0.5 to 2 mg/min. Peds: Start 0.3 to 1 mg/kg/dose (max 20 mg). May be used to manage BP during pregnancy. Alpha-1, beta-1, and beta-2 receptor blocker. ▶LK ♀C ▶+ © $$$ Generic/Trade: Tabs scored 100, 200, 300 mg. Blocks binding of catecholamines to postsynaptic alpha-1, beta-1, and beta-2 receptors. Serious: Bronchoconstriction, hepatotoxicity, masks hypoglycemic response and slow recovery, rebound hypertension/angina. Frequent: Bradycardia, fatigue, impotence, hypotension.

> Nursing Implications This medication is contraindicated in patients with dysrhythmias such as sinus bradycardia, second degree heart block, third degree heart block, cardiogenic shock, heart failure, asthma, pregnancy and lactation. This medication should be utilized cautiously in patients with diabetes mellitus or hypoglycemia, and pheochromocytoma. Patients need to have an EKG done prior to taking this medication. Patients need to monitor blood sugars carefully if they are diabetic as this medication can mask unusual symptoms of hypoglycemia. Patients need to have their blood pressure and heart rate monitored as this medication lowers blood pressure and heart rate. This medication may also decrease libido and may cause fatigue.

METOPROLOL (*Lopressor, Toprol-XL, ✚ Betaloc*) Acute MI: 50 to 100 mg PO q 12 h; or 5 mg increments IV q 5 to 15 min up to 15 mg followed by oral therapy. HTN (immediate-release): Start 100 mg PO daily or in divided doses, increase prn up to 450 mg/day; may require multiple daily doses to maintain 24-h BP control. HTN (extended-release): Start 25 to 100 mg PO daily, increase prn up to 400 mg/day. Heart failure: Start 12.5 to 25 mg (extended-release) PO daily, double dose q 2 weeks as tolerated up to max 200 mg/day. Angina: Start 50 mg PO two times per day (immediate-release) or 100 mg PO daily (extended-release), increase prn up to 400 mg/day. IV to PO conversion: 1 mg IV is equivalent to 2.5 mg PO (divided four times per day). The immediate- (metoprolol tartrate) and extended-release (metoprolol succinate) products may not give same clinical response on mg:mg basis; monitor response and side effects when interchanging between metoprolol products. Extended-release tabs may be broken in half, but do not chew or crush. Beta-1 receptor selective. Take with food. ▶L ♀C ▶? © $$ Generic/Trade: Tabs scored 50, 100 mg, extended-release 25, 50, 100, 200 mg. Generic only: Tabs scored 25 mg. Blocks binding of catecholamines to beta-1 receptors. Serious: Bronchoconstriction (high doses), masks hypoglycemic response and slow recovery, rebound hypertension/angina. Frequent: Bradycardia, fatigue, impotence.

> **Nursing Implications** Do not use in patients allergic to metoprolol, or who have a history of serious heart problems. Use cautiously in patients with history of congestive heart failure, circulation problems, asthma or other breathing problems, diabetes, depression, renal or liver dysfunction, thyroid disorders, or allergies. Promote avoidance of alcohol and the use of caution when operating heavy machinery. Promote following diet, medication, and exercise routines closely as prescribed by provider.

NADOLOL   (***Corgard***) HTN: Start 20 to 40 mg PO daily, max 320 mg/day. Prevent rebleeding esophageal varices: 40 to 160 mg PO daily; titrate dose to reduce heart rate to 25% below baseline. Beta-1 and beta-2 receptor blocker. ▶K ♀C ▶– © $$ Generic/Trade: Tabs scored 20, 40, 80, 120, 160 mg. Blocks binding of catecholamines to beta-1 and beta-2 receptors. Serious: Bronchoconstriction, masks hypoglycemic response and slow recovery, rebound hypertension/angina. Frequent: Bradycardia, fatigue, impotence.

> **Nursing Implications** Observe patients for severe allergic reactions such as hives, urticaria, shortness of breath, tightness in the chest, and swelling of the mouth, face, lips, or tongue. This medication may cause drowsiness or dizziness. Patients need to be advised not to drink alcohol or take other medications that can affect the central nervous system. This medication should be taken with food and/or milk. Patients need to be advised of this. This medication may have an effect on a patient's blood sugar level. These levels should be monitored periodically. Diabetic patients on this medication need more close monitoring of their blood sugars. Stopping this medication may induce withdrawal symptoms such as a fast heart rate, low blood pressure, chest pain, and nervousness.

PROPRANOLOL   (***Inderal, Inderal LA, InnoPran XL***) HTN: Start 20 to 40 mg PO two times per day or 60 to 80 mg PO daily, max 640 mg/day; extended-release (Inderal LA) max 640 mg/day; extended-release (InnoPran XL) 80 mg at bedtime (10 pm), max 120 mg at bedtime (chronotherapy). Supraventricular tachycardia or rapid atrial fibrillation/flutter: 1 mg IV q 2 min. Max of 2 doses in 4 h. Migraine prophylaxis: Start 40 mg PO two times per day or 80 mg PO daily (extended-release), max 240 mg/day. Prevent rebleeding esophageal varices: 20 to 180 mg PO two times per day; titrate dose to reduce heart rate to 25% below baseline. Beta-1 and beta-2 receptor blocker. ▶L ♀C ▶+ © $$ Generic/Trade: Tabs, scored 40, 60, 80. Caps, extended-release 60, 80, 120, 160 mg. Generic only: Soln 20, 40 mg/5 mL. Tabs, 10, 20 mg. Trade only: (InnoPran XL at bedtime) 80, 120 mg. Blocks binding of catecholamines to beta-1 and beta-2 receptors. Serious: Anaphylaxis, agranulocytosis, bronchoconstriction, masks hypoglycemic response and slows recovery, rebound hypertension/angina, Stevens-Johnson syndrome. Frequent: Bradycardia, fatigue, dizziness, impotence.

> **Nursing Implications** Nursing should observe for severe allergic reactions such as hives, urticaria, shortness of breath, tightness in the chest, and swelling of the mouth, face, lips, or tongue. The most common side effects are drowsiness, dizziness and lightheadedness. This medication may lower the blood sugar level. Blood sugar levels should be checked frequently in diabetic patients. This medication may interfere with certain tests such as glaucoma screening and dobutamine stress echocardiography. The elderly are more sensitive to this medication. Some patients also report decreased libido. Nursing should monitor patient's blood pressure and heart rate when patients are taking this medication.

Calcium Channel Blockers (CCBs)—Dihydropyridines

NOTE: *See also Antihypertensive Combinations.*

AMLODIPINE   (***Norvasc***) HTN: Start 5 mg PO daily, max 10 mg/day.. Elderly, small, frail, or with hepatic insufficiency: Start 2.5 PO daily. ▶L ♀C ▶? © $ Generic/Trade: Tabs unscored 2.5, 5, 10 mg. Blocks calcium-dependent contractions in cardiac and peripheral smooth muscle leading to vasodilation. Serious: None. Frequent: Peripheral edema, headache, palpitations.

> **Nursing Implications** Nursing should monitor patient's blood pressure and heart rate when they are on this medication. The most common side effect of this medication is swelling of the extremities, particularly the ankles and the feet. Nursing should educate patients to avoid over-the-counter nonprescription medications that can raise blood pressure, ie, medications for appetite control, asthma, colds, cough, hay fever, or sinus problems.

NICARDIPINE (***Cardene, Cardene SR***) HTN emergency: Begin IV infusion at 5 mg/h, titrate to effect, max 15 mg/h. HTN: Start 20 mg PO three times per day, max 120 mg/day. Sustained-release: Start 30 mg PO two times per day, max 120 mg/day. Short-term management of HTN, patient receiving PO nicardipine: If using 20 mg PO q 8 h, give 0.5 mg/h IV; if using 30 mg PO q 8 h, give 1.2 mg/h IV; if using 40 mg PO q 8 h, give 2.2 mg/h. ▶L ♀C ▶? © $$ Generic/Trade: Caps immediate-release 20, 30 mg. Trade only: Caps sustained-release 30, 45, 60 mg. Blocks calcium-dependent contractions in cardiac and peripheral smooth muscle leading to vasodilation. Serious: None. Frequent: Peripheral edema, headache, palpitations.

> **Nursing Implications** Administer PO by sustained-release capsules or by short-term IV infusion. Infusion rate should be reduced to 30/mL/h once BP goal is achieved. Do not expose IV bag to light. Do not combine with any other IV drug. If using series connections, do not use plastic containers. Change infusion site q 12 h to minimize irritation. Administer through large veins. If after completion of IV course, patient will take oral form, first oral dose should be given 1 h before IV is discontinued. Inspect IV soln for particulate matter and color. Store at room temp and do not freeze. Closely monitor pt for low BP and rapid HR. GI disturbances and headache may also occur. With IV administration monitor for development of DVTs, edema, confusion, hearing problems, and frequent urination. Cyclosporine levels can be elevated with concomitant administration of IV nicardipine; call prescriber to adjust dose. Edema of the lower extremities (ie, the feet and ankles) is common. Patients should be advised that this medication may cause decreased libido. Patients need to be educated not to drink grapefruit juice or to eat grapefruit because of potentiation of the drug's effect. Do not give to pts with aortic stenosis.

NIFEDIPINE (***Procardia, Adalat, Procardia XL, Adalat CC, Afeditab CR, ✦ Adalat XL, Adalat PA***) HTN/Angina: Extended-release: 30 to 60 mg PO daily, max 120 mg/day. Angina: Immediate-release: Start 10 mg PO three times per day, max 120 mg/day. Avoid sublingual administration, may cause excessive hypotension, acute MI, CVA. Do not use immediate-release caps for treating HTN, hypertensive emergencies, or ST-elevation MI. Preterm labor: Loading dose: 10 mg PO q 20 to 30 min if contractions persist, up to 40 mg within the first h. Maintenance dose: 10 to 20 mg PO q 4 to 6 h or 60 to 160 mg extended-release PO daily. ▶L ♀C ▶– © $$ Generic/Trade: Caps 10, 20 mg. Tabs extended-release (Adalat CC, Afeditab CR, Procardia XL) 30, 60 mg, (Adalat CC, Procardia XL) 90 mg. Blocks calcium-dependent contractions in cardiac and peripheral smooth muscle leading to vasodilation. Tocolytic. Serious: Hypotension, gastrointestinal obstruction (extended-release tab). Frequent: Peripheral edema, headache, flushing.

> **Nursing Implications** Patient should be advised to have their blood pressure checked frequently. A common side effect of this medication is edema of the lower extremities (ie, the feet and ankles.) Patients should be advised that this medication may cause decreased libido. Patients need to be educated not to drink grapefruit juice or to eat grapefruit when on this medication as grapefruit can potentiate the effects of this medication.

Calcium Channel Blockers (CCBs)—Non-Dihydropyridines

NOTE: *See also Antihypertensive Combinations.*

DILTIAZEM (***Cardizem, Cardizem LA, Cardizem CD, Cartia XT, Dilacor XR, Diltiazem CD, Diltzac, Diltia XT, Tiazac, Taztia XT***) Atrial fibrillation/flutter, PSVT: Bolus 20 mg (0.25 mg/kg) IV over 2 min. Rebolus 15 min later (if needed) 25 mg (0.35 mg/kg). Infusion 5 to 15 mg/h. HTN, once daily, extended-release: Start 120 to 240 mg PO daily, max 540 mg/day. HTN, once daily, graded extended-release (Cardizem LA): Start 180 to 240 mg PO daily, max 540 mg/day. HTN, twice daily, sustained-release: Start 60 to 120 mg PO two times per day, max 360 mg/day. Angina, immediate-release: Start 30 mg PO four times per day, max 360 mg/day divided three to four times per day; Angina, extended-release: Start 120 to 240 mg PO daily, max 540 mg/day. Angina, once daily, graded extended-release (Cardizem LA): start 180 mg PO daily, doses more than 360 mg may provide no additional benefit. ▶L ♀C ▶+ © $$ Generic/Trade:

Tabs immediate-release, unscored (Cardizem) 30 mg, scored 60, 90, 120 mg; Caps extended-release (Cardizem CD, Cartia XT daily) 120, 180, 240, 300, 360 mg, (Diltzac, Taztia XT, Tiazac daily) 120, 180, 240, 300, 360, 420 mg, (Dilacor XR, Diltia XT) 120, 180, 240 mg. Trade only: Tabs extended-release graded (Cardizem LA daily) 120, 180, 240, 300, 360, 420 mg. Blocks calcium-dependent contractions in cardiac and peripheral smooth muscle leading to vasodilation; slows cardiac conduction through the AV node. Serious: Bradycardia, heart block (rare). Frequent: Peripheral edema, headache.

> **Nursing Implications** Check all other drugs patient is taking since diltiazem interacts with many drugs; Monitor for dizziness or weakness, headache, slow heartbeat, vomiting or diarrhea, constipation, cough, slow heartbeat (teach patient to take pulse before taking drug), difficulty breathing, jaundice of skin or eyes, increased frequency or strength of angina pain, or unusual swelling should be immediately reported. Store medication in cool, dry place; BP should be checked regularly.

VERAPAMIL (*Isoptin SR, Calan, Covera-HS, Verelan, Verelan PM, ✦ Veramil*) SVT adults: 5 to 10 mg IV over 2 min; SVT peds (age 1 to 15 yo): 2 to 5 mg (0.1 to 0.3 mg/kg) IV, max dose 5 mg. Angina: Immediate-release, start 40 to 80 mg PO three to four times per day, max 480 mg/day; sustained to release, start 120 to 240 mg PO daily, max 480 mg/day (use twice daily dosing for doses greater than 240 mg/day with Isoptin SR and Calan SR); (Covera-HS) 180 mg PO at bedtime, max 480 mg/day. HTN: Same as angina, except (Verelan PM) 100 to 200 mg PO at bedtime, max 400 mg/day; immediate-release tabs should be avoided in treating HTN. Use cautiously with impaired renal/hepatic function. ▶L ♀C ▶– © $$ Generic/Trade: Tabs, immediate-release, scored (Calan) 40, 80, 120 mg; Tabs, sustained-release, unscored (Isoptin SR) 120, scored 180, 240 mg; Caps, sustained-release (Verelan) 120, 180, 240, 360 mg; Caps, extended-release (Verelan PM) 100, 200, 300 mg. Trade only: Tabs, extended-release (Covera-HS) 180, 240 mg. Blocks calcium-dependent contractions in cardiac and peripheral smooth muscle leading to vasodilation; slows cardiac conduction through the SA node. Serious: Bradycardia, heart block (rare). Frequent: Constipation, headache.

> **Nursing Implications** An ECG should be done to detect any heart abnormalities, if any are found, do not use verapamil; also do not give to patients with hypotension, second- or third-degree AV block, hypersensitivity to verapamil hydrochloride, or sick sinus syndrome. ECGs should be done regularly on patients taking verapamil to ensure no heart problems arise. The blood pressure and heart rate should be monitored periodically. A common side effect of this medication is edema in the feet and ankles.

Diuretics—Loop

BUMETANIDE (*Bumex, ✦ Burinex*) Edema: 0.5 to 1 mg IV/IM; 0.5 to 2 mg PO daily. 1 mg bumetanide is roughly equivalent to 40 mg furosemide. ▶K ♀C ▶? © $ Generic/Trade: Tabs scored 0.5, 1, 2 mg. Block chloride reabsorption by inhibiting the Na+/K+/Cl– cotransport system in the thick ascending limb of the loop of Henle. Serious: Electrolyte imbalances (hypokalemia, hyponatremia, hypochloremic alkalosis, hypomagnesemia, hypocalcemia, hyperuricemia), dehydration, ototoxicity (rare), skin reactions. Frequent: Dizziness, headache, fatigue, muscle cramps, impotence.

> **Nursing Implications** May be taken with food or milk at least 4 h before bedtime. Administer medication at same time every day. Do not use in patients with a history of severe renal or liver disease. Do not use in patients currently taking cisapride. Notify provider if patient is also using amphotericin B, any corticosteroids, digoxin, ginseng, lithium, any NSAID drugs, or probenecid. Use cautiously in patients with a history of diabetes, gout, sodium or potassium imbalance disorders, or irregular heart rhythms. Promote use of caution when operating heavy machinery. Avoid alcohol. Promote completion of entire course of therapy.

FUROSEMIDE (*Lasix*) HTN: Start 10 to 40 mg PO twice daily, max 600 mg daily. Edema: Start 20 to 80 mg IV/IM/PO, increase dose by 20 to 40 mg in 6 to 8 h until desired response is achieved, max 600 mg/day. Ascites: 40 mg PO daily in combination with spironolactone; may increase dose after 2 to 3 days if no response. ▶K ♀C ▶? © $ Generic/Trade: Tabs unscored 20, scored 40, 80 mg. Generic only: Oral soln 10 mg/mL, 40 mg/5 mL. Block chloride reabsorption by inhibiting the Na+/K+/Cl– cotransport system in the thick ascending limb of the loop of Henle. Serious: Electrolyte imbalances (hypokalemia, hyponatremia, hypochloremic alkalosis, hypomagnesemia, hypocalcemia, hyperuricemia), dehydration, pancreatitis (rare), photosensitivity (rare), hypersensitivity (rare), ototoxicity (rare), dermatologic hypersensitivity reactions. Frequent: Dizziness, headache, fatigue, muscle cramps, impotence.

> **Nursing Implications** In adults, do not exceed 4 mg per min infusion rate.

TORSEMIDE (*Demadex*) HTN: Start 5 mg PO daily, increase prn q 4 to 6 weeks, max 10 mg daily. Edema: 10 to 20 mg IV/PO daily, max 200 mg IV/PO daily. ▶LK ♀B ▶? © $ Generic/Trade: Tabs scored 5, 10, 20, 100 mg. Block chloride reabsorption by inhibiting the Na+/K+/Cl– cotransport system in the thick ascending limb of the loop of Henle. Serious: Electrolyte imbalances (hypokalemia, hyponatremia, hypochloremic alkalosis, hypomagnesemia, hypocalcemia, hyperuricemia), dehydration, pancreatitis (rare), photosensitivity (rare), hypersensitivity (rare). Frequent: Dizziness, headache, fatigue, muscle cramps, impotence.

> Nursing Implications Advise patients to increase dietary forms of potassium such as oranges, bananas, and potatoes. Patients need to have serum electrolytes monitored periodically.

Diuretics—Potassium Sparing

NOTE: *See also Antihypertensive Combinations and aldosterone antagonists. Beware of hyperkalemia. Use cautiously with other agents that may cause hyperkalemia (ie, ACE inhibitors, ARBs, aliskiren).*

TRIAMTERENE (*Dyrenium*) ▶LK ♀B ▶–© $$$ Trade only: Caps 50, 100 mg. Block sodium reabsorption and potassium excretion in the distal tubule. Serious: Hyperkalemia (rare). Frequent: Headache.

> Nursing Implications Do not administer at night as it may interrupt sleep pattern for urination. For patients who have difficulty taking pills, medication may be mixed with liquids or food.

Diuretics—Thiazide Type

NOTE: *See also Antihypertensive Combinations.*

CHLOROTHIAZIDE (*Diuril*) ▶L ♀C, D if used in pregnancy-induced HTN ▶+© $ Trade only: Susp 250 mg/5 mL. Generic only: Tabs, scored 250, 500 mg. Blocks sodium and chloride reabsorption in the distal tubules. Serious: Electrolyte imbalances (hypokalemia, hyponatremia, hypomagnesemia, hypercalcemia, hyperuricemia), pancreatitis (rare), photosensitivity (rare), hypersensitivity (rare). Frequent: Dizziness, headache, fatigue, muscle cramps, impotence.

> Nursing Implications Do not use in patients allergic to this drug or in those unable to urinate. Do not use in patients allergic to sulfa drugs, or in those with liver or kidney disease, asthma, other allergies, gout, lupus, or diabetes. Promote avoidance of alcohol and promote increased hydration.

CHLORTHALIDONE (*Thalitone*) HTN: 12.5 to 25 mg PO daily, max 50 mg/day. Edema: 50 to 100 mg PO daily, max 200 mg/day. Nephrolithiasis (unapproved use): 25 to 50 mg PO daily. ▶L ♀B, D if used in pregnancy-induced HTN ▶+© $ Trade only: Tabs unscored (Thalitone) 15 mg. Generic only: Tabs unscored 25, 50 mg. Blocks sodium and chloride reabsorption in the distal tubules and decreases urinary calcium excretion. Serious: Agranulocytosis, aplastic anemia, electrolyte imbalances (hypokalemia, hyponatremia, hypomagnesemia, hypercalcemia, hyperuricemia), pancreatitis (rare), photosensitivity (rare), hypersensitivity (rare), thrombocytopenia. Frequent: Dizziness, headache, fatigue, muscle cramps, impotence.

> Nursing Implications Do not use in patients allergic to this drug or in those unable to urinate. Do not use in patients allergic to sulfa drugs, or in those with liver or kidney disease, asthma, other allergies, gout, lupus, or diabetes. Promote avoidance of alcohol and promote increased hydration. Promote regular visits to provider for blood testing.

Nitrates

ISOSORBIDE DINITRATE (*Isordil, Dilatrate-SR, ✦Cedocard SR, Coronex*) Angina prophylaxis: 5 to 40 mg PO three times per day (7 am, noon, 5 pm), sustained-release: 40 to 80 mg PO two times per day (8 am, 2 pm). Acute angina, SL Tabs: 2.5 to 10 mg SL q 5 to 10 min prn, up to 3 doses in 30 min. ▶L ♀C ▶? © $ Generic/Trade: Tabs, scored 5, 10, 20, 30 mg. Trade only: Tabs, (Isordil) 40 mg, Caps, extended-release (Dilatrate-SR) 40 mg. Generic only: Tabs, sustained-release 40 mg, Tabs, sublingual 2.5, 5 mg. Relaxes cardiac and peripheral smooth muscle (venous greater than arterial). Serious: Hypotension, methemoglobinemia (rare). Frequent: Headache, tachycardia, dizziness, flushing.

> Nursing Implications Patients taking this medication should have their blood pressure monitored regularly.

Other

NESIRITIDE (*Natrecor*) Hospitalized patients with decompensated heart failure with dyspnea at rest: 2 mcg/kg IV bolus over 1 min, then 0.01 mcg/kg/min IV infusion for up to 48 h. Do not initiate at higher doses. Limited experience with increased doses. Mix 1.5 mg vial in 250 mL D5W (6 mcg/mL) a bolus of 23.3 mL is 2 mcg/kg for a 70 kg patient, infusion set at rate 7 mL/h delivers a 0.01 mcg/kg/min for a 70 kg patient. Symptomatic hypotension. May increase mortality. Not indicated for outpatient infusion, for scheduled repetitive use, to improve renal function, or to enhance diuresis. ▶K, plasma ♀C ▶? © $$$$$ Human B-type natriuretic peptide that relaxes cardiac smooth muscle (arterial and venous vasodilation). Serious: Arrhythmias, altered kidney function. Frequent: Hypotension, headache, insomnia, dizziness, nausea.

> Nursing Implications Administer by IV infusion. Monitor for severe allergic reaction/anaphylaxis. Call prescriber if pt experiences increased HR, chest pain, confusion immediately post-administration, faintness, blood in sputum, bruising, pallor, and fever. If BP drops call prescriber for dose adjustment. Draw bolus ONLY from the prepared infusion bag. Use within 24 h and inspect for particulate matter and color. Continuously monitor pt's HR, development of arrhythmias, and GI disturbances.

Pressors/Inotropes

EPHEDRINE ▶K ♀C ▶? © $ Generic only: Caps, 50 mg. Stimulates beta-1 receptors (increases cardiac contractility and chronotropic effect), stimulates alpha receptors (peripheral vasoconstriction), stimulates beta-2 receptors (mild peripheral vasodilation). Serious: Arrhythmias, tachycardia. Frequent: Hypertension, headache, palpitations, flushing, sweating, dizziness.

> Nursing Implications Cautionary use in elderly, children, pregnant women, and diabetics. Do not take with MAOIs, with high BP, or other cardiovascular problems. Interacts with many drugs including reserpine, beta-blockers, digoxin, and tricyclics. Avoid alcohol. Monitor for dizziness, shortness of breath, rash, headache, nausea, agitation, insomnia, and GI symptoms, and for elevated blood sugar in diabetics.

MIDODRINE (✦*Amatine*) Orthostatic hypotension: 10 mg PO three times per day. The last daily dose should be no later than 6 pm to avoid supine HTN during sleep. ▶LK ♀C ▶? © $$$$$ Generic: Tabs, scored 2.5, 5, 10 mg. Stimulates alpha receptors (peripheral vasoconstriction). Serious: Hypertension. Frequent: Paresthesia, piloerection, pruritus, dysuria, chills.

> Nursing Implications Observe patients for severe allergic reactions such as hives, urticaria, shortness of breath, tightness in the chest, and swelling of the mouth, face, lips, or tongue. Common side effects include chest pain, confusion or abnormal thinking, decreased urination, fainting, headache, increased or unusual dizziness, pounding in the ears or the chest, slow pulse, and vision changes. Patients need to be educated to take this medication in the morning after first arising and remaining in an upright position. Patients need to be educated to have their blood pressure assessed on a regular basis.

MILRINONE (*Primacor*) Systolic heart failure (NYHA class III, IV): Load 50 mcg/kg IV over 10 min, then begin IV infusion of 0.375 to 0.75 mcg/kg/min. ▶K ♀C ▶? © $$ Inhibits phosphodiesterase enzyme leading to increased intracellular cAMP (positive inotropic effect). Serious: Arrhythmias. Frequent: None.

CARDIAC PARAMETERS AND FORMULAS

> Cardiac output (CO) = heart rate × CVA volume [normal 4 to 8 L/min]
> Cardiac index (CI) = CO/BSA [normal 2.8 to 4.2 L/min/m^2]
> MAP (mean arterial press) = [(SBP − DBP)/3] + DBP [normal 80 to 100 mmHg]
> SVR (systemic vasc resis) = (MAP − CVP) × (80)/CO [normal 800 to 1200 dyne × sec/cm^5]
> PVR (pulm vasc resis) = (PAM − PCWP) × (80)/CO [normal 45 to 120 dyne × sec/cm^5]
> QTc = QT/square root of RR [normal 0.38 to 0.42]
> Right atrial pressure (central venous pressure) [normal 0 to 8 mmHg]
> Pulmonary artery systolic pressure (PAS) [normal 20 to 30 mmHg]
> Pulmonary artery diastolic pressure (PAD) [normal 10 to 15 mmHg]
> Pulmonary capillary wedge pressure (PCWP) [normal 8 to 12 mmHg (post-MI ~16 mmHg)]

THROMBOLYTIC THERAPY FOR ACUTE MI

Indications (if high-volume cath lab unavailable)	Clinical history and presentation strongly suggestive of MI within 12 h plus at least 1 of the following: 1 mm ST elevation in at least 2 contiguous leads; new left BBB; or 2 mm ST depression in V1–4 suggestive of true posterior MI.
Absolute contraindications	Previous cerebral hemorrhage, known cerebral aneurysm or arteriovenous malformation, known intracranial neoplasm, recent (<3 months) ischemic CVA (except acute ischemic CVA <3 h), aortic dissection, active bleeding or bleeding diathesis (excluding menstruation), significant closed head or facial trauma (<3 months).
Relative contraindications	Severe uncontrolled HTN (>180/110 mm Hg) on presentation or chronic severe HTN; prior ischemic CVA (>3 months), dementia, other intracranial pathology; traumatic/prolonged (>10 min) cardiopulmonary resuscitation; major surgery (<3 weeks); recent (within 2–4 weeks) internal bleeding; puncture of noncompressible vessel; pregnancy; active peptic ulcer disease; current use of anticoagulants. For streptokinase/anistreplase: prior exposure (>5 days ago) or prior allergic reaction.

Reference: *Circulation* 2004;110:588-636

> **Nursing Implications** Administer by IV infusion with continuous close ECG monitoring. Oral preparation also available. Monitor for ventricular tachycardia; sudden death can occur. Teach pt to comply with laboratory testing since kidney function and fluid and electrolyte balance can be affected. Do not inject furosemide into a milrinone infusion. Continuously assess pt for adverse reactions such as arrhythmias, low BP, chest pain. Headache, tremor, and low potassium can also occur. Monitor infusion site for reaction.

Pulmonary Arterial Hypertension

SILDENAFIL (***Revatio***) Pulmonary arterial hypertension: 20 mg PO three times per day; or 10 mg IV three times per day. Contraindicated with nitrates. Coadministration is not recommended with ritonavir, potent CYP3A inhibitors, or other phosphodiesterase-5 inhibitors. Teach patients to seek medical attention for vision loss, hearing loss, or erections lasting longer than 4 h. ▶LK ♀B ▶–© $$$$ Trade only (Revatio): Tabs 20 mg. Selectively inhibits phosphodiesterase-5 resulting in relaxation of pulmonary vascular smooth muscle bed. Serious: MI, CVA, hypotension, syncope, cerebral thrombosis, retinal hemorrhage, vision loss (nonarteritic ischemic optic neuropathy). Frequent: Dyspepsia, dyspnea, erythema, epistaxis, flushing, headache, insomnia, rhinitis.

> **Nursing Implications** Observe for signs and symptoms of severe allergic reactions such as: rash, hives, itching, difficulty breathing, tightness in the chest, swelling of the mouth, face, lips, or tongue. Do not prescribe if a patient is currently using nitrate medications for chest pain and heart problems/conditions. Patients should avoid alcohol when taking this medication. May increase the risk of heart-related and other side effects such as chest, shoulder, neck and jaw pain, paresthesia, dizziness, fainting, and vision changes.

Thrombolytics

ALTEPLASE (***tPA, Activase, Cathflo, ◆Activase rt-PA***) Acute MI: wt 67 kg or less, give 15 mg IV bolus, then 0.75 mg/kg (max 50 mg) over 30 min, then 0.5 mg/kg (max 35 mg) over the next 60 min; wt greater than 67 kg, give 15 mg IV bolus, then 50 mg over 30 min, then 35 mg over the next 60 min. Acute ischemic stroke with symptoms 3 h or less: 0.9 mg/kg (max 90 mg); give 10% of total dose as an IV bolus, and the remainder IV over 60 min. Multiple exclusion criteria. Acute pulmonary embolism: 100 mg IV over 2 h, then restart heparin when PTT twice normal or less. Occluded central venous access device: 2 mg/mL in catheter for 2 h. May use second dose if needed. ▶L ♀C ▶? © $$$$$ Enhances conversion of plasminogen to plasmin to achieve fibrinolysis. Serious: Bleeding, intracranial hemorrhage, hypersensitivity. Frequent: N/V, bleeding, hypotension, fever.

Nursing Implications Give only to pt with diagnosis of ischemic stroke. Do not give to pts with history or suspected intracranial bleeding or other internal hemorrhaging or uncontrolled hypertension greater than 180/110 at time of treatment, suspected aneurysm or pts taking heparin or Coumadin. Rapid intervention with activase is crucial, must be administered within the first 3 hours of the very first symptom of ischemic stroke. Give initial 10% of dose in infusion line over 60 minutes. Do not mix with any other medication. Do not use in pts with minor neurologic deficit or whose symptoms indicate rapid improvement.

Volume Expanders

ALBUMIN (*Albuminar, Buminate, Albumarc*, ✚ *Plasbumin*) Shock, burns: 500 mL of 5% soln IV infusion as rapidly as tolerated, repeat in 30 min if needed. ▶L ♀C ▶? © $$$$$ Expands plasma volume. Serious: Pulmonary edema (rapid infusion), hypersensitivity (rare), bleeding. Frequent: Hypotension (rapid infusion), fever, chills, itching.

Nursing Implications Administer by IV only, do not dilute or use if cloudy. Rapid administration may be necessary to restore normal blood volume. Do not use in patients with severe anemia, cardiac or renal failure, increased intravascular volume, nephritis, cirrhosis, malabsorption, and pancreatic insufficiency.

DERMATOLOGY

Antibacterials (Topical)

GENTAMICIN—TOPICAL (*Garamycin*) Apply three to four times per day. ▶K ♀D ▶? © $ Generic only: Ointment 0.1% 15, 30 g. Cream 0.1% 15, 30 g. Antibacterial, interferes with bacterial protein synthesis. Frequent: Neurotoxicity (when applied to large areas), gait instability, ototoxicity, nephrotoxicity.

Nursing Implications Do not administer to pregnant patients because it leads to hearing loss in fetus. Monitor for allergic reaction, especially in pediatric patients. Montior patient for other infections caused by nonsusceptible organisms. Monitor renal function in infants, neonates, and elderly patients. Promote reporting of hearing loss or other adverse reactions to prescriber.

MUPIROCIN (*Bactroban, Centany*) Impetigo/infected wounds: Apply three times per day. Nasal methicillin-resistant *S. aureus* eradication: 0.5 g in each nostril two times per day for 5 days. ▶Not absorbed ♀B ▶? © $$ Generic/Trade: Ointment 2% 22 g. Nasal ointment 2% 1 g single-use tubes (for MRSA eradication). Trade only: Cream 2% 15, 30 g. Antibacterial; inhibits protein and RNA synthesis. Frequent: Dryness, burning, erythema, stinging, tenderness.

Nursing Implications Avoid the eyes, nose, mouth, and lips when applying this drug. Promote hand washing after each dose. Promote completion of entire course of therapy.

Antifungals (Topical)

KETOCONAZOLE—TOPICAL (*Extina, Nizoral, Xolegel*, ✚ *Ketoderm*) Tinea/candidal infections: Apply daily. Seborrheic dermatitis: Apply cream one to two times per day for 4 weeks or gel daily for 2 weeks or foam two times per day for 4 weeks. Dandruff: Apply shampoo twice a week. Tinea versicolor: Apply shampoo to affected area, leave on for 5 min, rinse. ▶L ♀C ▶? © $$ Generic/Trade: Cream 2% 15, 30, 60 g. Shampoo 2% 120 mL. Trade only: Shampoo 1% 120, 210 mL (OTC Nizoral). Gel 2% 15 g (Xolegel). Foam 2% 50, 100 g (Extina). Antifungal; alters fungal cell wall permeability. Frequent: Burning, stinging, irritation, erythema.

Nursing Implications Use cautiously in patients with liver and renal disease, or if family has history of long QT syndrome. Do not give antacids for at least 2 h after administering drug. Promote avoidance of alcohol. Discontinue if patient displays fatigue, dyspnea, and peripheral edema.

NYSTATIN—TOPICAL (*Mycostatin*, ✚ *Nilstat, Nyaderm, Candistatin*) Candidiasis: Apply two to three times per day. ▶Not absorbed ♀C ▶? © $ Generic/Trade: Cream, Ointment 100,000 units/g 15, 30 g. Powder 100,000 units/g 15, 30, 60 g. Antifungal; alters fungal cell wall permeability. Frequent: Contact dermatitis, N/V, diarrhea, stomach pain. Severe: Stevens-Johnson syndrome, hypersensitivity.

Nursing Implications The most common side effects of this medication are gastrointestinal upset such as: nausea, vomiting and diarrhea. Uritcaria has been reported rarely as has Stevens-Johnson syndrome. Patients need to be aware that oral irritation and sensitization has been reported.

TERBINAFINE—TOPICAL   (*Lamisil, Lamisil AT*) Tinea: Apply one to two times per day. ▶L ♀B ▶? © $ OTC Trade only (Lamisil AT): Cream 1% 12, 24 g. Spray pump soln 1% 30 mL. Gel 1% 6, 12 g. Antifungal; alters fungal cell wall synthesis. Frequent: Contact dermatitis, burning, irritation, pruritus.

Nursing Implications Use cautiously in patients with liver and renal disease. Monitor for anorexia, dark urine, fatigue, jaundice, nausea, pale stools, right upper abdominal pain, and vomiting. Discontinue use if any of these symptoms occur. Discourage consumption of alcohol during therapy.

Antivirals (Topical)

ACYCLOVIR—TOPICAL   (*Zovirax*) Herpes genitalis: Apply ointment q 3 h (6 times per day) for 7 days. Recurrent herpes labialis: Apply cream 5 times per day for 4 days. ▶K ♀C ▶? © $$$$$ Trade only: Ointment 5% 15 g. Cream 5% 2, 5 g. Antiviral; inhibits DNA synthesis and viral replication. Frequent: Rash (oint). Skin irritation (cream). Severe: Cutaneous sensitization.

Nursing Implications Administer topically only. Use cautiously in patients with history of renal disease or dysfunction. Monitor for fever, diarrhea, nausea, vomiting, vision changes, and dizziness and report any symptoms to provider. Promote increased hydration for duration of treatment.

Corticosteroids (Topical)

NOTE: After long-term use, do not discontinue abruptly; switch to a less potent agent or alternate use of corticosteroids and emollient products. Monitor for hyperglycemia/adrenal suppression if used for long period of time or over a large area of the body, especially in children. Chronic administration may cause skin atrophy and interfere with pediatric growth and development.

HYDROCORTISONE—TOPICAL   (*Cortizone, Hycort, Hytone, Tegrin-HC, Dermolate, Synacort, Anusol-HC, Proctocream HC, ✦ Cortoderm, Prevex-HC, Cortate, Emo-Cort*) ▶L ♀C ▶? © $ Products available OTC and Rx depending on labeling. 2.5% preparation available Rx only. Generic/Trade: Ointment 0.5% 30 g. Ointment 1% 15, 20, 30, 60, 454 g. Ointment 2.5% 5, 20, 30, 454 g. Cream 0.5% 30 g. Cream 1% 5, 15, 20, 30, 120 g. Cream 2.5% 5, 20, 30, 454 g. Lotion 1% 120 mL. Lotion 2.5% 60 mL. Anal preparations: Generic/Trade: Cream 2.5% 30 g (Anusol HC, Proctocream HC). Suppositories 25 mg (Anusol HC). Anti-inflammatory; suppresses DNA synthesis, decreases WBC influx. Frequent: Burning, pruritus, dryness, irritation, erythema.

Nursing Implications Caution in patients with high BP and glaucoma and/or kidney, gastric, thyroid, liver, heart failure, or clotting disease. Monitor for increased intracranial pressure including seizures and general CNS symptoms including mood and personality changes; visual disturbances; nasopharyngeal irregularities including fungal infections; general gastric symptoms including rectal bleeding, stomach ulcers, and pancreatitis; fluid retention; endocrine disorders with prolonged use or failure to wean; muscle weakness; bronchospasm; skin conditions. Teach patient to self-monitor including regular checks of weight, BP, and electrolytes; to discontinue topical form if irritation develops; to take drug with food; to eat small and frequent meals. Patient must be carefully monitored during weaning.

ENDOCRINE AND METABOLIC

Bisphosphonates

ZOLEDRONIC ACID   (*Reclast, Zometa, ✦ Aclasta*) Treatment of osteoporosis: 5 mg (Reclast) once yearly IV infusion over 15 min or longer. Prevention and treatment of glucocorticoid-induced osteoporosis: 5 mg (Reclast) once a year IV infusion over 15 min or longer. Hypercalcemia (Zometa): 4 mg IV infusion over 15 min or longer. Wait at least 7 days before considering retreatment. Paget's disease (Reclast): 5 mg IV single dose infused over 15 min or longer. Multiple myeloma and metastatic bone lesions from solid tumors (Zometa): 4 mg IV infusion over 15 min or longer q 3 to 4 weeks. ▶K

♀D ▶? © $$$$$ A bisphosphonate that inhibits osteoclast-mediated bone resorption, increases bone mineral density, decreases serum calcium. Serious: Hypotension, renal impairment, granulocytopenia, thrombocytopenia, pancytopenia, osteonecrosis of the jaw, severe musculoskeletal pain, ocular inflammation, atypical femoral shaft fracture. Frequent: Electrolyte depletion (potassium, magnesium, calcium, phosphate), flu-like symptoms, fever, infusion site reaction, N/V, skeletal pain, constipation, diarrhea, conjunctivitis.

> **Nursing Implications** Alcohol and other medicines should not be taken with Zometa. Plenty of fluids should be ingested while on Zometa. Adequate hydration must be maintained while on this medication. There is a risk of jawbone problems. The highest risks for this problem are if the patient has cancer, poor dental hygiene, poorly fitting dentures, and is on other medications such as chemotherapy or corticosteroids. This medication is teratogenic. It is important to monitor CBC, electrolytes, and renal function.

Corticosteroids

NOTE: See also dermatology, ophthalmology.

DEXAMETHASONE   (*Decadron, Dexpak*, ✦*Dexasone*) Anti-inflammatory/immunosuppressive: 0.5 to 9 mg/day PO/IV/IM, divided two to four times per day. Cerebral edema: 10 to 20 mg IV load, then 4 mg IM q 6 h (off-label IV use common) or 1 to 3 mg PO three times per day. Bronchopulmonary dysplasia in preterm infants: 0.5 mg/kg PO/IV divided q 12 h for 3 days, then taper. Croup: 0.6 mg/kg PO or IM for one dose. Acute asthma: age older than 2 yo: 0.6 mg/kg to max 16 mg PO daily for 2 days. Fetal lung maturation, maternal antepartum: 6 mg IM q 12 h for 4 doses. Antiemetic, prophylaxis: 8 mg IV or 12 mg PO prior to chemotherapy; 8 mg PO daily for 2 to 4 days. Antiemetic, treatment: 10 to 20 mg PO/IV q 4 to 6 h. ▶L ♀C ▶– © $ Generic/Trade: Tabs 0.5, 0.75. Generic only: Tabs 0.25, 1.0, 1.5, 2, 4, 6 mg; elixir 0.5 mg/5 mL; Soln 0.5 mg/5 mL, 1 mg/1 mL (concentrate). Trade only: Dexpak 13 day (51 total 1.5 mg tabs for a 13-day taper), Dexpak 10 day (35 total 1.5 mg tabs for 10-day taper), Dexpak 6 days (21 total 1.5 mg tabs for 6-day taper). Long-acting glucocorticoid. Serious: Hypertension, diabetes, osteoporosis, immunosuppression, impaired wound healing, adrenal suppression, peptic ulcer disease, cataracts. Frequent: Cushingoid state, N/V, weight gain, myopathy, leukocytosis, skin atrophy, edema.

> **Nursing Implications** Since drug is a corticosteroid, a careful assessment of all patient's diseases, disorders, and other drug use is imperative. Teach patient to be alert for wt gain, increased BP, potassium loss, muscle weakness, headache, eye disorders, GI symptoms, and mood disturbances. Dexamethasone can depress adrenal gland production of natural steroids so withdrawal must be gradual. Monitor for infections since immunosuppression is a side effect. Calcium or vitamins dose/dosing may be indicated in prolonged use because of bone thinning. Teach pt to take at same time each day and not to abruptly stop drug even if feeling well. If taken in pregnancy drug passes into breastmilk. Infant should be monitored for persistent GI symptoms and weakness. Numerous, serious drug interactions warrant a thorough review.

CORTICOSTEROIDS	Approximate Equivalent Dose (mg)	Relative Anti-inflammatory Potency	Relative Mineralocorti-coid Potency	Biological Half-life (h)
betamethasone	0.6–0.75	20–30	0	36–54
cortisone	25	0.8	2	8–12
dexamethasone	0.75	20–30	0	36–54
fludrocortisone	n.a.	10	125	18–36
hydrocortisone	20	1	2	8–12
methylprednisolone	4	5	0	18–36
prednisolone	5	4	1	18–36
prednisone	5	4	1	18–36
triamcinolone	4	5	0	12–36

n.a.= not available.

HYDROCORTISONE   (*Cortef, Cortenema, Solu-Cortef*) Adrenocortical insufficiency: 100 to 500 mg IV/ IM q 2 to 6 h prn (sodium succinate) or 20 to 240 mg/day PO divided three to four times per day. Ulcerative colitis: 100 mg retention enema at bedtime (laying on side for 1 h or longer) for 21 days. ▶L ♀C ▶– © $ Generic/Trade: Tabs 5, 10, 20 mg; Enema 100 mg/60 mL. Short-acting glucocorticoid with mineralocorticoid activity at higher doses. Serious: Hypertension, diabetes, osteoporosis, immunosuppression, impaired wound healing, adrenal suppression, peptic ulcer disease, cataracts. Frequent: Cushingoid state, N/V, weight gain, myopathy, leukocytosis, skin atrophy, edema.

Nursing Implications   Give with food/milk; advise patient to eat small, frequent meals; rotate injection sites if using injectable; instruct patient against abrupt discontinuation of drug. Carefully monitor BP, weight gain, electrolyte levels, leg swelling, severe gastric symptoms, irregular menstruation, fever, infections, blood clots, fluid retention, bronchospasm. With prolonged use, regular eye exams should be conducted. Drug ID tag is advised.

DIABETES NUMBERS*

Criteria for diagnosis	Self-monitoring glucose goals
Pre-diabetes: Fasting glucose 100–125 mg/dL or A1C 5.7–6.4% or 140–199 mg/dL 2 h after 75 g oral glucose load	Preprandial: 70–130 mg/dL Postprandial: < 180 mg/dL
Diabetes:[†] A1C ≥ 6.5% Fasting glucose ≥ 126 mg/dL. Random glucose with symptoms: ≥ 200 mg/dL, or ≥ 200 mg/dL 2 h after 75 g oral glucose load	A1C goal: < 7% for most non-pregnant adults, individualize based on comorbid conditions, hypoglycemia, and other patient specific factors.

Hospitalized patients: may consider more stringent goal if safely achievable without hypoglycemia

Critically ill glucose goal: 140–180 mg/d

Non-critically ill glucose goal (hospitalized patients): premeal blood glucose < 140 mg/dL, random < 180 mg/dL

Estimated average glucose (eAG): eAG (mg/dL) = (28.7 × A1C) − 46.7

Complications prevention & management: ASA[‡] (75–162 mg/day) in Type 1 & 2 adults for primary prevention if 10-year cardiovascular risk > 10% (includes most men older than 50 yo or women older than 60 yo with at least one other major risk factor) and secondary prevention (those with vascular disease); statin therapy to achieve goal LDL regardless of baseline LDL (for those with vascular disease, those older than 40 yo and additional risk factor, or those younger than 40 yo but LDL > 100 mg/dL); ACE inhibitor or ARB if hypertensive or micro-/macro-albuminuria; pneumococcal vaccine (revaccinate one time if age 65 yo or older and previously received vaccine at age younger than 65 or older and more than 5 years ago).

Every visit: Measure wt & BP (goal < 130/80 mm Hg); visual foot exam; review self-monitoring glucose record; review/adjust meds; review self-mgmt skills, dietary needs, and physical activity; smoking cessation counseling.

Twice a year: A1C in those meeting treatment goals with stable glycemia (quarterly if not); dental exam.

Annually: Fasting lipid profile** [goal LDL < 100 mg/dL, cardiovascular disease consider LDL < 70 mg/dL; HDL > 40 mg/dL (> 50 mg/dL in women), TG < 150 mg/dL], q 2 years with low-risk lipid values; creatinine; albumin to creatinine ratio spot collection; dilated eye exam; flu vaccine.

*See recommendations at: care.diabetesjournals.org. Reference: *Diabetes Care* 2012;35(Suppl 1):S11-63. Glucose values are plasma.
[†]In the absence of symptoms, confirm diagnosis with glucose testing on subsequent day.
[‡]Avoid ASA if younger than 21 yo due to Reye's Syndrome risk; use if younger than 30 yo has not been studied.
**LDL is primary target of therapy, consider 30 to 40% LDL reduction from baseline as alternate goal if unable to reach targets on maximal tolerated statin.

METHYLPREDNISOLONE (*Solu-Medrol, Medrol, Depo-Medrol*) Anti-inflammatory/immunosuppressive: Oral (Medrol): Dose varies, 4 to 48 mg PO daily. Medrol Dosepak tapers 24 to 0 mg PO over 7 days. IM/Joints (Depo-Medrol): Dose varies, 4 to 120 mg IM q 1 to 2 weeks. Parenteral (Solu-Medrol): Dose varies, 10 to 250 mg IV/IM. Peds: 0.5 to 1.7 mg/kg PO/IV/IM divided q 6 to 12 h. ▶L ♀C ▶– © $ Trade only: Tabs 2, 16, 32 mg. Generic/Trade: Tabs 4, 8 mg. Medrol Dosepak (4 mg, 21 tabs). Intermediate-acting glucocorticoid. Serious: Cardiac arrest or arrhythmia (with IV), hypertension, osteoporosis, immunosuppression, impaired wound healing, adrenal suppression, peptic ulcers, cataracts, postinjection flare, HPA axis suppression. Frequent: Cushingoid state, N/V, weight gain, edema, hyperglycemia, hypokalemia, injection site hypo/hyperpigmentation, myopathy, dermal or subdermal changes, deltoid muscle atrophy with IM injection.

> Nursing Implications The most common side effects to this medication include: increased appetite, weight gain and moon facies. This medication needs to be weaned in patients on long-term therapy.

PREDNISONE (*Deltasone, Sterapred, ✦Winpred*) 1 to 2 mg/kg or 5 to 60 mg PO daily. ▶L ♀C ▶+ © $ Trade only: Sterapred (5-mg tabs: Tapers 30 to 5 mg PO over 6 days or 30 to 10 mg over 12 days), Sterapred DS (10-mg tabs: Tapers 60 to 10 mg over 6 days, or 60 to 20 mg PO over 12 days) taper packs. Generic only: Tabs 1, 2.5, 5, 10, 20, 50 mg. Soln 5 mg/5 mL, 5 mg/mL (Prednisone Intensol). Intermediate-acting glucocorticoid with mineralocorticoid activity; primarily used for its glucocorticoid effects. Serious: Hypertension, diabetes, osteoporosis, immunosuppression, impaired wound healing, adrenal suppression, peptic ulcer disease, cataracts, psychosis, depression. Frequent: Cushingoid state, N/V, weight gain, myopathy, leukocytosis, skin atrophy, edema.

> Nursing Implications Nursing needs to educate patients to take this medication with food. This medication may cause sodium and fluid retention. Patients may develop a "moon" facies. Patients may be more susceptible to infections. Patients should be educated to avoid contact with individuals who have colds and other infections. Prolonged use of this medication can cause calcium loss resulting in osteopenia and osteoporsis. Diabetic patients need to be educated that this medication may affect the blood sugar. Diabetic patient's blood sugar should be checked frequently. Women may experience a change in their menstrual cycle. This medication may also cause an increased appetite and excessive wt gain.

TRIAMCINOLONE (*Aristospan, Kenalog, Trivaris*) 4 to 48 mg PO/IM daily. Intra-articular 2.5 to 40 mg (Kenalog, Trivaris), 2 to 20 mg (Aristospan). ▶L ♀C ▶– © $ Trade only: Injection 10 mg/mL, 40 mg/mL (Kenalog), 5 mg/mL, 20 mg/mL (Aristospan), 8 mg (80 mg/mL) syringe (Trivaris). Intermediate-acting glucocorticoid. Serious: Hypertension, diabetes, osteoporosis, immunosuppression, impaired wound healing, adrenal suppression, peptic ulcer disease, cataracts, postinjection flare, anaphylaxis, angioedema. Frequent: Cushingoid state, N/V, wt gain, myopathy, leukocytosis, skin atrophy, injection site hyper/hypopigmentation, edema.

> Nursing Implications Inject into joint space or soft tissue ONLY. Assess for allergic reaction. Call prescriber if pt has HR changes, SOB, edema/wt gain, high BP, vision or eye problems, seizure, changes in behavior/mood, and muscular pain. Teach pt that minor side effects may occur such as GI disturbances, headache, changes in skin, insomnia, slow healing, bruising/swelling, or irregular menstruation. Since drug is a steroid, precautions should be taken as applied to long-term use and weaning from the drug. Assess pt for all prescription and OTC drugs used since many interact with this drug.

Diabetes-Related—"Gliptins" (DPP-4 inhibitors)

SITAGLIPTIN (*Januvia*) DM, Type 2: 100 mg PO daily. ▶K ♀B ▶? © $$$$$ Trade only: Tabs 25, 50, 100 mg. Dipeptidyl peptidase IV (DPP-IV) inhibitor that slows inactivation of incretin hormones, resulting in increased glucose-stimulated insulin secretion and decreased glucagon secretion. Serious: Hypersensitivity, anaphylaxis, angioedema, pancreatitis. Frequent: URI, nasopharyngitis, HA, increased serum transaminases, constipation, vomiting.

> Nursing Implications Lower dose must be utilized in patients with renal impairment. The serum creatinine and BUN levels must be monitored prior to administration of this medication.

Diabetes-Related—Combinations

DUETACT   (pioglitazone + glimepiride) DM, Type 2: Start 30/2 mg PO daily. Start up to 30/4 mg PO daily if prior glimepiride therapy, or 30/2 mg PO daily if prior pioglitazone therapy; max 30/4 mg/day. Obtain LFTs before therapy and periodically thereafter. ▶LK ♀C ▶– © $$$$ Trade only: Tabs 30/2, 30/4 mg pioglitazone/glimepiride. Combination product that stimulates pancreatic beta-cell insulin release and increases insulin sensitivity in adipose tissue, skeletal muscle, and liver. Serious: Potential hepatotoxicity, heart failure exacerbation, resumption of ovulation, hypoglycemia, hypersensitivity, SIADH, disulfiram-like reaction, cholestatic jaundice, marrow suppression, hemolytic anemia, eosinophilia, hepatic porphyria, increased LFTs, macular edema, fracture, bladder tumor. Frequent: Edema, wt gain, upper respiratory tract infection, headache, fatigue, N/V/D, dyspepsia, rash, pruritus, blurred vision. Fracture risk in PI for women; in men citation is: *Arch Intern Med.* 2008;168(8):820-825.

> Nursing Implications Caution in patients with kidney, liver, adrenal, or pituitary disease; heart failure; pregnancy; breastfeeding; or elderly. Monitor for cardiac symptoms, abnormal vision, dizziness/headache, blood dyscrasias, signs of hepatitis, low blood sugar, skin rash, photosensitivity. Frequent CBCs and blood chemistry, blood glucose and hemoglobin, LFTs. Teach patient to self-monitor blood sugar and signs of low blood sugar. Patient should wear medical ID, keep a sugar source available, avoid driving until drug effect is known. Promote avoidance of alcohol, reporting of symptoms to provider, such as visual changes, nausea, vomiting, stomach pain, tiredness, dizziness, swelling of legs or ankles, loss of appetite, dark urine, or yellowing of skin or eyes.

GLUCOVANCE   (glyburide + metformin) DM, Type 2, Initial therapy (drug-naive): Start 1.25/250 mg PO daily or two times per day with meals; max 10/2000 mg daily. Inadequate control with a sulfonylurea or metformin alone: Start 2.5/500 or 5/500 mg PO two times per day with meals; max 20/2000 mg daily. ▶KL ♀B ▶? © $$$ Generic/Trade: Tabs 1.25/250, 2.5/500, 5/500 mg. Combination product that stimulates pancreatic beta-cell insulin release, decreases hepatic gluconeogenesis, and increases insulin sensitivity. Serious: Hypoglycemia, hypersensitivity, SIADH, disulfiram-like reaction, cholestatic jaundice, aplastic anemia, hemolytic anemia, leukopenia, thrombocytopenia, agranulocytosis, pancytopenia, eosinophilia, hepatic porphyria, increased LFTs, hepatitis, liver failure, lactic acidosis, decreased serum vitamin B12. Frequent: Diarrhea, N/V, flatulence, abdominal discomfort, headache, fatigue, rash, weight gain or loss, taste disturbance.

> Nursing Implications Caution in elderly patients; patients with liver, adrenal, cardiac, renal, thyroid disease; and impaired adrenal and pituitary function, infection, and stress. Monitor for dizziness, heart failure, gastric symptoms, visual disturbances, hepatitis, blood dyscrasias, low blood sugar. Teach patient how to monitor and maintain normal blood sugar level including signs of high or low blood sugar, to carry medical ID and supplemental sugar source, and to drink fluids. Avoid driving until effect of drug is known. Regular blood tests required. Baseline creatinine before first dose. Give at breakfast. Promote avoidance of alcohol. Withhold metformin-containing medications before or at the time of studies requiring IV administration of iodinated contrast media and for 48 h after study.

JANUMET, JANUMET XR   (sitagliptin + metformin) DM, Type 2: Individualize based on patient's current therapy. Immediate-release: 1 tab PO two times per day. Extended-release: 1 tab PO daily. If inadequate control with metformin monotherapy: Immediate-release: Start 50/500 or 50/1000 two times per day based on current metformin dose. Extended-release: Start 100 mg sitagliptin daily plus current daily metformin. If inadequate control on sitagliptin: Immediate-release: start 50/500 two times per day. Extended-release: Start 100/1000 daily. Max 100/2000 mg/day. Give with meals. ▶K ♀B ▶? © $$$$ Trade only: Immediate-release tabs 50/500, 50/1000 mg, extended-release tabs 100/1000, 50/500, 50, 1000 mg sitagliptin/metformin. Combination product that decreases hepatic gluconeogenesis, increases insulin sensitivity, and slows inactivation of incretin hormones. Serious: Lactic acidosis, hypersensitivity, decreased serum vitamin B12, pancreatitis. Frequent: Diarrhea, N/V, flatulence, abdominal discomfort, headache, weight loss, taste disturbance, URI, nasopharyngitis, vomiting.

> Nursing Implications Administer with or without food. Caution in use with pts with renal impairment. Promote avoidance of alcohol. Withhold metformin before or at the time of studies requiring IV administration of iodinated contrast media and for 48 h after study. Instruct patient to reports signs and symptoms of lactic acidosis: hyperventilation, myalgia, malaise.

Diabetes-Related—Insulins

INSULIN—INJECTABLE INTERMEDIATE/LONG-ACTING   (*Novolin N, Humulin N, Lantus, Levemir*) Diabetes: Doses vary, but typically total insulin 0.3 to 0.5 unit/kg/day SC in divided doses (Type 1), and 1 to 1.5 unit/kg/day SC in divided doses (Type 2). Generally, 50 to 70% of insulin requirements are provided by rapid- or short-acting insulin and the remainder from intermediate- or long-acting insulin. Lantus: Start 10 units SC daily (same time every day) in insulin-naive patients. Levemir: Type 2 DM (inadequately controlled on oral meds): Start 0.1 to 0.2 units/kg once daily in evening or 10 units SC daily or two times per day. ▶LK ♀B/C ▶+ © $$$$ Trade only: Injection NPH (Novolin N, Humulin N). Insulin glargine (Lantus). Insulin detemir (Levemir). Insulin available in pen form: Novolin N InnoLet, Humulin N Pen, Lantus OptiClik (reusable), Lantus SoloStar (prefilled-disposable), Levemir InnoLet, Levemir FlexPen. Premixed preparations of NPH and regular insulin also available. Stimulates peripheral glucose uptake and inhibits hepatic gluconeogenesis. Serious: Hypoglycemia, allergic reaction, hypokalemia. Frequent: Weight gain, lipoatrophy, lipohypertrophy, injection site reaction.

> Nursing Implications   SC: Administer SC once daily at any time during the day, but at the same time each day. Do not administer IV or use with insulin pumps.

INSULIN—INJECTABLE SHORT-/RAPID-ACTING   (*Apidra, Novolin R, NovoLog, Humulin R, Humalog, ✚ NovoRapid*) Diabetes: Doses vary, but typically total insulin 0.3 to 0.5 unit/kg/day SC in divided doses (Type 1), and 1 to 1.5 unit/kg/day SC in divided doses (Type 2). Generally, 50 to 70% of insulin requirements are provided by rapid- or short-acting insulin and the remainder from intermediate- or long-acting insulin. Administer rapid-acting insulin (Humalog, NovoLog, Apidra) within 15 min before or immediately after a meal. Administer regular insulin 30 min before meals. Severe hyperkalemia: 5 to 10 units regular insulin plus concurrent dextrose IV. Profound hyperglycemia (eg, DKA): 0.1 unit regular/kg IV bolus, then initial infusion 100 units regular in 100 mL NS (1 unit/mL), at 0.1 units/kg/h. ▶LK ♀B/C ▶+ © $$$ Trade only: Injection regular 100 units/mL (Novolin R, Humulin R), Injection regular 500 units/mL (Humulin U-500, concentrated). Insulin glulisine (Apidra). Insulin lispro (Humalog). Insulin aspart (Novolog). Insulin available in pen form: Novolin R InnoLet, Humulin R, Apidra OptiClik, Humalog KwikPen, Novolog FlexPen. Stimulates peripheral glucose uptake, and inhibits hepatic gluconeogenesis. Serious: Hypoglycemia, allergic reaction, hypokalemia. Frequent: Weight gain, lipoatrophy, lipohypertrophy, injection site reaction.

INJECTABLE INSULINS*

		Onset (h)	Peak (h)	Duration (h)
Rapid-/short acting	Insulin aspart (NovoLog)	<0.2	1–3	3–5
	Insulin glulisine (Apidra)	0.30–0.4	1	4–5
	Insulin lispro (Humalog)	0.25–0.5	0.5–2.5	≤5
	Regular (Novolin R, Humulin R)	0.5–1	2–3	3–6
Intermediate-/long acting	NPH (Novolin N, Humulin N)	2–4	4–10	10–16
	Insulin detemir (Levemir)	n.a.	flat action profile	up to 23†
	Insulin glargine (Lantus)	2–4	peakless	24
Mixtures	Insulin aspart protamine susp/aspart (NovoLog Mix 70/30)	0.25	1–4 (biphasic)	up to 24
	Insulin lispro protamine susp/insulin lispro (Humalog Mix 75/25, Humalog Mix 50/50)	<0.25	1–3 (biphasic)	10–20
	NPH/Reg (Humulin 70/30, Novolin 70/30)	0.5–1	2–10 (biphasic)	10–20

*These are general guidelines, as onset, peak, and duration of activity are affected by the site of injection, physical activity, body temperature, and blood supply.
†Dose-dependent duration of action, range from 6 to 23 h.
n.a.= not available.

Nursing Implications By sub-cutaneous injection in abdominal wall, upper arm or thigh, rotating injection sites. Give 15 to 20 minutes pre meal. Teach patient to monitor blood glucose levels and to adjust dosage accordingly. Teach patient to self monitor for low blood sugar signs including hunger, confusion, headache, nausea, drowsiness/dizziness, rapid HR, sweating, tremors and seizures. Patient should always carry hard candy or glucose tablets to counteract hypoglycemia. Low potassium may also occur with muscle pain, irregular HR, increased urination and thirst. Patient should immediately report confusion.

Diabetes-Related—Meglitinides

REPAGLINIDE (*Prandin*, ✦ *Gluconorm*) DM, Type 2: Start 0.5 to 2 mg PO three times per day before meals, maintenance 0.5 to 4 mg three to four times per day, max 16 mg/day. ▶L ♀C ▶? © $$$$$ Trade only: Tabs 0.5, 1, 2 mg. Stimulates pancreatic beta-cell insulin release. Serious: Hypoglycemia, hypersensitivity, thrombocytopenia, leukopenia, increased serum transaminases. Frequent: Diarrhea, arthralgia, upper respiratory tract infection.

Nursing Implications Patients must be advised to take this medication with each meal (usually ½ hour prior to eating). A missed dose should only be taken if the patient is ready to eat a meal. Patients need to be educated to the signs and symptoms of hypoglycemia and hyperglycemia. Advise patients to keep a source of sugar available to them at all times in case of low blood sugar levels. This medication is contraindicated in pregnancy and lactation.

Diabetes-Related—Sulfonylureas—2nd Generation

GLIPIZIDE (*Glucotrol, Glucotrol XL*) DM, Type 2: Start 5 mg PO daily, usual 10 to 20 mg/day, max 40 mg/day (divide two times per day if more than 15 mg/day). Extended-release: Start 5 mg PO daily, usual 5 to 10 mg/day, max 20 mg/day. ▶LK ♀C ▶? © $ Generic/Trade: Tabs 5, 10 mg; Extended-release tabs 2.5, 5, 10 mg. Stimulates pancreatic beta-cell insulin release. Serious: Hypoglycemia, hypersensitivity, SIADH, disulfiram-like reaction, cholestatic jaundice, hepatocellular injury, aplastic anemia, hemolytic anemia, leukopenia, thrombocytopenia, agranulocytosis, pancytopenia, eosinophilia, hepatic porphyria, increased serum transaminases. Frequent: Weight gain, fatigue, diarrhea, nausea, dyspepsia, rash.

Nursing Implications Caution in patients with kidney, liver, adrenal, cardiac, or thyroid disease and impaired adrenal and pituitary function. Monitor for dizziness, heart failure, gastric symptoms, blood dyscrasias, low blood sugar, rash, and edema. Teach patient how to monitor and maintain normal blood sugar level including signs of high or low blood sugar, and to carry medical ID and supplemental sugar source. Avoid driving until effect of drug is known. Regular blood tests required. Promote avoidance of alcohol.

Diabetes-Related—Thiazolidinediones

PIOGLITAZONE (*Actos*) DM, Type 2: Start 15 to 30 mg PO daily, max 45 mg/day. Monitor LFTs. ▶L ♀C ▶– © $$$$$ Trade only: Tabs 15, 30, 45 mg. Increases insulin sensitivity in adipose tissue, skeletal muscle, and liver. Serious: Hepatotoxicity, liver failure, heart failure exacerbation, resumption of ovulation, macular edema, fracture, bladder tumor. Frequent: Edema, wt gain, upper respiratory tract infection, headache, myalgia.

Nursing Implications Do not use in patients with history of coronary conditions, renal disease, or liver disease. Promote avoidance of alcohol, reporting of symptoms to provider, such as visual changes, nausea, vomiting, stomach pain, tiredness, dizziness, swelling of legs or ankles, loss of appetite, dark urine, or yellowing of skin or eyes. Monitor liver function tests. Avoid in patients with history of heart failure.

Diabetes-Related—Other

METFORMIN (*Glucophage, Glucophage XR, Glumetza, Fortamet, Riomet*) DM, type 2: Immediate-release: Start 500 mg PO one to two times per day or 850 mg PO daily with meals, may gradually increase to max 2550 mg/day. Extended-release: Glucophage XR: 500 mg PO daily with evening meal; increase by

500 mg once a week to max 2000 mg/day (may divide two times per day). Glumetza: 1000 mg PO daily with evening meal; increase by 500 mg once a week to max 2000 mg/day (may divide two times per day). Fortamet: 500 to 1000 mg daily with evening meal; increase by 500 mg once a week to max 2500 mg/day. Polycystic ovary syndrome (unapproved, immediate-release): 500 mg PO three times per day. DM prevention, Type 2 (with lifestyle modifications, unapproved): 850 mg PO daily for 1 month, then increase to 850 mg PO two times per day. All products started at low doses to improve GI tolerability, gradually increase as tolerated. ▶K ♀B ▶? © $ Generic/Trade: Tabs 500, 850, 1000 mg, extended-release 500, 750 mg. Trade only, extended-release: Fortamet 500, 1000 mg; Glumetza 500, 1000 mg. Trade only: Oral soln 500 mg/5 mL (Riomet). Decreases hepatic gluconeogenesis and increases insulin sensitivity. Serious: Lactic acidosis, decreased serum vitamin B12. Frequent: Diarrhea, N/V, flatulence, abdominal discomfort, headache, weight loss, taste disturbance.

> Nursing Implications The most common side effects to this medication include diarrhea and lactic acidosis. This medication should be withheld when patients are having any type of contrast media study.

Gout-Related

COLCHICINE   (***Colcrys***) Rapid treatment of acute gouty arthritis: 1.2 mg (2 tabs) PO at signs of attack then 0.6 mg (1 tab) 1 h after initial administration. Gout prophylaxis: 0.6 mg PO two times per day if CrCl is 50 mL/min or greater, 0.6 mg PO daily if CrCl is 35 to 49 mL/min, 0.6 mg PO q 2 to 3 days if CrCl is 10 to 34 mL/min. Familial Mediterranean Fever: 1.2 to 2.4 mg PO daily or divided two times per day. ▶L ♀C ▶? © $$$$ Trade: Tabs 0.6 mg. Reduces the inflammatory response to deposited crystals, and diminishes phagocytosis. Serious: Peripheral neuritis, hepatotoxicity, renal failure, bone marrow depression, leukocytopenia, granulocytopenia, aplastic anemia, thrombocytopenia, purpura, myopathy, rhabdomyolysis, hypersensitivity. Frequent: Diarrhea, N/V, abdominal pain, dermatoses, hair loss.

> Nursing Implications Give with food/milk; monitor for CNS, respiratory depression, and GI symptoms (eg, cramps, constipation, nausea, or vomiting); instruct patient not to drive until adjusted to the drug; instruct patient to not drink alcohol and change positions slowly to avoid dizziness.

Minerals

CALCIUM ACETATE   (***PhosLo, Eliphos***) Phosphate binder to reduce serum phosphorous in end stage renal disease: Initially 2 tabs/caps PO with each meal. ▶K ♀C ▶? © $$$$ Generic/Trade: Gelcaps 667 mg (169 mg elem Ca). Trade: Tab 667 mg (169 mg elem Ca). Binds with dietary phosphate to form a nonabsorbable complex. Serious: Severe hypercalcemia (with confusion, delirium, stupor, coma), renal calculi. Frequent: Mild hypercalcemia, constipation, anorexia, N/V.

> Nursing Implications Administer with each meal. Do not use in patients with high levels of calcium in the blood or those taking digoxin. Promote avoidance of antacids during course of therapy. Monitor for nausea, vomiting, loss of appetite, constipation, dry mouth, increased thirst, or increased urination. Read manufacturer's instructions for list of drug interactions.

CALCIUM GLUCONATE 2.25 to 14 mEq slow IV. 500 to 2000 mg PO two to four times per day. ▶K ♀+ ▶+ © $ Generic only: Injectable 10% (1000 mg/10 mL, 4.65 mEq/10 mL) 1, 10, 50, 100, 200 mL. OTC Generic only: Tabs 50, 500, 650, 975, 1000 mg. Chewable tabs 650 mg. Essential mineral that maintains the nervous, muscular, and skeletal systems and cell membrane and capillary permeability; antagonizes the cardiotoxic effects of hyperkalemia. Serious: Severe hypercalcemia (with confusion, delirium, stupor, coma), renal calculi; with IV: vasodilation, hypotension, arrhythmia, syncope, and cardiac arrest. Frequent: Mild hypercalcemia, constipation, anorexia, N/V, irritation at infusion site (for IV).

> Nursing Implications Administer with 8 ounces of water and food. Promote avoidance of antacids during course of therapy. Monitor for nausea, vomiting, loss of appetite, constipation, dry mouth, increased thirst, or increased urination. Read manufacturer's instructions for list of drug interactions. IV: Monitor ECG. Assess IV for patency. Extravasation may cause tissue necrosis or cellulitis.

FLUORIDE SUPPLEMENTATION

Age	<0.3 ppm in drinking water	0.3–0.6 ppm in drinking water	>0.6 ppm in drinking water
0–6 mo	none	none	none
6 mo–3 yo	0.25 mg PO daily	none	none
3–6 yo	0.5 mg PO daily	0.25 mg PO daily	none
6–16 yo	1 mg PO daily	0.5 mg PO daily	none

JADA 2010;141:1480-1489

IV SOLUTIONS

Solution	Dextrose	Calories/ Liter	Na*	Ca*	Lactate*	Osm*
0.9 NS	0 g/L	0	154	0	0	310
LR	0 g/L	9	130	3	28	273
D5 W	50 g/L	170	0	0	0	253
D5 0.2 NS	50 g/L	170	34	0	0	320
D5 0.45 NS	50 g/L	170	77	0	0	405
D5 0.9 NS	50 g/L	170	154	0	0	560
D5 LR	50 g/L	179	130	2.7	28	527

* All given in mEq/L

FERRIC GLUCONATE COMPLEX　(**Ferrlecit**)　125 mg elemental iron IV over 10 min or diluted in 100 mL NS IV over 1 h. Peds age 6 yo or older: 1.5 mg/kg (max 125 mg) elemental iron diluted in 25 mL NS and administered IV over 1 h. ▶KL ♀B ▶? © $$$$$ Essential mineral needed for hemoglobin, myoglobin, and enzymatic function. Serious: Anaphylactic reaction, chest pain, hypotension, shock, cardiac arrest, iron overdose. Frequent: Arthralgia, backache, chills, dizziness, fever, flushing, headache, infusion site reaction, malaise, myalgia, N/V.

> Nursing Implications　Administer intravenously or by injection. Do not mix with other IV medications or parenteral nutrition solutions. Check solution for discoloration or particulate matter. Do not freeze. Monitor patient for hypersensitivity/anaphylactic reaction and low BP. Teach patient to recognize adverse reactions such as any changes in BP, GI symptoms, dizziness and cramps, rapid HR, headache and abnormal red blood cells as reported on blood tests.

IRON SUCROSE　(**Venofer**)　Iron deficiency with hemodialysis: 5 mL (100 mg elemental iron) IV over 5 min or diluted in 100 mL NS IV over 15 min or longer. Iron deficiency in nondialysis chronic kidney disease: 10 mL (200 mg elemental iron) IV over 5 min. ▶KL ♀B ▶? © $$$$$ Essential mineral needed for hemoglobin, myoglobin, and enzymatic function. Serious: Anaphylaxis, chest pain, hypotension, shock, cardiac arrest, iron overdose. Frequent: Arthralgia, backache, chills, dizziness, fever, flushing, headache, infusion site reaction, malaise, myalgia, N/V.

> Nursing Implications　The most common side effect to this medication is constipation. Patients should be advised to increase fiber intake while on this medication.

MAGNESIUM OXIDE　(**Mag-200, Mag-Ox 400**)　400 to 800 mg PO daily. ▶K ♀A ▶+ © $ OTC Generic/ Trade: Caps: 140 (84.5 mg elemental Mg), 250 (elemental), 400 (240 mg elemental Mg), 420 (253 mg elemental Mg), 500 mg (elemental). Essential mineral needed for muscle function, organ function, and potassium and calcium absorption. Serious: Potential magnesium intoxication. Frequent: Diarrhea, weakness, N/V.

> Nursing Implications　Instruct patient to take with a full glass of water.

MAGNESIUM SULFATE   Hypomagnesemia: 1 g of 20% soln IM q 6 h for 4 doses, or 2 g IV over 1 h (monitor for hypotension). Peds: 25 to 50 mg/kg IV/IM q 4 to 6 h for 3 to 4 doses, max single dose 2 g. Eclampsia: 4 to 6 g IV over 30 min, then 1 to 2 g/h. Drip: 5 g in 250 mL D5W (20 mg/mL), 2 g/h is a rate of 100 mL/h. Preterm labor: 6 g IV over 20 min, then 1 to 3 g/h titrated to decrease contractions. Monitor respirations and reflexes. If needed, may reverse toxic effects with calcium gluconate 1 g IV. Torsades de pointes: 1 to 2 g IV in D5W over 5 to 60 min. ▶K ♀A ▶+ © $ Essential mineral needed for muscle function, organ function, and potassium and calcium absorption; blocks neuromuscular transmission to prevent or control convulsions. Serious: Magnesium intoxication, cardiac depression, CNS depression, respiratory paralysis, hypotension, stupor, hypothermia, circulatory collapse. Frequent: Flushing, sweating, depressed reflexes.

> Nursing Implications   Administer by IV or IM. Monitor serum magnesium levels until normal. Give IV in 10 to 20% soln with great caution. Monitor for low BP, hypothermia, breathing problems and respiratory depression, flushing, and sweating. Have IV calcium gluconate on hand should antidote be needed. Give no more than 20 g in 48 h if pt has renal insufficiency. Cautionary use with barbiturates, anesthetics, and narcotics because of Mg sulfate's central depressive effect. Do not give to pts with heart block or heart damage.

PHOSPHORUS   (*Neutra-Phos, K-Phos*) 1 cap/packet PO four times per day. 1 to 2 tabs PO four times per day. Severe hypophosphatemia (eg, less than 1 mg/dL): 0.08 to 0.16 mmol/kg IV over 6 h. ▶K ♀C ▶? © $ OTC Trade only: (Neutra-Phos, Neutra-Phos K) tab/cap/packet 250 mg (8 mmol) phosphorus. Rx: Trade only: (K-Phos) tab 250 mg (8 mmol) phosphorus. Essential mineral needed for bone metabolism and enzymatic functions. Serious: Phosphate intoxication with reciprocal hypocalcemic tetany (with IV). Frequent: Laxative-like effect, nausea, abdominal pain, vomiting.

> Nursing Implications   Patients need to be advised that this medication may cause severe allergic reactions (rash; hives; itching; difficulty breathing; tightness in the chest; swelling of the mouth, face, lips, or tongue). This medication may lower the seizure threshold so patients may be more prone to seizures when taking this medication. This medication needs to be taken with meals and at bedtime. It should be taken with a full glass of water. The possibility of passing kidney stones is increased with this medication. Nursing needs to monitor lab values including renal function and serum electrolytes. This medication can be teratogenic to the fetus.

POTASSIUM   (*Cena-K, Effer-K, K+8, K+10, Kaochlor, Kaon, Kaon Cl, Kay Ciel, Kaylixir, K+Care, K+Care ET, K-Dur, K-G Elixir, K-Lease, K-Lor, Klor-con, Klorvess Effervescent, Klotrix, K-Lyte, K-Lyte Cl, K-Norm, Kolyum, K-Tab, K-vescent, Micro-K, Micro-K LS, SI*) IV infusion 10 mEq/h (diluted). 20 to 40 mEq PO one or two times per day. Use IV or immediate-release PO if rapid replacement needed. ▶K ♀C ▶? © $ Injectable, many different products in a variety of salt forms (ie, chloride, bicarbonate, citrate, acetate, gluconate), available in tabs, caps, liquids, effervescent tabs, packets. Potassium gluconate is available OTC. Intracellular cation that participates in numerous essential physiological processes. Serious: Hyperkalemia, gastrointestinal toxicity (obstruction, bleed, ulcer, perforation, esophagitis). Frequent: N/V, diarrhea, abdominal pain, infusion site irritation (IV).

> Nursing Implications   Serum potassium levels need to be monitored in patients on PO therapy. Elevated serum potassium levels or low serum potassium levels can cause cardiac dysrhythmias and death. Potassium administered intravenously can NEVER be administered by intravenous bolus or push method. Potassium IV must be administered via IV admixture in a 1 liter bag of IV fluid. Refer to manufacture guidelines for IV administration. Each hospital's pharmacy & therapeutics committee should have established guidelines for the administration of potassium intravenously.

Nutritionals

OMEGA-3-ACID ETHYL ESTERS   (*Lovaza*, fish oil, omega 3 fatty acids) Hypertriglyceridemia: 4 caps PO daily or divided two times per day. ▶L ♀C ▶? © $ Trade only: (Lovaza) 1 g cap (total 840 mg EPA plus DHA). Fish oil supplement that decreases serum triglycerides, mechanism not completely understood. Possible mechanisms include EPA and DHA inhibition of esterification of other fatty acids. Serious: Bleeding (rare), hypersensitivity, infection. Frequent: Nausea, belching, taste changes (fish), diarrhea, body odor, rash.

> Nursing Implications   May be taken as a single 4-g dose or as 2 g twice daily. May be administered with food.

Other

CINACALCET   (*Sensipar*) ▶LK ♀C ▶? © $$$$$ Trade only: Tabs 30, 60, 90 mg. Lowers parathyroid hormone levels and decreases serum calcium by increasing sensitivity of the calcium-sensing receptor to extracellular calcium. Serious: Seizures, adynamic bone disease, hypocalcemia, hypotension, worsening heart failure, arrhythmia, hypersensitivity. Frequent: N/V, diarrhea, myalgia, dizziness, rash.

> Nursing Implications Instruct patient to always swallow pills whole and to take medication shortly after eating. Monitor for signs and symptoms of hypocalcemia. Monitor serum calcium and phosphorous.

SODIUM POLYSTYRENE SULFONATE   (*Kayexalate*) Hyperkalemia: 15 g PO one to four times per day or 30 to 50 g retention enema (in sorbitol) q 6 h prn. Retain for 30 min to several hours. Irrigate with tap water after enema to prevent necrosis. ▶Fecal excretion ♀C ▶? © $$$$ Generic only: Susp 15 g/60 mL. Powdered resin. Cation exchange resin that reduces potassium in exchange for sodium. Serious: Hypokalemia, hypocalcemia, hypomagnesemia, intestinal obstruction, intestinal necrosis, serious GI events (bleeding, perforation). Frequent: Sodium and water retention, gastric irritation, anorexia, N/V, constipation.

> Nursing Implications Check labwork daily on potassium levels during treatment. Monitor minerals, electrolytes, and acid-based balances in patients who receive a repeated dose. ECGs are also recommended. Observe patients for early signs of hypokalemia. Potassium serum levels do not always reflect deficiency in potassium. This medication contains 100 mg of sodium per g. Consult with physician on restricting sodium content from dietary nutritional sources.

Phosphate Binders

SEVELAMER   (*Renagel, Renvela*) Hyperphosphatemia: 800 to 1600 mg PO three times per day with meals. ▶Not absorbed ♀C ▶? © $$$$$ Trade only (Renagel—sevelamer hydrochloride): Tabs 400, 800 mg. (Renvela—sevelamer carbonate): Tabs 800 mg; Powder: 800, 2400 mg packets. Binds intestinal phosphate preventing absorption. Serious: Hypophosphatemia, intestinal obstruction, dysphagia, bowel perforation. Frequent: N/V, dyspepsia, diarrhea, flatulence, constipation.

> Nursing Implications Administer by tab. Monitor for severe allergic reaction/anaphylaxis. Notify prescriber if symptoms worsen such as mood changes, panic, insomnia, impulsiveness, agitation, aggression, hyperactivity, restlessness, or suicidal thoughts. Adverse reactions may occur such as headache, dry mouth, GI symptoms, insomnia, wt gain. Assess pt for preexisting WBC and teach pt to comply with frequent blood monitoring in first months of therapy. In pts with preexisting hypertension, Seroquel may enhance effects of antihypertensive drugs. Death can occur if given to elderly pts with dementia-related psychosis. Teach pt.to report suicidal thoughts and increased depression. Consult prescriber before discontinuing drug—weaning is necessary.

Thyroid Agents

LEVOTHYROXINE   (*L-Thyroxine, Levolet, Levo-T, Levothroid, Levoxyl, Novothyrox, Synthroid, Thyro-Tabs, Tirosint, Unithroid, T4, ✦ Eltroxin, Euthyrox*) Start 100 to 200 mcg PO daily (healthy adults) or 12.5 to 50 mcg PO daily (elderly or CV disease), increase by 12.5 to 25 mcg/day at 3- to 8-week intervals. Usual maintenance dose 100 to 200 mcg/day, max 300 mcg/day. ▶L ♀A ▶+ © $ Generic/Trade: Tabs 25, 50, 75, 88, 100, 112, 125, 137, 150, 175, 200, 300 mcg. Trade only: Caps: 25, 50, 75, 100, 125, 150 mcg in 7-day blister packs, Tabs: 13 mcg (Tirosint). Synthetic thyroid derivative that increases metabolic rate of body tissues. Serious: Hyperthyroidism (arrhythmia, heart failure, angina, cardiac arrest), pseudotumor cerebri. Frequent: Palpitations, tachycardia, tremor, headache, nervousness, insomnia, diarrhea, vomiting, weight loss, menstrual irregularity, sweating, heat intolerance.

> Nursing Implications PO by tab. Before use assess pt for thyrotoxicosis, adrenal insufficiency, heart disease, high BP, and diabetes. Teach pt to notify prescriber if the following adverse reactions occur: insomnia, headache, agitated feeling, fever, flushing or sweating, changes in menstruation, appetite, or wt. Should be taken 30 min to 1 h before breakfast. Many drug and food interactions are associated with drug—check carefully and assess pts, drug and food intake patterns. Teach pt to comply with periodic lab tests to assess drug level. May affect bone density in postmenopausal women.

PEDIATRIC REHYDRATION SOLUTIONS									
Brand	**Glucose**	**Calories/ Liter**	**Na***	**K***	**Cl***	**Citrate***	**Phos***	**Ca***	**Mg***
CeraLyte 50†	0 g/L	160	50	20	40	30	0	0	0
CeraLyte 70†	0 g/L	160	70	20	60	30	0	0	0
CeraLyte 90†	0 g/L	160	90	20	80	30	0	0	0
Infalyte	30 g/L	140	50	25	45	34	0	0	0
Kao Lectrolyte†	20 g/L	90	50	20	40	30	0	0	0
Lytren (Canada)	20 g/L	80	50	25	45	30	0	0	0
Naturalyte	25 g/L	100	45	20	35	48	0	0	0
Pedialyte and Pedialyte Freezer Pops	25 g/L	100	45	20	35	30	0	0	0
Rehydralyte	25 g/L	100	75	20	65	30	0	0	0
Resol	20 g/L	80	50	20	50	34	5	4	4

* All given in mEq/L
† Premeasured powder packet

METHIMAZOLE (*Tapazole*) Start 5 to 20 mg PO three times per day or 10 to 30 mg PO daily, then adjust. ▶L ♀D ▶+ © $$$ Generic/Trade: Tabs 5, 10. Generic only: Tabs 15, 20 mg. Inhibits synthesis of thyroid hormones. Serious: Agranulocytosis, granulocytopenia, thrombocytopenia, aplastic anemia, leukopenia, interstitial pneumonitis, dermatitis, hepatotoxicity, periarteritis, nephritis, hypoprothrombinemia. Frequent: N/V, rash, pruritus, headache, dizziness, vertigo, drowsiness, alopecia, constipation, paresthesia, neuritis, hyperpigmentation.

Nursing Implications Administer at the same time each day with a meal. Food can effect absorption (either an increase or decrease is possible). Food may either increase or decrease absorption. Monitor for signs/symptoms of hypothyroidism: cold intolerances, fatigue, constipation, weakness.

PROPYLTHIOURACIL (*PTU*, ✦ *Propyl Thyracil*) Hyperthyroidism: Start 100 mg PO three times per day, then adjust. Thyroid storm: 200 to 300 mg PO four times per day, then adjust. ▶L ♀D (but preferred over methimazole in first trimester) ▶+ © $ Generic only: Tabs 50 mg. Inhibits synthesis of thyroid hormones. Serious: Agranulocytosis, granulocytopenia, thrombocytopenia, aplastic anemia, leukopenia, interstitial pneumonitis, exfoliative dermatitis, vasculitis, hepatotoxicity. Frequent: N/V, rash, pruritus, headache, dizziness, drowsiness, alopecia, constipation, paresthesia, neuritis, hyperpigmentation.

Nursing Implications Observe for severe allergic reactions such as hives, urticaria, shortness of breath, tightness in the chest, and swelling of the mouth, face, lips, or tongue. More common side effects of this medication are dizziness, drowsiness, headache, mild hair loss, mild muscle pain, and taste changes or loss. This medication can have a profound effect on the blood inclusive of blood clotting and liver function. This medication can lower the platelet count. Nursing needs to monitor lab values including thyroid values (TSH), CBC, and liver function studies. Patients should be advised not to drink alcohol or take other medications that can affect the central nervous system when on this medication. Patients should be advised to avoid activities that may cause injury, bruising, or bleeding. This medication is teratogenic.

Vitamins

FOLIC ACID (folate, *Folvite*) 0.4 to 1 mg IV/IM/PO/SC daily. ▶K ♀A ▶+ © $ OTC Generic only: Tabs 0.4, 0.8 mg. Rx Generic 1 mg. Water-soluble vitamin that stimulates red blood cell, white blood cell, and platelet production, and is a cofactor for transformylation reactions. Serious: Masking pernicious anemia. Frequent: None.

Nursing Implications Safe for adults with regular dosage, few side effects. High doses may cause gastric symptoms and high doses with prolonged use may increase risk of heart attack.

MULTIVITAMINS (*MVI*) Dose varies with product. Tabs come with and without iron. ▶LK ♀+ ▶+ © $ OTC and Rx: Many different brands and forms available with and without iron (tabs, caps, chewable tabs, gtts, liquid). Combination vitamin that usually contains vitamins A, D, E, B1, B2, B3, B5, B6, B12, and C; biotin; and folic acid. Usually no adverse effects in recommended doses (see individual vitamins).

> Nursing Implications Multivitamins should be discontinued if signs/symptoms of severe allergic reaction occur such as: urticaria, hives, shortness of breath, difficulty breathing, and swelling of the lips, face, mouth and tongue.

NIACIN (**vitamin B3, nicotinic acid, *Niacor, Nicolar, Slo-Niacin, Niaspan***) Niacin deficiency: 10 to 500 mg PO daily. Hyperlipidemia: Start 50 to 100 mg PO two to three times per day with meals, increase slowly, usual maintenance range 1.5 to 3 g/day, max 6 g/day. Extended-release (Niaspan): Start 500 mg at bedtime, increase monthly up to max 2000 mg. Extended-release formulations not listed here may have greater hepatotoxicity. Start with low doses and increase slowly to minimize flushing; 325 mg aspirin (non-EC) 30 to 60 min prior to niacin ingestion will minimize flush. ▶K ♀C ▶? © $ OTC Generic only: Tabs 50, 100, 250, 500 mg; Timed-release cap 125, 250, 400 mg; Timed-release tab 250, 500 mg; Liquid 50 mg/5 mL. Trade only: 250, 500, 750 mg (Slo-Niacin). Rx: Trade only: Tabs 500 mg (Niacor), Timed-release caps 500 mg, Timed-release tabs 500, 750, 1000 mg (Niaspan, $$$$). Water-soluble vitamin that serves as a coenzyme for oxidation-reduction reactions. Decreases lipoproteins associated with high LDL-cholesterol and triglycerides and increases lipoproteins associated with low HDL cholesterol. Serious: Hepatotoxicity, diabetes, peptic ulcer disease, gout, hypotension, myopathy, creatine kinase increase, hepatitis. Frequent: Flushing, dyspepsia, vomiting, abdominal pain, rash, burning paresthesias.

> Nursing Implications Patients should be advised to take this medication with food, a low-fat snack, and/or milk. Medications that are also utilized to lower blood cholesterol levels should not be taken at the same time of day as this medication (eg, colestipol or cholestyramine). Nursing needs to monitor laboratory values that assess cholesterol and triglyceride serum levels. Nursing needs to educate patients about the possible flushing that results from this medication. Patients should be advised to avoid hot beverages such as coffee, alcohol, and spicy foods around the time that this medication is taken. Patients should be advised to check with their healthcare provider to see if aspirin should be taken with this medication in order to lessen the side effects of flushing.

PHYTONADIONE (**vitamin K, *Mephyton, AquaMephyton***) Single dose of 0.5 to 1 mg IM within 1 h after birth. Excessive oral anticoagulation: Dose varies based on INR. INR 4.5 to 10: 2012 CHEST guidelines recommend AGAINST routine vitamin K administration; INR greater than 10 with no bleeding: 2012 CHEST guidelines recommend giving vitamin K, but do not specify a dose, 2008 guidelines previously recommended 5 to 10 mg PO; serious bleeding and elevated INR: 5 to 10 mg slow IV infusion. Adequate daily intake: 120 mcg (males) and 90 mcg (females). ▶L ♀C ▶+ © $ Trade only: Tabs 5 mg. Fat-soluble vitamin that promotes formation of clotting factors. Serious: Anaphylactic reaction. Frequent: Injection-site reaction, flushing sensation, "peculiar" taste sensation.

> Nursing Implications Patients need to be observed for severe allergic reactions (rash; hives; difficulty breathing; tightness in the chest; swelling of the mouth, face, lips, or tongue). A blue tinge to the skin, fingernails, or toenails may occur in some patients. Other adverse reactions include a fast or week pulse, dizziness, shortness of breath, and skin lesions. It has been noted to cause yellowing of the skin and/or eyes in newborns. This medication contains benzyl alcohol and toxic reactions can occur in newborn children. Laboratory values need to be monitored by nursing, in particular, INR and PT/PTT values.

THIAMINE (**vitamin B1**) 10 to 100 mg IV/IM/PO daily. ▶K ♀A ▶+ © $ OTC Generic only: Tabs 50, 100, 250, 500 mg; Enteric-coated tab 20 mg. Water-soluble vitamin needed for carbohydrate metabolism, normal growth maintenance, nerve impulse transmission, and acetylcholine synthesis. Serious: Hypersensitivity, anaphylaxis, cyanosis, pulmonary edema, GI hemorrhage, cardiovascular shock. Frequent: Injection site reaction, feeling of warmth, pruritus, sweating, N/V, restlessness, angioedema.

> Nursing Implications Thiamine should be discontinued if signs/symptoms of severe allergic reaction occur, such as urticaria, hives, shortness of breath, difficulty breathing, and swelling of the lips, face, mouth and tongue. Less serious side effects of Thiamine are the following: a feeling of warmth; flushing; hives; itching; nausea; restlessness; sweating; tingling; weakness, and retention of fluid.

Antihistamines—Non-Sedating

LORATADINE   (*Claritin, Claritin Hives Relief, Claritin RediTabs, Alavert, Tavist ND*)   10 mg PO daily for age older than 6 yo, 5 mg PO daily for age 2 to 5 yo.   ▶LK   ♀B   ▶+   © $ OTC Generic/Trade: Tabs 10 mg. Fast-dissolve tabs (Alavert, Claritin RediTabs) 5, 10 mg. Syrup 1 mg/mL. Rx Trade only (Claritin): Chewable tabs 5 mg, Liquigel caps 10 mg. Antihistamine. Serious: None. Frequent: None.

> Nursing Implications This medication is contraindicated in patients with an allergy to antihistamines, narrow-angle glaucoma, symptomatic BPH, bladder neck obstruction, stenosing peptic ulcer, and asthma. Patients need to be advised not to drink alcohol and not to drive or perform tasks that require alertness. Assess patient for thickening of bronchial secretions and dryness of nasal mucosa when on this medication.

Antihistamines—Other

CETIRIZINE   (*Zyrtec, ✦ Reactine, Aller-Relief*)   5 to 10 mg PO daily for age older than 6 yo. Peds: Give 2.5 mg PO daily for age 6 to 23 mo, give 2.5 mg PO daily to two times per day for age 2 to 5 yo.   ▶LK   ♀B   ▶– © $$$ OTC Generic/Trade: Tabs 5, 10 mg. Syrup 5 mg/5 mL. Chewable tabs, grape flavored 5, 10 mg. Antihistamine. Serious: None. Frequent: Sedation in 14%.

> Nursing Implications Can be taken with or without food. Do not use in patients allergic to this drug. Promote caution while driving or using heavy machinery. Promote avoidance of alcohol. Monitor for irregular heartbeat, weakness, tremors, sleep problems, confusion, vision problems, and problems with urination. Refer to manufacturer's list of drug and herbal supplement interactions.

HYDROXYZINE   (*Atarax, Vistaril*)   25 to 100 mg IM/PO one to four times per day or prn.   ▶L   ♀C   ▶– © $$ Generic only: Tabs 10, 25, 50, 100 mg; Caps 100 mg; Syrup 10 mg/5 mL. Generic/Trade: Caps 25, 50 mg, Susp 25 mg/5 mL (Vistaril). (Caps = Vistaril, Tabs = Atarax). Antihistamine. Serious: None. Frequent: Sedation.

> Nursing Implications Caution in liver disease and in elderly patients. Monitor for dizziness, drowsiness, headache, general gastric symptoms, urine retention, wheezing, oversedation. Teach patient to self-monitor and report these side effects to provider, to avoid driving until effect of drug is known, and to avoid alcohol.

Antitussives/Expectorants

BENZONATATE   (*Tessalon, Tessalon Perles*)   100 to 200 mg PO three times per day. Swallow whole. Do not chew. Numbs mouth; possible choking hazard.   ▶L   ♀C   ▶? © $$ Generic/Trade: Softgel caps: 100, 200 mg. Local anesthetic. Serious: None. Frequent: None.

> Nursing Implications Administer with 8 ounces of water. Do not crush, chew, or break pill. Dosage must be swallowed whole. Do not use in patients allergic to this drug or other numbing medications such as procaine or tetracaine. Do not use in patients under the age of 10 yo. Promote immediate reporting of side effects to provider, such as rash, dizziness, choking, chest pain, numbness, lightheadedness, confusion, or hallucinations.

Decongestants

NOTE: *See ENT—Nasal Preparations for nasal spray decongestants (oxymetazoline, phenylephrine). Deaths have occurred in children younger than 2 yo attributed to toxicity from cough and cold medications; the FDA does not recommend their use in this age group.*

PSEUDOEPHEDRINE   (*Sudafed, Sudafed 12 Hour, Efidac/24, Dimetapp Decongestant Infant Drops, PediaCare Infants' Decongestant Drops, Triaminic Oral Infant Drops, ✦ Pseudofrin*)   Adult: 60 mg PO q 4 to 6 h. Extended-release tabs: 120 mg PO two times per day or 240 mg PO daily. Peds: Give 15 mg PO q 4 to 6 h for age 2 to 5 yo, give 30 mg PO q 4 to 6 h for age 6 to 12 yo.   ▶L   ♀C   ▶+ © $ OTC Generic/Trade: Tabs 30, 60 mg, Tabs, extended-release 120 mg (12 h), Soln 15, 30 mg/5 mL. Trade only: Chewable tabs 15 mg, Tabs, extended-release 240 mg (24 h). Rx only in some states. Decongestant. Serious: None. Frequent: Insomnia, palpitations.

ENT COMBINATIONS (selected)	Decong estant	Antihist amine	Anti- tussive	Typical Adult Doses
OTC				
Actifed Cold & Allergy	PE	CH	–	1 tab q 4–6 h
Actifed Cold & Sinus‡	PS	CH	–	2 tabs q 6 h
Allerfrim, Aprodine	PS	TR	–	1 tab or 10 mL q 4–6 h
Benadryl Allergy/Cold‡	PE	DPH	–	2 tabs q 4 h
Benadryl-D Allergy/Sinus Tablets	PE	DPH		1 tab q 4 h
Claritin-D 12-h, Alavert D-12	PS	LO	–	1 tab q 12 h
Claritin-D 24-h	PS	LO	–	1 tab daily
Dimetapp Cold & Allergy Elixir	PE	BR	–	20 mL q 4 h
Dimetapp DM Cold & Cough	PE	BR	DM	20 mL q 4 h
Drixoral Cold & Allergy	PS	DBR	–	1 tab q 12 h
Mucinex-DM Extended-Release	–	–	GU, DM	1–2 tabs q 12 h
Robitussin CF	PE	–	GU, DM	10 mL q 4 h*
Robitussin DM, Mytussin DM	–	–	GU, DM	10 mL q 4 h*
Robitussin PE, Guiatuss PE	PE	–	GU	10 mL q 4 h*
Triaminic Cold & Allergy	PE	CH		10 mL q 4 h
Rx Only				
Allegra-D 12-h	PS	FE	–	1 tab q 12 h
Allegra-D 24-h	PS	FE	–	1 tab daily
Bromfenex	PS	BR	–	1 cap q 12 h
Clarinex-D 24-h	PS	DL	–	1 tab daily
Deconamine	PS	CH	–	1 tab or 10 mL tid-qid
Deconamine SR, Chlordrine SR	PS	CH	–	1 tab q 12 h
Deconsal I	PE	–	GU	1-2 tabs q 12 h
Dimetane-DX	PS	BR	DM	10 mL PO q 4 h
Duratuss	PE	–	GU	1 tab q 12 h
Duratuss HD©III	PE	–	GU, HY	5-10 mL q 4–6 h
Entex PSE, Guaifenex PSE 120	PS	–	GU	1 tab q 12 h
Histussin D ©III	PS	–	HY	5 mL qid
Histussin HC ©III	PE	CH	HY	10 mL q 4 h
Humibid DM	–	–	GU, DM	1 tab q 12 h
Hycotuss ©III	–	–	GU, HY	5 mL after meals & at bedtime
Phenergan/Dextromethorphan	–	PR	DM	5 mL q 4–6 h
Phenergan VC	PE	PR	–	5 mL q 4–6 h
Phenergan VC w/codeine ©V	PE	PR	CO	5 mL q 4–6 h
Robitussin AC ©V (generic only)	–	–	GU, CO	10 mL q 4 h*
Robitussin DAC ©V (generic only)	PS	–	GU, CO	10 mL q 4 h*
Rondec Syrup	PE	CH	–	5 mL qid†
Rondec DM Syrup	PE	CH	DM	5 mL qid†
Rondec Oral Drops	PE	CH	–	0.75 to 1 mL qid
Rondec DM Oral Drops	PE	CH	DM	0.75 to 1 mL qid
Rynatan	PE	CH	–	1–2 tabs q 12 h
Rynatan-P Pediatric	PE	CH	–	2.5–5 mL q 12 h*
Semprex-D	PS	AC	–	1 c ap q 4–6 h
Tanafed (generic only)	PS	CH	–	10–20 mL q 12 h*
Tussionex ©III	–	CH	HY	5 mL q 12 h

tid=three times per day; qid=four times per day

©=class	DL= desloratadine	FE=fexofenadine	PE=phenylephrine
AC=acrivastine	DM=dextromethorphan	GU=guaifenesin	PR=promethazine
BR=brompheniramine	DBR=dexbrompheniramine	HY=hydrocodone	PS=pseudoephedrine
CH=chlorpheniramine	DPH=diphenhydramine	LO=loratadine	TR=triprolidine
CO=codeine			

*5 mL/dose if 6–11 yo. 2.5 mL if 2–5 yo.
†2.5 mL/dose if 6–11 yo. 1.25 mL if 2–5 yo.
‡Also contains acetaminophen.

Nursing Implications Take 30 minutes prior to traveling. Do not drive or operate machinery. Frequent sips of water for dry/cotton mouth. Patients need to be advised not to take diet or appetite-control medications. Blood sugar levels need to be monitored in diabetic patients as this medication may cause elevation in blood sugar levels. The elderly are more sensitive to this medication.

GASTROENTEROLOGY

Antidiarrheals

LOPERAMIDE (*Imodium, Imodium AD*, ✢ *Loperacap, Diarr-eze*) 4 mg PO initially, then 2 mg PO after each unformed stool to a maximum of 16 mg per day. Peds: 1 mg PO three times per day for wt 13 to 20 kg, 2 mg PO two times per day for wt 21 to 30 kg, 2 mg PO three times per day for wt greater than 30 kg. ▶L ♀C ▶+ © $ OTC Generic/Trade: Tabs 2 mg. Oral soln 1 mg/5 mL. OTC Trade only: Oral soln 1 mg/7.5 mL. Antidiarrheal, inhibits peristalsis of intestinal muscles. Frequent: Sedation in children.

> Nursing Implications Loperamide is not recommended to be utilized in children up to the age of 6 years. The preferred treatment in this population is rehydration. Loperamide should not be utilized in patients with infectious diarrhea, if diarrhea is accompanied by fever or if there is blood and mucus in the stool. Concomitant use of opioid narcotics with loperamide my cause sever diarrhea.

Antiemetics—5-HT3 Receptor Antagonists

ONDANSETRON (*Zofran*) Nausea with chemo: IV: 32 mg IV over 15 min, or 0.15 mg/kg dose 30 min prior to chemo and repeated at 4 and 8 h after 1st dose for age 6 mo or older. PO: 4 mg PO 30 min prior to chemo and repeat at 4 and 8 h for age 4 to 11 yo, 8 mg PO and repeated 8 h later for age 12 yo or older. Prevention of postop nausea: 4 mg IV over 2 to 5 min or 4 mg IM or 16 mg PO 1 h before anesthesia. Give 0.1 mg/kg IV over 2 to 5 min as a single dose for age 1 mo to 12 yo if wt 40 kg or less; 4 mg IV over 2 to 5 min as a single dose if wt greater than 40 kg. Prevention of N/V associated with radiotherapy: 8 mg PO three times per day. ▶L ♀B ▶? © $$$$$ Generic/Trade: Tabs 4, 8, 24 mg. Orally disintegrating tabs 4, 8 mg. Oral soln 4 mg/5 mL. Generic only: Tabs 16 mg. Antiemetic, serotonin antagonist blocking chemoreceptor trigger zone. Frequent: Headache, fever, diarrhea, constipation, transient increases in LFTs. Severe: Transient blindness, especially with IV, arrhythmia, QT prolongation.

> Nursing Implications This medication is contraindicated in those patients allergic to Ondansetron. This medication must be utilized cautiously in pregnancy and lactation. Patients need to be advised to change position slowly as this medication can cause vertigo. Patients need to be advised to peel the foil back on the tablets rather than pushing the tablet through the foil. Patients need to be advised not to drink alcohol and not to drive or perform tasks that require alertness.

Antiemetics—Other

METOCLOPRAMIDE (*Reglan, Metozolv ODT*, ✢ *Maxeran*) 10 mg IV/IM q 2 to 3 h prn. 10 to 15 mg PO four times per day, 30 min before meals and at bedtime. Caution with long-term (more than 3 months) use. ▶K ♀B ▶? © $ Generic/Trade: Tabs 5, 10 mg. Trade: Orally disintegrating tabs 5, 10 mg (Metozolv). Generic only: Oral soln 5 mg/5 mL. Dopamine blockade; inhibits chemoreceptor trigger zone. Frequent: Restlessness, drowsiness, diarrhea, asthenia.

> Nursing Implications Patients need to be advised that this medication must be taken exactly as prescribed and MUST NOT be taken for longer than 12 weeks as a severe movement disorder can result with long term use. Symptoms of this disorder include uncontrollable muscle movements of the lips, tongue, eyes, face, arms, and legs. Symptoms are more likely to develop the longer that one is on this medication. The risk of this side effect is increased in women, diabetics, and the elderly.Patients allergic to metoclopramide should not take this medication. Patients with bleeding or a blockage in the stomach or intestines should not take this medication. This medication is also contraindicated in those patients with epilepsy or other seizure disorders, a perforation in the stomach or intestines, or a pheochromocytoma (adrenal gland tumor). Diabetic patients need to be advised that their insulin dose may need to be adjusted when taking this medication.

PROCHLORPERAZINE (*Compazine*, ✢ *Stemetil*) 5 to 10 mg IV over at least 2 min. 5 to 10 mg PO/ IM three to four times per day. 25 mg PR q 12 h. Sustained-release: 15 mg PO q am or 10 mg PO q 12 h. Peds: 0.1 mg/kg/dose PO/PR three to four times per day or 0.1 to 0.15 mg/kg/dose IM three to four times per day. ▶LK ♀C ▶? © $ Generic only: Tabs 5, 10, 25 mg. Supp 25 mg. Blocks post-synaptic dopaminergic receptors. Frequent: None. Severe: Cardiac arrest, hypotension, extrapyramidal signs.

> **Nursing Implications** Administered PO by tabs or capsules, by rectal suppository, or by IM or IV infusion. Should not be given subcutaneously because of irritation. Call prescriber if uncontrolled twitching occurs. Monitor pt for all side effects associated with the phenothiazines including the development of extrapyramidal symptoms and Tardive Dyskinesia with long-term use. Teach patient to report sore throat, other infections, or flu-like symptoms. Sleepiness, vision problems, low BP, and skin reactions can also occur.

PROMETHAZINE (*Phenergan*) Adults: 12.5 to 25 mg PO/IM/PR q 4 to 6 h. Peds: 0.25 to 1 mg/kg PO/IM/PR q 4 to 6 h. Contraindicated if age younger than 2 yo; caution in older children. IV use common but not approved. ▶LK ♀C ▶– © $ Generic only: Tabs/Supp 12.5, 25, 50 mg. Syrup 6.25 mg/5 mL. Antihistamine; blocks post-synaptic dopaminergic receptors. Frequent: Sedation, dry mouth. Severe: Cardiac arrest, hypotension, extrapyramidal signs, cholestatic jaundice.

> **Nursing Implications** Observe for severe allergic reactions such as hives, urticaria, shortness of breath, tightness in the chest, and swelling of the mouth, face, lips, or tongue. The more common side effects to this medication are dizziness, drowsiness, dry mouth, nausea, vomiting, and weakness. Patients need to be educated that if they are taking this medication for motion sickness, they should take a dose at least 30 to 60 minutes prior to traveling. Patients should avoid alcohol or other medications that affect the central nervous system when on this medication. The most serious side effect is neuroleptic malignant syndrome, which is manifested by fever, still muscle, mental confusion, abnormal thinking, a fast and/or irregular heart rate, and sweating. There are serious side effects in children under the age of 2 inclusive of drowsiness and coma. The elderly are more sensitive to this medication (ie, more drowsiness). The medication may affect the blood sugar, so diabetic patients should have their blood sugar monitored closely.

Antiulcer—H2 Antagonists

FAMOTIDINE (*Pepcid, Pepcid AC, Maximum Strength Pepcid AC*) 20 mg IV q 12 h, 20 to 40 mg PO at bedtime, or 20 mg PO two times per day. ▶LK ♀B ▶? © $ Generic/Trade: Tabs 10 mg (OTC, Pepcid AC Acid Controller), 20 mg (Rx and OTC, Maximum Strength Pepcid AC), 40 mg. Rx Generic/Trade: Susp 40 mg/5 mL. Histamine-2 receptor blocker. Frequent: Dizziness, headache, nausea. Severe: Convulsion in renal impairment, interstitial pneumonia, Stevens-Johnson syndrome.

> **Nursing Implications** Caution in elderly pts, in pts with renal disease, and in pregnant or breastfeeding mothers. Avoid alcohol, smoking, caffeine-containing foods. Give with food or liquids; if given IV may cause temporary irritation at IV site. Monitor for dizziness, headache, rapid pulse, general GI symptoms, eye edema red conjunctiva, tinnitus. Instruct pt to take at bedtime; drug effect may take several days. May be used in anaphylaxis.

RANITIDINE (*Zantac, Zantac Efferdose, Zantac 75, Zantac 150, Peptic Relief*) 150 mg PO two times per day or 300 mg PO at bedtime. 50 mg IV/IM q 8 h, or continuous infusion 6.25 mg/h (150 mg/day). ▶K ♀B ▶? © $$$ Generic/Trade: Tabs 75 mg (OTC: Zantac 75), 150 mg (OTC and Rx: Zantac 150), 300 mg. Syrup 75 mg/5 mL. Rx Trade only: Effervescent tabs 25 mg. Rx Generic only: Caps 150, 300 mg. Histamine-2 receptor blocker. Frequent: Dizziness, headache, nausea, constipation, taste changes, stool or tongue darkening.

> **Nursing Implications** Observe patients for severe allergic reactions such as hives, urticaria, shortness of breath, tightness in the chest, unusual hoarseness, and swelling of the mouth, face, lips, or tongue. Assess patients for abdominal pain and/or blood in stools, emesis, or gastric aspiration. Can cause false-positive results for urine protein. May cause dizziness and drowsiness. Inform pts that increased fiber and fluid intake may minimize constipation. Report onset of tarry/black stools, sore throat, fever, rash, diarrhea, confusion, hallucinations, and dizziness. Medication can temporarily cause tongue and stools to appear greyish black. Common side effects are nausea, diarrhea, stomach upset, and headache. This medication may cause drug-induced hepatitis and may interfere with certain laboratory tests inclusive of urine protein testing. Cases of chemically induced hepatitis have been reported. Advise pt not to drink alcohol while taking this medication.

Antiulcer—Proton Pump Inhibitors

ESOMEPRAZOLE (*Nexium*) Erosive esophagitis: 20 to 40 mg PO daily for 4 to 8 weeks. Maintenance of erosive esophagitis: 20 mg PO daily. Zollinger-Ellison: 40 mg PO two times per day for 4 to 8 weeks. GERD: 20 mg PO daily for 4 weeks. GERD with esophagitis: 20 to 40 mg IV daily for 10 days until taking PO. Prevention of NSAID-associated gastric ulcer: 20 to 40 mg PO daily for up to 6 months. *H. pylori* eradication: 40 mg PO daily with amoxicillin 1000 mg PO two times per day and clarithromycin 500 mg PO two times per day for 10 days. ▶L ♀B ▶? © $$$$ Trade only: Caps delayed-release 20, 40 mg. Delayed-release granules for oral susp 10, 20, 40 mg per packet. H-K ATPase proton pump inhibitor. Frequent: Headache, dizziness, rash, diarrhea, N/V, taste perversion. Severe: Anaphylaxis, toxic epidermal necrolysis, Stevens-Johnson syndrome, erythema multiforme, pancreatitis, hepatitis.

> Nursing Implications Instruct patient to always swallow capsules whole. Administer 1 h before meals. Can mix granules inside 1 tablespoon of apple sauce for patients with difficulty swallowing. Nasogastric tube: Mix intact granules with 50 mL of water in 60 mL syringe, mix, and administer; flush tube with additional water.

LANSOPRAZOLE (*Prevacid*) Heartburn: 15 mg PO daily. Duodenal ulcer or maintenance therapy after healing of duodenal ulcer: 15 mg PO daily for up to 12 months. NSAID–induced gastric ulcer: 30 mg PO daily for 8 weeks (treatment), 15 mg PO daily for up to 12 weeks (prevention). GERD: 15 mg PO daily. Gastric ulcer: 30 mg PO daily. Erosive esophagitis: 30 mg PO daily for up to 8 weeks or 30 mg IV daily for 7 days or until taking PO. ▶L ♀B ▶? © $$$ OTC Trade only: Caps 15 mg. Rx Generic/Trade: 15, 30 mg. Rx Trade only: Orally disintegrating tabs 15, 30 mg. Prevacid NapraPac: 7 lansoprazole 15 mg caps packaged with 14 naproxen tabs 375 mg or 500 mg. H-K ATPase proton pump inhibitor. Frequent: Fatigue, dizziness, headache, abdominal pain, diarrhea, nausea, increased appetite. Severe: Pancreatitis, severe skin reactions, myositis, interstitial nephritis.

> Nursing Implications The most common side effects of this medication are abdominal pain and cramping and other gastrointestinal side effects such as nausea and diarrhea. Patients need to be advised to take this medication 30 min prior to their first meal of the day. They need to swallow the capsule whole. Capsules should not be cut or broken. This medication may cause hypomagnesemia and affect calcium levels. Patients may have an increased risk of fractures of the hip, wrist, and spine. Benign gastric polyps have been reported.

OMEPRAZOLE (*Prilosec*, ✦*Losec*) GERD, duodenal ulcer, erosive esophagitis: 20 mg PO daily. Heartburn (OTC): 20 mg PO daily for 14 days. Gastric ulcer: 40 mg PO daily. Hypersecretory conditions: 60 mg PO daily. ▶L ♀C ▶? © OTC $, Rx $$$$ Rx Generic/Trade: Caps 10, 20, 40 mg. Trade only: Granules for oral susp 2.5 mg, 10 mg. OTC Trade only: Cap 20 mg. H-K ATPase proton pump inhibitor. Frequent: Headache, dizziness, rash, diarrhea, N/V, taste perversion. Severe: Stevens-Johnson syndrome, erythema multiforme, stomatitis, agitation, pancytopenia, agranulocytosis, other blood dyscrasias, pancreatitis, psychiatric disturbances.

> Nursing Implications The most common side effects are headache, diarrhea, nausea, flatulence, abdominal pain, constipation, dry mouth. Serious side effects include: bradycardia, peripheral edema, severe skin reactions, pancreatitis, and interstitial nephritis. This medication should not be utilized with clopidogrel (Plavix) as it may decrease its effectiveness.

PANTOPRAZOLE (*Protonix*, ✦*Pantoloc*) GERD: 40 mg PO daily. Zollinger-Ellison syndrome: 80 mg IV q 8 to 12 h for 7 days until taking PO. GERD associated with a history of erosive esophagitis: 40 mg IV daily for 7 to 10 days until taking PO. ▶L ♀B ▶? © $$$$ Generic/Trade: Tabs 20, 40 mg. Trade only: Granules for susp 40 mg/packet. H-K ATPase proton pump inhibitor. Frequent: Headache. Serious: Rhabdomyolysis, anaphylaxis, angioedema, severe dermatologic reactions, hepatocellular damage, interstitial nephritis, pancreatitis, pancytopenia.

> Nursing Implications This medication may cause abdominal bloating, increased flatulence, and abdominal pain and cramping. Taking this medication for a prolonged period of time may decrease vitamin B12 absorption. There may be an increased risk of fractures. Hypomagnesemia may result from taking this medication. Patients need to be advised to take this medication 30 min prior to eating breakfast.

RABEPRAZOLE (*AcipHex*, ✦*Pariet*) 20 mg PO daily. ▶L ♀B ▶? © $$$$ Trade: Tabs 20 mg. H-K ATPase proton pump inhibitor. Frequent: Headache. Serious: rhabdomyolysis, anaphylaxis, angioedema, severe dermatologic reactions, hepatocellular damage, interstitial nephritis, pancreatitis, pancytopenia.

Nursing Implications Use cautiously in patients who have experienced adverse reactions to other —azole drugs. Monitor for increases in INR and prothrombin time in patients also being treated with warfarin. Report occurrence of headache, diarrhea, nausea, vomiting, and abdominal pain to provider.

Antiulcer—Other

SIMETHICONE (***Mylicon, Gas-X, Phazyme, ✦ Ovol***) 40 to 360 mg PO four times per day prn, max 500 mg/day. Infants: 20 mg PO four times per day prn. ▶Not absorbed ♀C but + ▶? © $ OTC Generic/Trade: Chewable tabs 80, 125 mg. Gtts 40 mg/0.6 mL. Trade only: Softgels 166 mg (Gas-X) 180 mg (Phazyme). Strips, oral (Gas-X) 62.5 mg (adults), 40 mg (children). Theoretically, relieves gas pressure and bloating. Frequent: None.

Nursing Implications Advise patient to take this medication after each meal and at bedtime. Patients need to be observed for extreme abdominal pain and an increase in symptoms.

SUCRALFATE (***Carafate, ✦ Sulcrate***) 1 g PO 1 h before meals (2 h before other medications) and at bedtime. ▶Not absorbed ♀B ▶? © $$ Generic/Trade: Tabs 1 g. Susp 1 g/10 mL. Forms synthetic barrier against peptic acid. Frequent: Constipation.

Nursing Implications This medication is contraindicated in patients with renal failure and those undergoing dialysis treatments. This medication decreases the efficacy of several medications (refer to product literature). Advise patients not to use aluminum containing antacids while on this medication as aluminum toxicity could result. Advise patients to take this medication on an empty stomach, 1 hour prior to a meal; 2 hours after a meal. Antacids, if utilized, should be taken 30 minutes before or after taking this medication. Severe epigastric pain needs to be reported to the health provider.

Laxatives—Osmotic

LACTULOSE (***Enulose, Kristalose***) Constipation: 15 to 30 mL (syrup) or 10 to 20 g (powder for oral soln) PO daily. Hepatic encephalopathy: 30 to 45 mL (syrup) PO three to four times per day, or 300 mL retention enema. ▶Not absorbed ♀B ▶? © $$ Generic/Trade: Syrup 10 g/15 mL. Trade only (Kristalose): 10, 20 g packets for oral soln. Converts NH3 to NH4+ to prevent rediffusion into plasma. Frequent: Flatulence, diarrhea.

Nursing Implications Patients need to be educated that this medication usually causes diarrhea. This medication will lower serum ammonia levels in patients with impaired liver function. Serum ammonia levels should be monitored periodically in these patients.

POLYETHYLENE GLYCOL (***MiraLax, GlycoLax***) 17 g (1 heaping tablespoon) in 4 to 8 oz water, juice, soda, coffee, or tea PO daily. ▶Not absorbed ♀C ▶? © $ OTC Trade only: Powder for oral soln 17 g/scoop. Rx Generic/Trade: Powder for oral soln 17 g/scoop. Osmotic and cathartic effect in intestinal lumen. Frequent: Nausea, fullness, bloating. Serious: Risk of aspiration in children.

Nursing Implications Dissolve in 8 oz. water before administering to patient. May need to remain near bathroom; evacuation urge may be sudden.

Laxatives—Stimulant

BISACODYL (***Correctol, Dulcolax, Feen-a-Mint, Fleet***) 5 to 15 mg PO prn, 10 mg PR prn, 5 to 10 mg PR prn if 2 to 11 yo. ▶L ♀C ▶? © $ OTC Generic/Trade: Tabs 5 mg, suppository 10 mg. OTC Trade only (Fleet): Enema, 10 mg/30 mL. Direct colonic stimulant. Frequent: None.

Nursing Implications Teach pt to avoid if nausea, vomiting, or abdominal pain occurs. Discontinue if no bowel movement after 1 week or if rectal bleeding occurs. Assess pt for history of kidney disease, intestinal disorders, swallowing problems. Dulcolax combined with a diuretic may cause electrolyte depletion. Teach pt not to take biscodyl until 2 h before bedtime after taking other medication and to immediately report decreased urination, confusion or mood changes, rectal bleeding, breathing problems, severe cramps, ongoing diarrhea or vomiting, and symptoms of low potassium.

SENNA (*Senokot, SenokotXTRA, Ex-Lax, Fletcher's Castoria, ♣Glysennid*) 2 tabs or 1 teaspoon granules or 10 to 15 mL syrup PO. Max 8 tabs, 4 teaspoon granules, 30 mL syrup/day. Take granules with full glass of water. ▶L ♀C ▶+ © $ OTC Generic/Trade (All dosing is based on sennosides content; 1 mg sennosides is equivalent to 21.7 mg standardized senna concentrate): Syrup 8.8 mg/5 mL, Liquid 33.3 mg senna concentrate/mL (Fletcher's Castoria), Tabs 8.6, 15, 17, 25 mg, Chewable tabs 10, 15 mg. Enhances GI motility. Frequent: Potential for severe diaper rash in children wearing diapers.

> Nursing Implications Instruct patient to take with a full glass of water. Administer at bedtime for evacuation 6 to 12 h later. Administer on an empty stomach for more rapid results. Shake oral solution well before administering.

Laxatives—Stool Softener

DOCUSATE (*Colace, Surfak, Kaopectate Stool Softener, Enemeez*) Docusate calcium: 240 mg PO daily. Docusate sodium: 50 to 500 mg/day PO divided in 1 to 4 doses. Peds: 10 to 40 mg/day for age younger than 3 yo, give 20 to 60 mg/day for age 3 to 6 yo, give 40 to 150 mg/day for age 6 to 12 yo. In all cases doses are divided up to four times per day. Cerumen impaction: 1 mL in affected ear. ▶L ♀C ▶? © $ Docusate calcium OTC Generic/Trade: Caps 240 mg. Docusate sodium OTC Generic/Trade: Caps 50, 100, 250 mg. Liquid 50 mg/5 mL. Syrup 20 mg/5 mL. Docusate sodium OTC Trade only (Enemeez): Enema, rectal 283 mg/5 mL. Softens stool, cerumen. Frequent: Abdominal cramping.

> Nursing Implications Monitor for abdominal pain, diarrhea, rectal bleeding, rash, dizziness, unusual swelling, or breathing problems. Caution with use in pregnancy.

Other GI Agents

ALVIMOPAN (*Entereg*) Short-term (up to 15 doses) in hospitalized patients undergoing partial large or small bowel resection surgery with primary anastomosis: 12 mg PO 30 min to 5 h prior to surgery, then 12 mg PO two times per day starting the day after surgery for up to 7 days. ▶Intestinal flora ♀B ▶? © ? Trade only: Caps 12 mg. Peripherally acting mu-opioid receptor antagonist used for postoperative ileus. Frequent: Anemia, dyspepsia, hypokalemia, back pain, urinary retention. Severe: Myocardial infarction.

> Nursing Implications Drug can be used only in hospitals registered for use and meeting registration requirements. Monitor pt for allergic reactions: hives, breathing difficulties, and anaphylaxis, and for serious side effects such as pallor, bleeding/bruising, urination problems, confusion, general and muscle weakness, abnormal HR, thirst, and leg discomfort. Do not give to pts who have had narcotics/opioids in last 7 days. Pts should not receive more than 15 doses.

BUDESONIDE (*Entocort EC*) 9 mg PO daily for up to 8 weeks (remission induction) or 6 mg PO daily for 3 months (maintenance). ▶L ♀C ▶? © $$$$$ Trade only: Caps 3 mg. Affects cell motility and protein synthesis; anti-inflammatory. Frequent: Palpitations, nervousness, dizziness, headache, pruritus, rash, GI irritation, nausea, bitter taste, hyperglycemia, increased infection rate. Severe: Anaphylaxis.

> Nursing Implications Use cautiously in patients with liver and heart disease, diabetes, glaucoma, depressed immune system, pts receiving steroids, pregnant and breastfeeding women, and children. Monitor for increased intracranial pressure, high BP, thrombophlebitis and embolism, high blood sugar, general GI symptoms, bronchospasm, adrenal insufficiency. Teach patient to immediately report rash, fever, swelling of face or neck, labored breathing, fungal infections of mouth. Patients should avoid high fat-meals and grapefruit in any form.

GLYCOPYRROLATE (*Robinul, Robinul Forte, Cuvposa*) Peptic ulcer disease: 1 to 2 mg PO two to three times per day. Chronic drooling in children (Cuvposa): 0.02 mg/kg PO three times per day. ▶K ♀B ▶? © $$$$ Trade: Solution 1 mg/5 mL (480 mL, Cuvposa). Generic/Trade: Tabs 1, 2 mg. Inhibits effects of acetylcholine. Frequent: Dry skin, dry mouth/throat, constipation, vomiting, flushing, nasal congestion, urinary retention, dry nose, local irritation.

> Nursing Implications IM or IV administration. Assess pt for allergies, glaucoma, urinary/prostate problems, GI problems, heart problems, and high BP. Stability of the drug may be compromised if put in same syringe with other drugs. Use clean syringe. Monitor pt for dry mouth, urinary problems, eye problems, heart palpitations, headache, dizziness, nausea and vomiting, sleep problems, constipation, skin rash, and any signs of hypersensitivity. Use in elderly may cause confusion. Extreme caution or best not to use in pts with glaucoma. Teach pt not to engage in activities requiring high mental alertness (ie, driving, operating machinery).

NEOMYCIN—ORAL (**Neo-Fradin**) Hepatic encephalopathy: 4 to 12 g/day PO divided q 4 to 6 h. Peds: 50 to 100 mg/kg/day PO divided q 6 to 8 h. ▶Minimally absorbed ♀D ▶? © $$$ Generic only: Tabs 500 mg. Trade only: Soln 125 mg/5 mL. Inhibits bacterial protein synthesis. Frequent: None.

> Nursing Implications Observe patients for severe allergic reactions such as: rash, hives, itching, trouble breathing, tightness in the chest, and swelling of the mouth, face, lips, or tongue. A hearing evaluation should be conducted prior to taking this medication. The most significant side effects to observe for ototoxicity and nephrotoxicity. Serum creatinine and BUN levels should be monitored periodically. This medication can cause a neuromuscular blockade with resultant involuntary muscle movements or muscle tremor.

OCTREOTIDE (**Sandostatin, Sandostatin LAR**) Variceal bleeding: Bolus 25 to 50 mcg IV followed by infusion 25 to 50 mcg/h. AIDS diarrhea: 25 to 250 mcg SC three times per day. ▶LK ♀B ▶? © $$$$$ Generic/Trade: Injection vials 0.05, 0.1, 0.2, 0.5, 1 mg. Trade only: Long-acting injectable susp (Sandostatin LAR) 10, 20, 30 mg. Mimics natural somatostatin. Frequent: Sinus bradycardia, chest pain, fatigue, headache, malaise, fever, dizziness, pruritus, hyperglycemia, abdominal pain, nausea, diarrhea. Severe: Hepatitis, progressive abdominal distension, severe epigastric pain.

> Nursing Implications Administer by subcutaneous injection at rotated sites or by IV infusion. Do NOT administer concurrent with TPN (total parenteral nutrition). Inspect soln for particulate matter and discoloration and do not use if either present. Refrigerate and protect from light. Monitor for severe allergic reaction/anaphylaxis. Call prescriber if pt experiences gall bladder pain/problems; GI disturbances, especially symptoms of pancreatitis; high or low blood sugar symptoms; and thyroid problems. Milder GI side effects and irritation at injection site are common. Assess pt for prior history of heart, kidney, liver; or gallbladder disease; diabetes; or thyroid disorder. Teach pt to recognize jaundice and report immediately.

ORLISTAT (**Alli, Xenical**) Weight loss: 60 to 120 mg PO three times per day with meals. ▶Gut ♀X ▶? © $$$ OTC Trade only (Alli): Caps 60 mg. Rx Trade only (Xenical): Caps 120 mg. Inhibits gastric and pancreatic lipases. Frequent: CNS effects, oily stool, fecal incontinence, flatus with discharge. Severe: Cholelithiasis, nephrolithiasis, nephropathy, pancreatitis, severe liver injury with hepatocellular necrosis, or acute hepatic failure.

> Nursing Implications The most common side effect to this medication is flatulence and diarrhea. Some patients state that they cannot control bowel function while on this medication.

PANCRELIPASE (**Creon, Pancrease, Viokase, Pancrease, Pancrease, Pancrecarb, Cotazym, Ku-Zyme HP, Ultressa, Viokace, Zenpep**) Varies by wt. Initial infant dose 2000 to 4000 lipase units PO per 120 mL formula or breastmilk. 12 mo or older to younger than 4 yo: 1000 lipase units/kg PO. 4 yo or older: 500 lipase units/kg per meal PO, max 2500 lipase units/kg per meal. ▶Gut ♀C ▶? © $$$ Tabs, Caps, Powder with varying amounts of lipase, amylase, and protease. Replaces endogenous enzymes. Frequent: None.

> Nursing Implications Patients need to be advised not to take this medication if they are allergic to pork proteins. This medication needs to be swallowed immediately. The capsule should not be held in the mouth. This medication should be taken with a snack and a full glass of water or juice. Common sides effects manifest in the gastrointestinal system such as nausea, vomiting, diarrhea, greasy stools, and bloating.

URSODIOL (**Actigall, URSO, URSO Forte**) Gallstone solution (Actigall): 8 to 10 mg/kg/day PO divided two to three times per day. Prevention of gallstones associated with rapid wt loss (Actigall): 300 mg PO two times per day. Primary biliary cirrhosis (URSO): 13 to 15 mg/kg/day PO divided in 2 to 4 doses. ▶Bile ♀B ▶? © $$$$ Generic/Trade: Caps 300 mg, Tabs 250, 500 mg. Decreases cholesterol content of bile and bile stones. Frequent: Diarrhea, constipation, nausea, vomiting, dizziness. Serious: Thrombocytopenia, hypersensitivity reactions.

> Nursing Implications Observe for signs and symptoms of severe allergic reactions such as hives, urticaria, shortness of breath, tightness in the chest, and swelling of the mouth, face, lips, or tongue. This medication is indicated for patients when surgery is contraindicated. An obstruction or inflammation of the bile duct, inflammation of the gallbladder, inflammation of the pancreas, calcified gall stones, or bleeding from the veins in the esophagus are problems in which ursodiol is contraindicated. Do not use estrogens when taking this medication. Patients should be educated that it may take several months for this medication to work. Liver function should be monitored. Common side effects are gastrointestinal in nature, such as consitpation or diarrhea. Patients need to be advised that they may experience a metallic taste when on this medication.

Ulcerative Colitis

MESALAMINE   (*5-aminosalicylic acid, Apriso, 5-Aspirin, Asacol, Lialda, Pentasa, Canasa, Rowasa, ✦ Mesasal, Salofalk*) Apriso: 1.5 g (4 caps) PO q am. Asacol: 800 to 1600 mg PO three times per day. Pentasa: 1000 mg PO four times per day. Lialda: 2.4 to 4.8 g PO daily with a meal. Canasa: 500 mg PR two to three times per day or 1000 mg PR at bedtime Susp: 4-g enema PR at bedtime (retain 8 h) for 3 to 6 weeks. ▶Gut ♀C ▶? © $$$$$ Trade only: Delayed-release tab 400 mg (Asacol), 800 mg (Asacol HD). Controlled-release cap 250, 500 mg (Pentasa). Delayed-release tabs 1200 mg (Lialda). Rectal suppository 1000 mg (Canasa). Controlled-release caps 0.375 g (Apriso). Generic/Trade: Rectal susp 4 g/60 mL (Rowasa). Unknown. Frequent: Headache, malaise, abdominal pain, cramps, flatulence, gas, hair loss. Severe: Cytopenias, myo- and pericarditis, hepatitis, pneumonitis, nephritis.

> **Nursing Implications** Do not use in patients allergic to mesalamine or other aspirin drugs. Use cautiously in patients with history of renal or liver dysfunction, stomach conditions, congestive heart failure, or history of sulfa-drug allergies. Do not crush, break, or chew tab. Discontinue medication and notifiy provider immediately if patient experiences severe stomach pain, cramping, fever, headache, or bloody diarrhea. The patient may also experience increased flatulence while taking this medication.

SULFASALAZINE   (*Azulfidine, Azulfidine EN-tabs, ✦ Salazopyrin En-tabs, S.A.S.*) Colitis: 500 to 1000 mg PO four times per day. Peds: 30 to 60 mg/kg/day PO divided q 4 to 6 h. RA: 500 mg PO two times per day after meals up to 1 g PO two times per day. May turn body fluids, contact lenses, or skin orange-yellow. ▶L ♀D ▶– © $$ Generic/Trade: Tabs 500 mg, scored. Enteric-coated, delayed-release (EN-tabs) 500 mg. Immunosuppressant, decreases colonic inflammation. Serious: Agranulocytosis, hemolytic anemia, nephro/hepatotoxicity, hepatic failure, drug rash. Frequent: Nausea, dyspepsia, rash.

> **Nursing Implications** To minimize side effects, instruct patient to take with food. Capsules should always be swallowed whole with a full glass of water. Shake oral suspension well before administration. Use a calibrated measuring device to measure liquid preparations.

HEMATOLOGY

Anticoagulants—Direct Thrombin Inhibitors

ARGATROBAN   HIT: Start 2 mcg/kg/min IV infusion. Get PTT at baseline and 2 h after starting infusion. Adjust dose (max dose: 10 mcg/kg/min) until PTT is 1.5 to 3 times baseline (not more than 100 sec). ACCP recommends starting at max of 2 mcg/kg/min with lower doses of 0.5 to 1.2 mcg/kg/min in patients with heart failure, multi-organ failure, anasarca, or post-cardiac surgery. ▶L ♀B ▶– © $$$$$ Direct thrombin inhibitor, synthetic derivative of L-arginine. Serious: Major bleeding, hypotension. Frequent: Fever, diarrhea.

> **Nursing Implications** Administered IV; aPTT must be done before administering; pt must not be on heparin therapy; check aPPT 2 h before bedtime after initial therapy. Monitor for signs of hemorrhage including general bleeding, GI or GU bleeding, decreased hemoglobin and hematocrit, intracranial bleeding. Monitor for breathing difficulties, GI or GU symptoms, fever, rapid heart rate, pain, or cerebrovascular symptoms. Check groin for bleeding or hematoma. Breathing problems, rash, or vasodilation may indicate allergic reaction.

BIVALIRUDIN   (*Angiomax*) Anticoagulation during PCI (patients with or at risk of HIT): 0.75 mg/kg IV bolus prior to intervention, then 1.75 mg/kg/h for duration of procedure (with provisional Gp IIb/IIIa inhibition). For CrCl less than 30 mL/min, reduce infusion dose to 1 mg/kg/h after bolus. For patients on dialysis, reduce infusion to 0.25 mg/kg/h after bolus. Use with aspirin 300 to 325 mg PO daily. Additional bolus of 0.3 mg/kg if activated clotting time is less than 225 sec. ▶proteolysis/K ♀B ▶? © $$$$$ Direct thrombin inhibitor (reversible). Serious: Major bleeding. Frequent: Back pain, nausea.

> **Nursing Implications** Administer by IV infusion ONLY. Intended for use with aspirin. Swirl until fully dissolved; do not mix with the following drugs: altepase, amiodarone HCL, amphotericin B, chlorpromazine, diazepam, prochlorpromazine, edisylate, reteplase, streptokinase, and vancomycin. Call prescriber if pt experiences numbness or one-sided body weakness; confusion, vision, balance, or speech problems; leg pain/swelling; uncontrolled bleeding including bloody stools. Bleeding is the most common adverse reaction and needs to be closely monitored. GI disturbances may also occur. Concomitant use of angiomax with other blood thinners increases risk of major bleeding events.

WEIGHT-BASED HEPARIN DOSING FOR DVT/PE*

Initial dose	80 units/kg IV bolus, then 18 units/kg/h. Check PTT in 6 h
PTT less than 35 sec (less than 1.2 × control)	80 units/kg IV bolus, then increase infusion rate by 4 units/kg/h
PTT 35–45 sec (1.2–1.5 × control)	40 units/kg IV bolus, then increase infusion by 2 units/kg/h
PTT 46–70 sec (1.5–2.3 × control)	No change
PTT 71–90 sec (2.3–3 × control)	Decrease infusion rate by 2 units/kg/h
PTT greater than 90 sec (greater than 3 × control)	Hold infusion for 1 h, then decrease infusion rate by 3 units/kg/h

*PTT = Activated partial thromboplastin time. Reagent-specific target PTT may differ; use institutional nomogram when available. Consider establishing a max bolus dose/max initial infusion rate or use an adjusted body wt in obesity. Monitor PTT 6 h after heparin initiation and 6 h after each dosage adjustment. When PTT is stable within therapeutic range, monitor every morning. Therapeutic PTT range corresponds to anti-factor Xa activity of 0.3–0.7 units/mL. Check platelets between days 3 and 5. Can begin warfarin on first day of heparin; continue heparin for at least 4 to 5 days of combined therapy. Adapted from *Ann Intern Med* 1993;119:874. *Chest* 2012;141:e28S, e154S. *Circulation* 2001;103:2994.

DABIGATRAN (*Pradaxa*, ✚ *Pradax*) Stroke prevention in atrial fibrillation: CrCl greater than 30 mL/min: 150 mg PO two times per day; CrCL between 15 to 30 mL/min: 75 mg PO two times per day; CrCl less than 15 mL/min: contraindicated. Per ACCP CHEST guidelines, not recommended if CrCl is less than 30 mL/min. ▶K ♀C ▶? © $$$$$ Trade only: caps 75, 150 mg. Direct thrombin inhibitor. Serious: Bleeding, hypersensitivity (anaphylaxis). Frequent: Dyspepsia, gastritis, hypersensitivity (urticaria, rash, and pruritus).

Nursing Implications Need to monitor patient for signs of bleeding, upper abdominal pain, dyspepsia, and diarrhea. Potential overdose is a concern because there is no antidote available. Sources of bleeding need investigation, discontinuation of the medication through ordering practitioner. Consider drug–drug interactions of amiodarone, NSAID use; therefore, increasing patient education of signs/symptoms of bleeding (gums, occult blood, urine) is indicated. For capsules, usual dose 150 mg two times per day. A missed dose should be taken as close to possible scheduled dose the next day. If, for example, the missed morning dose is not taken 6 h before the second dose of the day, then skip the missed morning dose. Do not attempt to "make up" the missed dose by doubling the dose the following day.

LEPIRUDIN (*Refludan*) Anticoagulation in HIT and associated thromboembolic disease: Bolus 0.4 mg/kg up to 44 mg IV over 15 to 20 seconds, then infuse 0.15 mg/kg/h up to 16.5 mg/h. Alternate initial dosing recommended by ACCP: Bolus 0.2 mg/kg IV (bolus only if life- or limb-threatening thrombosis) then infuse 0.1 mg/kg/h or less. Adjust dose to maintain PTT ratio of 1.5 to 2 times baseline. Dose reduction for renal insufficiency. ▶K ♀B ▶? © $$$$$ Direct thrombin inhibitor (irreversible). Serious: Severe anaphylactic reactions resulting in death have been reported upon initial or re-exposure. May have higher risk of bleeding than reversible thrombin inhibitors. Post-marketing reports of intracranial bleeding in absence of thrombolytics. Frequent: Abnormal LFTs.

Nursing Implications Administer by injection or IV infusion. Call for emergency help for allergic reaction. Call prescriber if pt experiences one-sided weakness/numbness; vision, speech, or balance problems; bloody/tarry stools; hematuria; nosebleed or other hemorrhagic events; confusion or sudden headache; or leg swelling and pain. Monitor prothrombin time during course of therapy. Prior to use assess pt for renal impairment and consult with prescriber. Inspect vial for particulate matter and use immediately at room temp. Should not be used with other thrombolytics or in pts with active peptic ulcers or recent major surgery.

Anticoagulants—Low Molecular Weight Heparins (LWMH)

DALTEPARIN (*Fragmin*) DVT prophylaxis, acute medical illness with restricted mobility: 5000 units SC daily. DVT prophylaxis, abdominal surgery: 2500 units SC 1 to 2 h preop and daily postop. DVT prophylaxis, abdominal surgery in patients with malignancy: 5000 units SC evening before surgery and daily postop, or 2500 units 1 to 2 h preop and 12 h later, then 5000 units daily. DVT prophylaxis, hip replacement: Preop start (day of surgery): 2500 units SC given 2 h preop, 4 to 8 h postop, then 5000 units daily starting at least 6 h after 2nd dose, or 5000 units 10 to 14 h preop, 4 to 8 h postop, then daily (approximately 24 h between doses). Preop start (evening before surgery): 5000 units SC given evening before surgery then 5000 units daily starting at least 4 to 8 h postop (approximately 24 h between doses). Postop start: 2500 units 4 to 8 h postop, then 5000 units daily starting at least 6 h after first dose. Treatment of DVT/PE in cancer: 200 units/kg SC daily for 1 month, then 150 units/kg SC daily for 5 months; max 18,000 units/day. Unstable angina or non-Q-wave MI: 120 units/kg up to 10,000 units SC q 12 h with aspirin (75 to 165 mg/day PO) until clinically stable. ▶KL ♀B ▶+ © $$$$$ Trade only: Single-dose syringes 2500, 5000 units/0.2 mL, 7500 units/0.3 mL, 10,000 units/1 mL, 12,500 units/0.5 mL, 15,000 units/0.6 mL, 18,000 units/0.72 mL; multidose vial 10,000 units/mL, 9.5 mL and 25,000 units/mL, 3.8 mL. Low molecular weight heparin, antithrombin activator that preferentially inhibits factor Xa and inhibits factor IIa. Serious: Major bleeding, HIT (rare), spinal/epidural hematomas associated with neuraxial anesthesia/spinal punctures before/during treatment. Frequent: Asymptomatic increase in hepatic transaminases, injection site pain.

> **Nursing Implications** Avoid in pts with liver or kidney disease, bleeding disorders, low platelets, stroke, uncontrolled high BP, stomach ulcers, recent surgery, Consider patient history of sensitivity to heparin, pork products, or enoxaparin. May cause blood clot in brain or spinal cord with spinal tap or epidural or when taken with other drugs that can affect clotting (eg, aspirin). Monitor for unusual bleeding, bleeding that will not stop, or blood in stools or vomit; cloudy or dark urine; bruising, pallor, dizziness; shortness of breath; rapid heart rate; red pinpoint spots under pt's skin; numbness or muscle weakness in limbs; paralysis; confusion; speech; vision, or balance problems. Medication is not interchangeable "unit for unit" with other LMWH or unfractionated heparin. Do not massage injection sites. Caution in pregnant or breastfeeding patients—rationale: may cross placenta; may enter breastmilk.

ENOXAPARIN (*Lovenox*) See table. ▶KL ♀B ▶+ © $$$$$ Generic/Trade: Syringes 30, 40 mg; graduated syringes 60, 80, 100, 120, 150 mg. Concentration is 100 mg/mL except for 120, 150 mg, which are 150 mg/mL. All strengths also available preservative free. Trade only: Multidose vial 300 mg. Low molecular weight heparin, antithrombin activator that preferentially inhibits factor Xa and inhibits factor IIa. Serious: Major bleeding, thrombocytopenia (rare), spinal/epidural hematomas associated with neuraxial anesthesia/spinal punctures before/during treatment. Reports of valve thrombosis when used for thromboprophylaxis in patients with prosthetic heart valves, especially pregnant women (maternal and fetal deaths reported). Frequent: Asymptomatic increase in hepatic transaminases, injection site reactions, peripheral edema.

> **Nursing Implications** Administered by injection. Notify prescriber if any of the following occur: uncontrolled bleeding, pallor, weakness, bruising, swelling, bruising or bleeding at incision site of surgical/medical procedure; vision problems; sudden numbness; breathing problems; decreased HR and weak pulse; tingling. Assess pt for allergies; liver; kidney, or heart disease/infection; bleeding/clotting disorders; high BP; recent surgery especially brain or spinal; GI ulcers; and diabetes. Teach pt to comply with periodic blood tests and appointments with provider and to notify dentist or surgeon of taking drug before any procedure. Teach pt that drug can interact with aspirin, other NSAIDs, and salicylates, all of which should be avoided.

Anticoagulants-Factor Xa Inhibitors

NOTE: *See cardiovascular section for antiplatelet drugs and thrombolytics.*

FONDAPARINUX (*Arixtra*) DVT prophylaxis, hip/knee replacement or hip fracture surgery, abdominal surgery: 2.5 mg SC daily starting 6 to 8 h postop. DVT/PE treatment based on wt: wt less than 50 kg: 5 mg SC daily; wt between 50 and 100 kg: 7.5 mg SC daily; wt greater than 100 kg: 10 mg SC daily for at least 5 days and therapeutic oral anticoagulation. ▶K ♀B ▶? © $$$$$ Generic/Trade: Prefilled syringes 2.5 mg/0.5 mL, 5 mg/0.4 mL, 7.5 mg/0.6 mL, 10 mg/0.8 mL. Synthetic pentasaccharide sequence of heparin that binds with antithrombin III to inactivate factor Xa. Serious: Major bleeding (especially in elderly, low body weight, or renal dysfunction), thrombocytopenia (rare), spinal/epidural hematomas associated with neuraxial anesthesia/spinal punctures before/during treatment. Frequent: None.

> Nursing Implications Monitor for neurologic impairment and report immediately. Skin rash; breathing difficulty; swelling of face, lips, tongue, and throat indicate severe allergic reaction. Assess pt for all allergies and for bleeding disorders, GU disease, low platelets, or bacterial endocarditis. Solution must be clear and free of any matter; inject in fatty tissue. Monitor for bleeding postadministration. Caution in use with other drugs that may cause bleeding. Initial dose should not be administered earlier than 6–8 h after surgery. Monitor renal function and low platelets while on drug. Packaging needle contains latex that may cause allergic reaction in pts with latex sensitivity.

Anticoagulants—Other

HEPARIN Venous thrombosis/pulmonary embolus treatment: Load 80 units/kg IV, then initiate infusion at 18 units/kg/h. Adjust based on coagulation testing (PTT)—see Table. DVT prophylaxis: 5000 units SC q 8 to 12 h. Acute coronary syndromes with or without PCI: 60 units/kg IV, then 12 units/kg/h infusion, adjust according to aPTT or antiXa. See Table. Peds: Load 50 units/kg IV, then infuse 25 units/kg/h. ▶Reticuloendothelial system ♀C but + ▶+ © $$ Generic only: 1000, 5000, 10,000, 20,000 units/mL in various vial and syringe sizes. Antithrombin activator that inhibits factors Xa and IIa. Serious: Major bleeding, HIT, elevated LFTs, hyperkalemia/hypoaldosteronism, osteoporosis (with long-term use). Frequent: None.

> Nursing Implications IV administration. Assess pt for allergy to drug. Call prescriber immediately if easy bruising/bleeding occurs; blood in stools or urine, nosebleed, or any uncontrolled bleeding. Cautionary use in pts with high BP, recent surgery, blood disorders, or cardiac disorders. Course of therapy must include periodic blood tests, coagulation/prothrombin time, platelet counts, occult blood in stool, and hematocrit. Carefully follow preparation–administration interactions. Flexible container should not be used with series connections. Monitor closely for signs of hemorrhage such as drop in BP or hematocrit or in diseases where hemorrhage is likely. Extreme caution should be used in pts with peptic ulcers, bacterial endocarditis, hemophilia, and for those who have had major surgery or spinal tap.

WARFARIN (*Coumadin, Jantoven*) Individualize dosing. Start 2 to 5 mg PO daily for 1 to 2 days, then adjust dose to maintain therapeutic INR. For healthy outpatients, 2012 ACCP CHEST guidelines recommend starting at 10 mg PO daily for 2 days, then adjust dose to maintain therapeutic INR. See product information if CYP2C9 or VKOR1C genotypes are known. ▶L ♀X, (D for mechanical heart valve replacement) ▶+ © $ Generic/Trade: Tabs 1, 2, 2.5, 3, 4, 5, 6, 7.5, 10 mg. Inhibits vitamin K–dependent coagulation factors II, VII, IX, X. Also inhibits biologic anticoagulant proteins C and S. Serious: Major bleeding, tissue necrosis in protein C or S deficiency (rare), systemic cholesterol microembolization, purple toe syndrome. Frequent: Bruising.

> Nursing Implications Carefully monitor for bleeding, hemorrhage, hematuria, skin rashes, purple toes. A poorly compliant patient needs close monitoring; vitamin K can reverse effects of this drug; health provider should be consulted before taking any OTC drugs; Patient should avoid rough sports—any activities that can cause bleeding; alcohol should be avoided.

Colony-Stimulating Factors

EPOETIN ALFA (*Epogen, Procrit,* erythropoietin alpha, *Eprex*) Anemia: 1 dose IV/SC 3 times a week. Initial dose if renal failure is 50 to 100 units/kg, zidovudine-induced anemia is 100 units/kg,

THERAPEUTIC GOALS FOR ANTICOAGULATION

INR Range*	Indication
2.0–3.0	Atrial fibrillation, deep venous thrombosis, pulmonary embolism, bioprosthetic heart valve (mitral position), mechanical prosthetic heart valve (aortic position)
2.5–3.5	Mechanical prosthetic heart valve (mitral position)

*Aim for an INR in the middle of the INR range (eg, 2.5 for range of 2 to 3 and 3.0 for range of 2.5 to 3.5).
Adapted from: *Chest* 2012; 141:e422S, e425S, e533S, e578S; see these guidelines for additional information and other indications.

chemo–associated anemia is 150 units/kg. Alternate for chemo–associated anemia: 40,000 units SC once a week. Adjust dose based on Hb. ▶L ♀C ▶? © $$$$$ Trade only: Single-dose 1-mL vials 2000, 3000, 4000, 10,000, 40,000 units/mL. Multidose vials 10,000 units/mL 2 mL, 20,000 units/mL 1 mL. Stimulates erythroid progenitor cells to increase red blood cell production. Serious: Hypertension in patients with chronic renal failure, seizures, pure red cell aplasia, thrombotic events, severe anemia secondary to antibodies. Frequent: Latrogenic iron deficiency, headache, arthralgia, fever.

> **Nursing Implications** Administer IV or SC Pts can be taught self-administration. Assess pt's iron status and maintain during treatment. Monitor pts for serious adverse CV reactions, stroke, and the development of thromboemboli. Pt must comply with lab tests for hemoglobin levels. Assess pt for development of DVTs. Monitor for high BP, joint pain, headache, GI disturbances, dizziness and fatigue, injection site reactions, and adverse reactions specific to pts with HIV, cancer, or those undergoing surgery. Store in dark. Do not use if drug has been frozen or shaken. Inspect for discoloration or particulate matter. Do not shake, dilute, or mix with other drugs. Monitor infusion site for clotting.

FILGRASTIM (**G-CSF, Neupogen**) Neutropenia: 5 mcg/kg SC/IV daily. Bone marrow transplant: 10 mcg/kg/day SC/IV infusion. ▶L ♀C ▶? © $$$$$ Trade only: Single-dose vials: 300 mcg/1 mL, 480 mcg/1.6 mL. Single-dose syringes: 300 mcg/0.5 mL, 480 mcg/0.8 mL. Granulocyte colony-stimulating factor, a colony-stimulating factor that stimulates neutrophil production. Serious: Allergic-type reactions, cutaneous vasculitis, osteoporosis. Frequent: Bone pain, increased levels of LDH and alkaline phosphatase.

> **Nursing Implications** Administer no earlier than 24 h after cytotoxic chemotherapy, at least 24 h after bone marrow infusion, and not during the 24 h before administration of chemotherapy. SC: If dose requires more than 1mL of solution, may be divided into 2 injection sites. May be administered as continuous SC infusion over 24 h after bone marrow transplantation. Continuous Infusion: After chemotherapy dose is administered via infusion over 15 to 60 minutes or as a continuous infusion. After bone marrow transplant dose should be administered as an infusion over 4 to 24 h. Do not shake. Store refrigerated; allow to reach room temperature but discard any vial that has been at room temperature for more than 6 h.

PEGFILGRASTIM (**Neulasta**) 6 mg SC once each chemo cycle. ▶Plasma ♀C ▶? © $$$$$ Trade only: Single-dose syringes 6 mg/0.6 mL. Long-acting form of filgrastim that is conjugated to polyethylene glycol (pegylated). Serious: Cutaneous vasculitis. Frequent: Bone pain, reversible increases in LDH, alkaline phosphatase, uric acid.

> **Nursing Implications** Neulasta must not be shaken. Neulasta should not be used if it contains particles, is cloudy in appearance or discolored, or if the vial is cracked or damaged in any way. Nursing should assess patients for splenic problems by carefully assessing for splenic enlargement and/or pain. Left-sided upper abdominal pain and/or left-sided shoulder pain can be signs of splenic rupture.

SARGRAMOSTIM (**GM-CSF, Leukine**) Specialized dosing for bone marrow transplant. ▶L ♀C ▶? © $$$$$ Granulocyte-macrophage colony-stimulating factor, a colony-stimulating factor that stimulates the production of neutrophils, monocytes, and eosinophils. Serious: Capillary leak syndrome, dyspnea due to sequestration of WBCs in lungs (rare). Frequent: Fluid retention, fever, asthenia, bone pain, chills, myalgia.

> **Nursing Implications** IV or SC administration. Call prescriber if allergic reaction, fainting, fever greater than 100.5 degrees, chills, respiratory congestion, sore throat, foot or leg edema including wt gain,or pain in chest and rapid irregular HB occurs. Pt can be taught to administer own injection including rotation of site, compliance with periodic lab tests and storage of medication. Pt should be assessed and prescriber called if pt on other medications such as lithium, steroids, OTC or herbal drugs, and chemotherapy.

Other Hematological Agents

AMINOCAPROIC ACID (**Amicar**) Hemostasis: 4 to 5 g PO/IV over 1 h, then 1 g/h prn. ▶K ♀D ▶? © $ IV $$$$$ Oral Generic/Trade: Syrup 250 mg/mL, Tabs 500 mg. Trade only: Tabs 1000 mg. Inhibits fibrinolysis. Serious: Skeletal muscle weakness and necrosis with prolonged use. Rapid IV administration can cause hypotension, bradycardia, arrhythmia. Frequent: None.

Nursing Implications Follow directions provided by manufacturer for infusion as prescribed by primary healthcare provider. May be infused at 4 to 5 g the first hour, then 1 g/h. Not recommended for undiluted rapid infusion. Infuse slowly (rationale: to avoid hypotension, bradycardia, dysrhythmias) over 8 h or until bleeding is controlled. Do not use in patients allergic to this drug or to benzyl alcohol. Use cautiously in patients with history of heart disease, renal or liver dysfunction, and any bleeding disorders. Notify prescriber if patient experiences pain at the injection site, headache, stomach pain, nausea, vomiting, diarrhea, dizziness, or unusual tiredness. Monitor for rash, muscle pain or weakness, changes in urination, confusion, sore throat, or unusual bleeding or bruising, and notify prescriber if any of these symptoms occur.

PROTAMINE Reversal of heparin: Within 30 minutes of IV heparin: 1 mg antagonizes about 100 units heparin. If more than 30 minutes since IV heparin: 0.5 mg antagonizes about 100 units heparin. Due to short half-life of heparin (60 to 90 min), use IV heparin doses only from last several hours to calculate dose of protamine. SC heparin may require prolonged administration of protamine. Reversal of low-molecular-weight heparin: If within 8 h of LMWH dose: Give 1 mg protamine per 100 anti-Xa units of dalteparin or 1 mg protamine per 1 mg enoxaparin. Smaller doses advised if more than 8 h since LMWH administration. Give IV (max 50 mg) over 10 min. May cause allergy/anaphylaxis. ▶Plasma ♀C ▶? © $ Binds with and neutralizes heparin and partially reverses LMWHs. Serious: Severe hypotension/anaphylactoid reaction with too rapid administration, allergic reactions in patients with fish allergy, previous exposure to protamine (including insulin), pulmonary edema, circulatory collapse. Frequent: Back pain, transient flushing.

Nursing Implications Observe for severe reactions such as anaphylaxis. Should not be used for bleeding without previous exposure to heparin. Monitor pulse and BP. Continue monitoring for 2-3 h after each dose, or by patient's response. Be prepared to treat for hemorrhaging and shock. Monitor protamine effects by PTT or ACT values. Perform coagulation test 5 to 15 minutes after drug administration. Observe patients who have had cardiac surgery or undergoing dialysis. Check carefully for bleeding. This can happen 30 minutes to 18 h after the surgery. Please note that additional protamine may be necessary for some patients.

HERBAL & ALTERNATIVE THERAPIES

Herbal & Alternative Therapies

NOTE: *In the United States, herbal and alternative therapy products are regulated as dietary supplements, not drugs. Premarketing evaluation and FDA approval are not required unless specific therapeutic claims are made. Because these products are not required to demonstrate efficacy, it is unclear whether many of them have health benefits. In addition, there may be considerable variability in content from lot to lot or between products. See www.tarascon.com/herbals for the evidence-based efficacy ratings used by Tarascon editorial staff.*

GLUCOSAMINE (*Cosamin DS, Dona*) OA: Glucosamine HCl 500 mg PO three times per day or glucosamine sulfate (Dona $$) 1500 mg PO once daily. Appears ineffective overall for OA pain, but glucosamine plus chondroitin may improve pain in moderate to severe knee OA. ▶L ♀– ▶– © $ Not by prescription. May stimulate production of cartilage matrix. GI complaints, allergic skin reactions (rare). Well tolerated in the GAIT study.

Nursing Implications Caution in use with diabetics, may increase blood sugar levels; Monitor for GI symptoms, headache, drowsiness, rapid heartbeat, sleeplessness. Teach pt that aspirin may interfere with glucosamine effect and diuretics may decrease effects.

IMMUNOLOGY

Immunosuppression

BASILIXIMAB (*Simulect*) Specialized dosing for organ transplantation. ▶Plasma ♀B ▶? © $$$$$ Immunosuppressant, prophylaxis of acute organ rejection. Frequent: Administration did not increase the incidence or severity of adverse events over placebo in immunosuppressed patients.

Nursing Implications For IV injection ONLY. Call for emergency help for allergic reaction. Call prescriber if pt experiences SOB, rales, irregular pulse, muscle weakness, or sudden muscular immobility. Assess pt for myasthenia gravis or kidney, liver, or heart disease, especially long QT syndrome. Assess other drugs including OTC drugs that pt is taking. Should not be taken with lithium, certain antibiotics, or magnesium. Consult with provider.

MYCOPHENOLATE MOFETIL   (*CellCept, Myfortic*) Specialized dosing for organ transplantation. ▶?
♀D ▶? © $$$$$ Generic/Trade: Caps 250 mg. Tabs 500 mg. Trade only (CellCept): Susp 200 mg/mL (175 mL). Trade only (Myfortic): Tabs Extended-release: 180, 360 mg. Immunosuppressant, prophylaxis of acute organ rejection. Frequent: GI upset, thrombophlebitis, thrombosis (with IV administration). Severe: Infection, GI bleeding, nephrotic syndrome, bone marrow suppression, leukopenia, lymphoma, malignancy, progressive multifocal leukoencephalopathy, pure red cell aplasia.

Nursing Implications Initial dose should be given within 24 h post-transplant (typically IV); must be diluted to 6mg/mL in D5W, never administer as rapid IV bolus; handle IV similarly to a chemotherapeutic drug as it is genotoxic. Child-bearing age women should have neg serum or urine pregnancy test within 1 week prior to therapy. Give on empty stomach. IV route used only for patients unable to take oral (switch to oral as soon as can be tolerated). IV via infusion pump over 2 h. Do not crush or open capsules. Avoid contact with skin or mucous membranes. If contact occurs, rinse and wash area thoroughly.

SIROLIMUS   (*Rapamune*) Specialized dosing for organ transplantation. ▶L ♀C ▶– © $$$$$ Trade only: Soln 1 mg/mL (60 mL). Tabs 1, 2 mg. Immunosuppressant, prophylaxis of acute organ rejection in solid organ transplant. Frequent: Hypertension, edema, chest pain, fever, headache, pain, insomnia, rash, abdominal pain, renal dysfunction, nausea, diarrhea, anemia, thrombocytopenia, arthralgia, dyspnea. Hyperlipidemia in up to 90% of patients. Severe: Hepatic artery thrombosis in liver transplant patients, hypersensitivity reactions, progressive multifocal leukoencephalopathy, nephrotic syndrome, exfoliative dermatitis, impaired wound healing, angioedema, vasculitis, interstitial lung disease, hemolytic uremic syndrome/thrombotic thrombocytopenic purpura/thrombotic microangiopathy, increased risk of infections such as tuberculosis, especially when used with calcineurin inhibitor.

Nursing Implications Observe for signs and symptoms of severe allergic reactions such as hives, urticaria, shortness of breath, tightness in the chest, unusual hoarseness, wheezing, and swelling of the mouth, face, lips, or tongue. Patients should be advised to take this medication on an empty stomach or with food. This medication should be taken in the same manner each time. Patients need to be advised to wash their hands immediately after taking the medication. Patients need to be educated not to eat grapefruits or drink grapefruit juice. Patients should avoid sunlamps and tanning booths. This medication lowers the patient's ability to fight infection. Signs and symptoms of infection need to be reported immediately. Patients are at an increased risk for develoment of certain types of cancers such as lymphoma and skin cancer.

TACROLIMUS   (*Prograf, FK 506*) Specialized dosing for organ transplantation. ▶L ♀C ▶– © $$$$$ Generic/Trade: Caps 0.5, 1, 5 mg. Immunosuppressant, prophylaxis of acute organ rejection. Frequent: Hypertension, peripheral edema, headache, insomnia, pain, fever, pruritus, N/V, diarrhea, abdominal pain, tremors, paresthesias. Severe: Anaphylaxis, edema, hypertrophic cardiomyopathy, myocardial hypertrophy, ECG abnormalities and arrhythmias, paralysis, stroke, hemolytic uremic syndrome, nephrotoxicity, secondary malignancy.

Nursing Implications Patients need to be advised to either take this medication on an empty stomach or with food, but to take the medication the same way each time. Patients should be advised not to drink grapefruit juice and not to eat grapefruits as this may potentiate the effects of this medication. Patients need to be advised to limit their exposure to the sun and to avoid using sunlamps or tanning booths. This medication may also lower the ability of the immune system to fight infection. Patients should be advised to avoid contact with individuals who have colds or infections accompanied by symptoms such as a sore throat, rash, or chills. Nursing needs to monitor laboratory values such as the CBC with differential.

Anticonvulsants

CARBAMAZEPINE (*Tegretol, Tegretol XR, Carbatrol, Epitol, Equetro*) Epilepsy: 200 to 400 mg PO divided into two to four doses per day. Extended-release: 200 mg PO twice per day. Age younger than 6 yo: 10 to 20 mg/kg/day PO divided into two to four doses per day. Age 6 to 12 yo: 100 mg PO twice per day or 50 mg PO four times per day (susp); increase by 100 mg/day at weekly intervals divided three to four doses per day (immediate-release), twice per day (extended-release), or four times per day (susp). Bipolar disorder, acute manic/mixed episodes (Equetro): Start 200 mg PO two times per day; increase by 200 mg/day to max 1600 mg/day. Trigeminal neuralgia: Start 100 mg PO two times per day (regular and XR tabs) or 50 mg PO four times per day (susp). May increase by 200 mg/day to pain relief or max 1200 mg/day. Aplastic anemia, agranulocytosis, many drug interactions. ▶LK ♀D ▶+ © $$ Generic/Trade: Tabs 200 mg, Chewable tabs 100 mg, Susp 100 mg/5 mL. Extended-release tabs (Tegretol XR) 100, 200, 400 mg. Generic only: Tabs 100, 300, 400 mg, Chewable tabs 200 mg. Trade only: Extended-release caps (Carbatrol and Equetro): 100, 200, 300 mg. Anticonvulsant, sodium channel blocker. Serious: Aplastic anemia and other blood dyscrasias, hepatotoxicity, SIADH/hyponatremia, rash, Stevens-Johnson syndrome, toxic epidermal necrolysis, hypersensitivity reactions, suicidality. Frequent: Drowsiness, ataxia, dizziness, confusion, N/V, blurred vision, nystagmus.

> Nursing Implications Observe patients closely when medication is first initiated. Serum levels of this medication can rise when utilized in patients with impaired liver function. Serum levels should be monitored 5 days after initiation of therapy and periodically thereafter. Changes in mental status are a sign of elevated serum levels.

GABAPENTIN (*Neurontin, Horizant, Gralise*) Partial seizures, adjunctive therapy: Start 300 mg PO at bedtime. Increase gradually to 300 to 600 mg PO three times per day. Max 3600 mg/day divided three times per day. Postherpetic neuralgia, immediate-release tabs: Start 300 mg PO on day 1; increase to 300 mg two times per day on day 2, and to 300 mg three times per day on day 3. Max 1800 mg/day divided three times per day. Postherpetic neuralgia (Gralise): Start 300 mg PO once daily with evening meal. Increase to 600 mg on day 2, 900 mg on days 3 to 6, 1200 mg on days 7 to 10, 1500 mg on days 11 to 14, and 1800 mg on day 15. Max 1800 mg/day. Postherpetic neuralgia (Horizant): Start 600 mg PO every morning for 3 days, then increase to 600 mg PO twice per day. Max 1200 mg/day. Partial seizures, initial monotherapy: Titrate as above. Usual effective dose is 900 to 1800 mg/day. Restless legs syndrome (Horizant): 600 mg PO once daily around 5:00 pm, taken with food. ▶K ♀C ▶? © $$$$ Generic only: Tabs 100, 300, 400 mg. Generic/Trade: Caps 100, 300, 400 mg. Tabs scored 600, 800 mg. Soln 50 mg/mL. Trade only: Tabs, extended-release 600 mg (gabapentin enacarbil, Horizant). Trade only (Gralise): Tabs 300, 600 mg. Unknown. Does not appear to be a GABA analog. Serious: Leukopenia. Frequent: Fatigue, drowsiness, dizziness, ataxia, nystagmus, tremor, peripheral edema, weight gain, suicidality. Peds only: Emotional lability, hostility, hyperactivity.

> Nursing Implications Caution in elderly, pts with renal disease, pregnant, or breastfeeding. Monitor WBC for leukopenia, high BP and edema, dizziness, tremors, behavior changes (eg, hostility, labile emotions), abnormal vision, rhinitis and cough, GI symptoms, loss of appetite, sexual dysfunction, joint pain, and fractures. First dose at bedtime; avoid driving until drug effect is known; joint pain or muscle aches may curtail physical activity.

LACOSAMIDE (*Vimpat*) Partial onset seizures, adjunctive (17 yo and older): Start 50 mg PO/IV twice daily. Increase by 50 mg twice daily to recommended dose of 100 to 200 mg twice daily. Max 600 mg/day or 300 mg/day in mild to moderate hepatic or severe renal impairment. ▶KL ♀C ▶? © $$$$$ Trade only: Tabs 50, 100, 150, 200 mg. Enhances slow inactivation of voltage-gated sodium channels. Severe: Increased PR interval, AV block, suicidality, syncope. Frequent: Dizziness, ataxia, nausea/vomiting, diplopia, vertigo, blurred vision, headache.

> Nursing Implications Observe for severe allergic reactions such as: urticaria, shortness of breath, tightness in the chest, and swelling of the mouth, face, lips, or tongue. Side effects include: fever, cardiac problems, jaundice, severe drowsiness and fainting. Patients should be assessed frequently for changes in mental health status as well as suicide ideation.

LAMOTRIGINE (*Lamictal, Lamictal CD, Lamictal ODT*) Partial seizures, Lennox-Gastaut syndrome, or generalized tonic-clonic seizures adjunctive therapy with a single enzyme-inducing anticonvulsant. Age 2 to 12 yo: dosing is based on wt and concomitant meds (see package insert). Age older than 12 yo: 50 mg PO daily for 2 weeks, then 50 mg twice per day for 2 weeks, then gradually increase to 150 to 250 mg PO twice per day. Conversion to monotherapy (age 16 yo or older): See package insert. Drug interaction with valproate (see package insert for adjusted dosing guidelines). Potentially life-threatening rashes reported in 0.3% of adults and 0.8% of children; discontinue at first sign of rash. ▶LK ♀C (see notes) ▶– © $$$$ Generic/Trade: Tabs, 25, 100, 150, 200 mg. Trade only: Chewable dispersible tabs (Lamictal CD) 2, 5, 25 mg. Trade only: Orally disintegrating tabs (Lamictal ODT) 25, 50, 100, 200 mg. Chewable dispersible tabs (Lamictal CD) 2 mg may not be available in all pharmacies; obtain through manufacturer representative, or by calling 888-825-5249. Blocks sodium channels and inhibits the release of glutamate. Serious: Stevens-Johnson syndrome, toxic epidermal necrolysis, hypersensitivity reactions, blood dyscrasias, multiorgan failure, suicidality, aseptic meningitis. Frequent: Rash, dizziness, diplopia, ataxia, drowsiness, headache, blurred vision, N/V, somnolence, insomnia.

> Nursing Implications This medication is contraindicated in pregnant patients, patients who are lactating, and patients with an allergy to this medication. The most common side effects are nausea, vomiting, diarrhea, abdominal pain and constipation. Patients need to be observed for vertigo, blurred vision and diplopia. A Stevens-Johnson syndrome has been reported in some patients.

LEVETIRACETAM (*Keppra, Keppra XR*) Partial seizures, juvenile myoclonic epilepsy (JME), or primary generalized tonic-clonic seizures (GTC), adjunctive: Start 500 mg PO/IV twice per day (Keppra) or 1000 mg/day (Keppra XR, partial seizures only); increase by 1000 mg/day q 2 weeks prn to max 3000 mg/day (partial seizures) or to target dose of 3000 mg/day (JME or GTC). IV route not approved for GTC or if younger than 16 yo. ▶K ♀C ▶? © $$$$$ Generic/Trade: Tabs 250, 500, 750, 1000 mg, Oral soln 100 mg/mL, Tabs extended-release 500, 750 mg. Unknown but may involve opposition of negative modulators of GABA and glycine-gated currents and inhibition of N-type calcium currents. Serious: Pancytopenia, pancreatitis, psychosis, depression, suicidality. Frequent: Drowsiness, dizziness, fatigue, asthenia, nervousness, emotional lability, hostility, ataxia.

> Nursing Implications This medication should not be utilized in patients allergic to this medication, patients who are pregnant or lactating. This medication must be utilized cautiously in patients with renal impairment. Patients need to be advised that this medication must be weaned down and not stopped abruptly in an effort to prevent seizures. Safety precautions should be taken in patients who experience dizziness while on this medication. Patients of child bearing age need to be advised to use contraception. Patients need to be advised to take this medication exactly as prescribed.

OXCARBAZEPINE (*Trileptal*) Start 300 mg PO two times per day. Titrate to 1200 mg/day (adjunctive) or 1200 to 2400 mg/day (monotherapy). Peds 2 to 16 yo: Start 8 to 10 mg/kg/day divided two times per day. Life-threatening rashes and hypersensitivity reactions. ▶LK ♀C ▶– © $$$$$ Generic/Trade: Tabs (scored) 150, 300, 600 mg. Trade only: Oral susp 300 mg/5 mL. Unknown. May inhibit sodium channels, increase potassium conductance, and modulate calcium channels. Serious: Stevens-Johnson syndrome, toxic epidermal necrolysis, hyponatremia/SIADH, bone marrow depression, leukopenia, agranulocytosis, aplastic anemia, angioedema, suicidality. Frequent: Dizziness, drowsiness, fatigue, headache, ataxia, diplopia, nystagmus, gait disturbance, tremor, N/V, abdominal pain.

> Nursing Implications Patients need to be advised that this medication can reduce the efficacy of birth control pills. Patients need to utilize other forms of birth control, (eg, a condom with a spermicide). This medication can significantly reduce serum sodium levels, which can cause grand mal seizures. Patients need to be assessed for suicide ideation and a plan as increased thoughts of suicide may occur when takng this medication. Common side effects of this medication are headache; mental slowness; trouble concentrating; problems with speech, balance, or walking; drowsiness; and a tired feeling. This medication lowers the seizure threshold. This medication should not be utilized in patients with an underlying seizure disorder.

PHENOBARBITAL (*Luminal*) Load: 20 mg/kg IV at rate no faster than 60 mg/min. Maintenance: 100 to 300 mg/day PO given once daily or divided two times per day. Peds 3 to 5 mg/kg/day PO divided two to three times per day. Many drug interactions. ▶L ♀D ▶–©IV $ Generic only: Tabs 15, 16.2, 30, 32.4, 60, 100 mg. Elixir 20 mg/5 mL. Nonselective CNS depressant. Serious: Respiratory and CNS depression, blood dyscrasias, anemia, thrombocytopenia, Stevens-Johnson syndrome, angioedema, suicidality. Frequent: Drowsiness, fatigue, N/V, bradycardia, ataxia, nystagmus, dizziness, cognitive symptoms, paradoxical CNS excitation.

Patients need to be advised that severe allergic reactions (rash; hives; itching; difficulty breathing; tightness in the chest; swelling of the mouth, face, lips, or tongue) may develop when taking this medication. Patients may experience dizziness, drowsiness, and lightheadedness when taking this medication. Patients need to be advised that hormonal birth control may not work as well and should utilize additional birth control methods such as condoms with a spermicide. This medication is teratogenic. This medication may be habit forming and is a controlled substance. Patients should be advised not to drink alcohol and not to take other sedative type medications while on this medication. The elderly are more sensitive to the side effects of this medication.

PHENYTOIN (*Dilantin, Phenytek*) Status epilepticus: Load 15 to 20 mg/kg IV no faster than 50 mg/min, then 100 mg IV/PO q 6 to 8 h. Epilepsy: Oral load: 400 mg PO initially, then 300 mg in 2 h and 4 h. Maintenance: 5 mg/kg (or 300 mg PO) given once daily (extended-release) or divided three times per day (susp and chew tabs) and titrated to a therapeutic level. Limit dose increases to 10% or less due to saturable metabolism. ▶L ♀D ▶+ © $$ Generic/Trade: Extended-release caps 30, 100 mg (Dilantin). Susp 125 mg/5 mL. Trade only: Extended-release caps 200, 300 mg (Phenytek). Chewable tabs 50 mg (Dilantin Infatabs). Generic only: Extended-release caps 200, 300 mg. Increases seizure threshold through modulation of sodium and calcium channels. Serious: Arrhythmias, blood dyscrasias, Stevens-Johnson syndrome, toxic epidermal necrolysis, hypotension, cardiovascular collapse, thrombocytopenia, anemia, hypersensitivity, local skin necrosis (IV only), suicidality. Frequent: Rash, nystagmus, tremor, ataxia, dizziness, sedation, lymphadenopathy. Frequent (chronic use): gingival hyperplasia, osteomalacia, coarse facies.

Administer PO by capsules. Call prescriber if agitation, confusion, behavior or mood changes, hostility, restlessness, or suicidal thoughts occur or if pt experiences bleeding/bruising, swollen glands, involuntary eye movements, or slurred speech. Teach pt to monitor and report skin reactions and GI disturbances, to avoid alcohol, and to report all prescription and OTC drugs for possible interactions with Dilantin. Monitor serum levels. Adverse reactions result when the serum level of Dilantin is either too high or too low. Low serum levels could be cause for the patient to have seizures. High serum levels can result in confusion, nausea, and vomiting. Common side effects are gingival hyperplasia, a decrease in the serum folate level resulting in anemia. Patients need to have the serum Dilantin level as well as the CBC and serum folate levels monitored periodically.

PREGABALIN (*Lyrica*) Painful diabetic peripheral neuropathy: Start 50 mg PO three times per day; may increase within 1 week to max 100 mg PO three times per day. Postherpetic neuralgia: Start 150 mg/day PO divided two to three times per day. May increase within 1 week to 300 mg/day divided two to three times per day; max 600 mg/day. Partial seizures (adjunctive): Start 150 mg/day PO divided two to three times per day; increase prn to max 600 mg/day divided two to three times per day. Fibromyalgia: Start 75 mg PO two times per day; may increase to 150 mg two times per day within 1 week; max 225 mg two times per day. Neuropathic pain associated with spinal cord injury: Start 75 mg PO two times per day; may increase to 150 mg two times per day within 1 week and then to 300 mg two times per day after 2 to 3 weeks if tolerated. ▶K ♀C ▶? ©V $$$$$ Trade only: Caps 25, 50, 75, 100, 150, 200, 225, 300 mg. Oral solution 20 mg/mL (480 mL). Unknown. Binds to alpha-2-delta subunit of voltage-gated calcium channels and reduces neurotransmitter release. Serious: Visual field changes, reduced visual acuity, thrombocytopenia, suicidality. Frequent: Dizziness, somnolence, dry mouth, decreased concentration/attention, blurred vision, peripheral edema, weight gain, ataxia, withdrawal reactions.

This medication can be taken with or without food.

TOPIRAMATE (*Topamax*) Partial seizures or primary generalized tonic-clonic seizures, monotherapy: Start 25 mg PO two times per day (week 1), 50 mg two times per day (week 2), 75 mg two times per day (week 3), 100 mg two times per day (week 4), 150 mg two times per day (week 5), then 200 mg two times per day as tolerated. Partial seizures, primary generalized tonic-clonic seizures or Lennox-Gastaut syndrome, adjunctive therapy: Start 25 to 50 mg PO at bedtime. Increase weekly by 25 to 50 mg per day to usual effective dose of 200 mg PO two times per day. Doses greater than 400 mg per day not shown to be more effective. Migraine prophylaxis: Start 25 mg PO at bedtime (week 1), then 25 mg two times per day (week 2), then 25 mg q am and 50 mg q pm (week 3), then 50 mg two times per day (week 4 and thereafter). Bipolar disorder (unapproved): Start 25 to 50 mg per day PO. Titrate prn to max 400 mg per day divided two times per day. ▶K ♀D ▶? © $$$$$ Trade: Tabs 25, 50, 100, 200 mg. Sprinkle Caps 15, 25 mg. Unknown. May modulate sodium channels and enhance GABA action.

Serious: Acute angle-closure glaucoma, nephrolithiasis, oligohidrosis, hyperthermia, metabolic acidosis, suicidality, hyperammonemia. Frequent: Somnolence, fatigue, ataxia, psychomotor slowing, cognitive symptoms, confusion, diplopia, nystagmus, dizziness, depression, nervousness, weight loss, paresthesia.

> Nursing Implications This medication may cause a decrease in appetite with a resultant decrease in weight. Patients should be advised not to drink alcohol when on this medication. Patients of child bearing age need to use other barrier forms of contraception when on this medication as it decreases the effects of hormonal contraception.

ZONISAMIDE   (*Zonegran*) Start 100 mg PO daily. Titrate q 2 weeks to 200 to 400 mg/day given once daily or divided two times per day. Max 600 mg/day. Drug interactions. Contraindicated in sulfa allergy. ▶LK ♀C ▶? © $$$$ Generic/Trade: Caps 25, 50, 100 mg. Unknown. May involve inhibition of sodium and calcium channels. Serious: Toxic epidermal necrolysis, Stevens-Johnson syndrome, hepatic necrosis, agranulocytosis, aplastic anemia, hypersensitivity, nephrolithiasis, psychosis, suicidality, oligohidrosis, hyperthermia. Frequent: Abdominal pain, headache, somnolence, fatigue, N/V, anorexia, dizziness, drowsiness, cognitive symptoms, ataxia, diplopia, confusion, depression, irritability, agitation, insomnia, weight loss.

> Nursing Implications Instruct patient to always swallow capsules whole. Can be taken with or without food.

Myasthenia Gravis

NEOSTIGMIDE   (*Prostigmin*) 15 to 375 mg/day PO in divided doses, or 0.5 mg IM/SC. ▶L ♀C ▶? © $$$$ Trade only: Tabs 15 mg. Reversible cholinesterase inhibitor. Serious: Cholinergic toxicity, respiratory paralysis, bronchospasm, arrhythmias, cardiac arrest, seizures. Frequent: N/V, diarrhea, abdominal cramping, dizziness, headache, muscle cramps/weakness, fasciculations, hypersalivation, increased bronchial secretions, miosis.

> Nursing Implications Administer with food or milk. IV: Administer doses undiluted. May be given through Y-site of an IV of D5W, 0.9% NaCL, NaCL, NSS, Ringers Lactate.

Other Agents

DEXTROMETHORPHAN/QUINIDINE   (*Nuedexta*) Start one cap PO daily for 7 days, then increase to maintenance dose of 1 cap PO twice daily. ▶LK– ♀C ▶? ⊚IV Trade only: Caps 10 mg dextromethorphan plus 20 mg quinidine. Dextromethorphan: sigma-1 agonist and uncompetitive NMDA antagonist. Quinidine: included to increase DM concentrations by CYP2D6 inhibition. Serious: thrombocytopenia, hypersensitivity, lupus-like syndrome, respiratory failure, muscle spasticity. Frequent: diarrhea, dizziness, cough, vomiting, asthenia, peripheral edema.

> Nursing Implications Advise patients to report any over the counter medications that they are taking to their health provider prior to starting this medication. Observe patients for signs and symptoms of allergic reactions. Advise patients to avoid eating grapefruit and drinking grape fruit juice when taking this medication. Observe patients for dizziness, which is a very common side effect of this medication. Patients should be advised to allow 12 hours between doses.

MANNITOL   (*Osmitrol, Resectisol*) Intracranial HTN: 0.25 to 2 g/kg IV over 30 to 60 min. ▶K ♀C ▶? © $$ Osmotic diuretic. Serious: Congestive heart failure, pulmonary edema, seizures, electrolyte changes, CNS depression, acute renal failure. Frequent: Headache, dizziness, N/V, polydipsia.

> Nursing Implications This is an osmotic diuretic. This medication is contraindicated in patients with anuria secondary to severe renal disease. This medication must be utilized cautiously in patients with pulmonary congestion, intracranial bleeding (exception is during craniotomy), dehydration, renal disease, heart failure, pregnancy and lactation. Patients should be observed closely during administration of this medication. Solution must not be exposed to cold temperatures as the solution may crystallize. Electrolyte-free mannitol should not be administered with blood. A filter system must be utilized with concentrated mannitol. Electrolytes require monitoring with prolonged treatment. Patients should be advised that they may experience increased urination when on this medication.

NIMODIPINE (*Nimotop*) Subarachnoid hemorrhage: 60 mg PO q 4 h for 21 days. ▶L ♀C ▶– © $$$$$
Generic only: Caps 30 mg. Calcium channel blocker. Serious: Heart failure, disseminated intravascular coagulation, deep vein thrombosis, neurological deterioration. Frequent: Hypotension, N/V, diarrhea, flushing, edema, headache.

> Nursing Implications Administer PO ONLY. If pt cannot swallow, gel may be extracted from soft capsule, transferred to a needleless syringe and given orally or through nasogastric tube. Monitor for several allergic reaction/anaphylaxis. Call prescriber if pt has rapid or slow HR, bruising/bleeding, swelling in legs, or fainting. Assess pt for previous cardiac history including use of calcium channel blockers, recent head injury, or liver disease. Caution pt to avoid driving or other complex activity until used to drug. Constantly monitor for decrease in BP. Monitor for less serious side effects such as rash, swelling, GI disturbances, and headache.

Parkinsonian Agents—COMT Inhibitors

TOLCAPONE (*Tasmar*) ▶LK ♀C ▶? © $$$$$ Trade only: Tabs 100, 200 mg. Blocks dopamine breakdown by inhibiting catechol-o-methyltransferase. Serious: fulminant hepatotoxicity, orthostatic hypotension, hallucinations, severe diarrhea, impulse control disorders. Frequent: dyskinesia, dystonia, anorexia, N/V, diarrhea, constipation, confusion, sleep disorders.

> Nursing Implications Administer with 8 ounces of water. Use only in conjunction with the drug levodopa. Do not use in patients taking MAO inhibitor drugs, those with a history of narrow-angle glaucoma, or malignant melanoma. Use cautiously in patients with history of heart disease, respiratory disease, renal or liver dysfunction, endocrine diseases, stomach or intestinal ulcers, or depression and psychiatric disorders. Promote caution while driving or using heavy machinery. Promote regular visits to provider for blood testing and monitor for allergic reaction, seizures, persistent nausea, vomiting and diarrhea, irregular heartbeat, behavioral changes, or suicidal thoughts.

Parkinsonian Agents—Dopaminergic Agents and Combinations

CARBIDOPA (*Lodosyn*) ▶LK ♀C ▶? © $$$ Trade only: Tabs 25 mg. Blocks the peripheral conversion of levodopa to dopamine. Serious: None. Frequent: None. The adverse effects of carbidopa/levodopa are due to the levodopa component.

> Nursing Implications Administer with 8 ounces of water. Use only in conjunction with the drug levodopa. Do not use in patients taking MAO inhibitor drugs, those with a history of narrow-angle glaucoma, or malignant melanoma. Use cautiously in patients with history of heart disease, respiratory disease, renal or liver dysfunction, endocrine diseases, stomach or intestinal ulcers, or depression and psychiatric disorders. Promote caution while driving or using heavy machinery. Promote regular visits to provider for blood testing and monitor for allergic reaction, seizures, persistent nausea, vomiting and diarrhea, irregular heartbeat, behavioral changes, or suicidal thoughts.

OB/GYN

Contraceptives—Other

NUVARING (ethinyl estradiol vaginal ring + etonogestrel) Contraception: 1 ring intravaginally for 3 weeks each month. ▶L ♀X ▶– © $$$ Trade only: Flexible intravaginal ring, 15 mcg ethinyl estradiol/0.120 mg etonogestrel/day in 1, 3 rings/box. Contraceptive steroid combination. Serious: DVT/PE, stroke, MI, hepatic neoplasia, and gallbladder disease. Frequent: Nausea, breast tenderness, breakthrough bleeding, asymptomatic vaginal discharge.

> Nursing Implications Patients need to be made aware to utilize alternate forms of contraception (eg, condom with spermicide) when on this medicated device. A diahpragm must be avoided. Patients need to be educated that smoking increases the risk for blood clots, stroke, and/ or heart attack, especially after the age of 35 years. This medicated device does not protect against sexually transmitted diseases such as HIV. Birth defects can result from use of this medicated device.

ORAL CONTRACEPTIVES* ▶L CX	Estrogen (mcg)	Progestin (mg)
Monophasic		
Necon 1/50, Norinyl 1+50	50 mestranol	1 norethindrone
Ovcon-50		
Demulen 1/50, Zovia 1/50E	50 ethinyl estradiol	1 ethynodiol
Ogestrel		0.5 norgestrel
Necon 1/35, Norinyl 1+35, Nortrel 1/35, Ortho-Novum 1/35		1 norethindrone
Brevicon, Modicon, Necon 0.5/35,Nortrel 0.5/35		0.5 norethindrone
Balziva, Femcon Fe, Ovcon-35, Zenchent, Zeosa	35 ethinyl estradiol	0.4 norethindrone
Previfem		0.18 norgestimate
MonoNessa, Ortho-Cyclen, Sprintec-28		0.25 norgestimate
Demulen 1/35, Kelnor 1/35, Zovia 1/35E		1 ethynodiol
Junel 1.5/30, Junel 1.5/30 Fe, Loestrin 211.5/30, Loestrin Fe 1.5/30, Microgestin Fe 1.5/30		1.5 norethindrone
Cryselle, Lo/Ovral, Low-Ogestrel		0.3 norgestrel
Apri, Desogen, Ortho-Cept, Reclipsen	30 ethinyl estradiol	0.15 desogestrel
Levora, Nordette, Portia, Solia		0.15 levonorgestrel
Ocella, Safyral, Yasmin, Zarah		3 drospirenone
Generess Fe	25 ethinyl estradiol	0.8 norethindrone
Junel 1/20, Junel Fe 1/20, Loestrin 211/20, Loestrin Fe 1/20, Loestrin 24 Fe, Microgestin Fe 1/20		1 norethindrone
Aviane, Lessina, Lutera, Sronyx	20 ethinyl estradiol	0.1 levonorgestrel
Amethyst†, Lybrel†		0.09 levonorgestrel
Gianvi, Yaz		3 drospirenone
Beyaz		2 drospirenone
Azurette, Kariva, Mircette	20/10 ethinyl estradiol	0.15 desogestrel
Progestin only		
Camila, Errin, Jolivette, Micronor, Nor-Q.D., Nora-BE	none	0.35 norethindrone
Biphasic (estrogen and progestin contents vary)		
Necon 10/11	35 ethinyl estradiol	0.5/1 norethindrone
Triphasic (estrogen and progestin contents vary)		
Caziant, Cesia, Cyclessa, Velivet	25 ethinyl estradiol	0.100/0.125/0.150 desogestrel
Ortho-Novum 7/7/7, Necon 7/7/7, Nortrel 7/7/7	35 ethinyl estradiol	0.5/0.75/1 norethindrone
Aranelle, Leena, Tri-Norinyl		0.5/1/0.5 norethindrone
Enpresse, Trivora-28	30/40/30 ethinyl estradiol	0.5/0.75/0.125 levonorgestrel
Ortho Tri-Cyclen, Trinessa, Tri-Previfem, Tri-Sprintec	35 ethinyl estradiol	0.18/0.215/0.25 norgestimate
Ortho Tri-Cyclen Lo	25 ethinyl estradiol	
Estrostep Fe, Tilia Fe, Tri-Legest, Tri-Legest Fe	20/30/35 ethinyl estradiol	1 norethindrone
Quadphasic		
Natazia	3 mg/2 mg estradiol valerate	2/3/0 dienogest
Extended Cycle††		
Jolessa, Quasense, Seasonale	30 ethinyl estradiol	0.15 levonorgestrel
Amethia, Seasonique	30/10 ethinyl estradiol	0.15 levonorgestrel
LoSeasonique	20 ethinyl estradiol	0.1 levonorgestrel

*All: Not recommended in smokers. Increases risk of thromboembolism, CVA, MI, hepatic neoplasia, and gallbladder disease. Nausea, breast tenderness, and breakthrough bleeding are common transient side effects. Effectiveness reduced by hepatic enzyme-inducing drugs such as certain anticonvulsants and barbiturates, rifampin, rifabutin, griseofulvin, and protease inhibitors. Coadministration with St. John's wort may decrease efficacy. Vomiting or diarrhea may also increase the risk of contraceptive failure. Consider an additional form of birth control in above circumstances. See product insert for instructions on missing doses. Most available in 21-and 28-day packs.
Progestin only: Must be taken at the same time every day. Because much of the literature regarding OC adverse effects pertains mainly to estrogen/progestin combinations, the extent to which progestin-only contraceptives cause these effects is unclear. No significant interaction has been found with broad-spectrum antibiotics. The effect of St. John's wort is unclear. No placebo days, start new pack immediately after finishing current one. Available in 28-day packs. Readers may find the following website useful: www.managingcontraception.com.
† Approved for continuous use without a "pill-free" period.
†† 84 active pills and 7 placebo pills.

Labor Induction/Cervical Ripening

OXYTOCIN (*Pitocin*) Labor induction: 10 units in 1000 mL NS (10 milliunits/mL), start at 6 to 12 mL/h (1 to 2 milliunits/min). Postpartum bleeding: 10 units IM or 10 to 40 units in 1000 mL NS IV, infuse 20 to 40 milliunits/min. ▶LK ♀? ▶– © $ Uterine stimulant. Serious: Anaphylaxis, water intoxication. Frequent: N/V.

> Nursing Implications Administer by IV infusion or IM injection only in settings where uterine contractions can be monitored. Monitor mother for irregular HR, chest pain, difficulty with breathing or urination, swelling, headache confusion, seizures, or excessive vaginal bleeding. Monitor mother also for GI disturbances for excessive blood loss, cardiac problems, uterine spasm or rupture. Monitor fetus for slow HR, seizures, heart arrhythmias, low Apgar score at 5 minutes, jaundice, and retinal hemorrhage.

Progestins

MEGESTROL (*Megace, Megace ES*) Endometrial hyperplasia: 40 to 160 mg PO daily for 3 to 4 months. AIDS anorexia: 800 mg (20 mL) susp PO daily or 625 mg (5 mL) ES daily. ▶L ♀D ▶? © $$$$$ Generic/Trade: Tabs 20, 40 mg. Susp 40 mg/mL in 240 mL. Trade only: Megace ES susp 125 mg/mL (150 mL). Gonadal steroid. Serious: Thrombophlebitis, cerebrovascular disorders, retinal thrombosis, DVT/PE. Frequent: Breakthrough bleeding, weight gain.

> Nursing Implications Administer by mouth. Do not store near heat. Monitor for severe allergic reaction/ anaphylaxis including swelling/numbness in extremities, vision problems and sudden, severe headache. Assess patient for clotting tendencies, CHF, High BP, kidney disease, and diabetes which can be exacerbated with use of Megace. Call prescriber at signs of high blood sugar. Teach patient that the following may occur: GI disturbances, faintness, mild SOB, sweating/hot flashes, menstrual bleeding, or insomnia. Respiratory infections may increase with long-term use.

Selective Estrogen Receptor Modulators

TAMOXIFEN (*Nolvadex, Soltamox, Tamone*, ✦ *Tamofen*) Breast cancer prevention: 20 mg PO daily for 5 years. Breast cancer: 10 to 20 mg PO two times per day. ▶L ♀D ▶– © $$ Generic/Trade: Tabs 10, 20 mg. Trade only (Soltamox): Sugar-free soln 10 mg/5 mL (150 mL). Selective estrogen receptor modulator. Serious: DVT/PE, retinal thrombosis, hepatotoxicity, endometrial cancer. Frequent: Hot flashes, leg cramps, vaginal discharge.

> Nursing Implications This medication is contraindicated in pregnancy, lactation, and patients on anticoagulation therapy or in patients with a history of DVT, PE, and other thromboembolic events. Patients need to have periodic assessments. An initial ophthalmologic examination needs to be done and then periodically thereafter if visual changes occur. Initial screening lab work inclusive of a CBC with differential and LFTs need to be done and should be done periodically throughout treatment. Patients need to be advised to use contraceptive methods when on this medication. Patients should also be advised not to drink grapefruit juice or eat grapefruit while on this medication.

ONCOLOGY

Alkylating Agents

BUSULFAN (*Myleran, Busulfex*) ▶LK ♀D ▶– © $ varies by therapy. Trade only (Myleran) Tabs 2 mg. Busulfex injection for hospital/oncology clinic use; not intended for outpatient prescribing. Alkylating agent. Serious: Bone marrow suppression, adrenal insufficiency, seizures, pulmonary fibrosis, hepatic veno-occlusive disease, febrile neutropenia; severe bacterial, viral (eg, cytomegaloviraemia), and fungal infections; sepsis; tumor lysis syndrome; thrombotic micro angiopathy (TMA); hyperpigmentation.

> Nursing Implications Since drug is immunosuppressant, monitor for signs of infection including flu-like symptoms, mouth sores, wt loss, and weakness. Teach pt to comply with regular blood tests. Assess patient for seizure disorder, post-head injury, or breathing problems. Teach pt signs of allergic reaction and to immediately report weakness, pallor, bruising, bleeding, or petechiae;

coughing up blood; GI symptoms, muscle tightness, involuntary movements or contraction; rapid or slow HR; seizures; or persistent cough. Advise pt that hair loss and darkened skin color may occur. Interacts with many other drugs. Check interactions and pt's medications before administering.

MELPHALAN (*Alkeran*) ▶Plasma ♀D ▶– © $ varies by therapy, Trade only: Tabs 2 mg. Injection for hospital/clinic use; not intended for outpatient prescribing. Alkylating agent. Serious: Bone marrow suppression, anaphylaxis. Frequent: Bone marrow suppression, N/V.

> **Nursing Implications** Assess for history of allergies and blood problems. Administer under supervision of physician who is expert in chemotherapeutic drugs. Severe immunosuppression possible— observe for bleeding, bruising, fever, chills, aches, and weakness. Flu-like symptoms, low-grade fever may also occur. Observe for jaundice, nausea and vomiting, appetite loss, and clay stools. Platelet and WBC counts, differential, and hemoglobin must be tested before first dose and subsequent treatments. Teach patient to call physician if rash, bleeding, vasculitis, nausea and vomiting, amenorrhea, wt loss, or persistent coughing occurs.

Antibiotics

DOXORUBICIN LIPOSOMAL (*Doxil*, ✦ *Caelyx, Myocet*) ▶L ♀D ▶– © $ varies by therapy. Antibiotic. Serious: Cardiac toxicity, bone marrow suppression, infusion-associated reactions, necrotizing colitis, palmar-plantar erythrodysesthesia, secondary malignancies. Frequent: Cardiac toxicity, bone marrow suppression, hyperuricemia, fatigue, fever, anorexia, N/V, stomatitis, diarrhea, urine discoloration.

> **Nursing Implications** This medication should be prepared in the pharmacy under a laminar flow hood. Precautions must be taken in the preparation of this medication. Medication devices must be properly discarded after use. Refer to product literature for complete instructions. Each hospital's pharmacy & therapeutics committee should have established guidelines for the administration of this medication.

Antimetabolites

AZACITIDINE (*Vidaza*) ▶K ♀D ▶– © $ varies by therapy. Antimetabolite. Serious: Bone marrow suppression, hepatotoxicity, renal failure. Frequent: N/V, bone marrow suppression, fever, diarrhea, fatigue, constipation.

> **Nursing Implications** Monitor pt for pallor, bruising, dizziness or weakness, bleeding, flu-like symptoms, increased heart rate, dry mouth or thirst, increased urination, pain, itching, or burning. Pt should be premedicated for nausea and vomiting before first dose. Monitor hematologic values and renal function; carefully follow directions for preparation and injection of the susp that will be cloudy for subcutaneous injection but must be clear for IV admin. Adverse reactions differ by route of injection. Blood disorders and nausea are the most common adverse reactions. High caution in patients with liver disease. May cause fetal harm in pregnant patients.

CYTARABINE (*Cytosar-U, Tarabine, Depo-Cyt, AraC*) ▶LK ♀D ▶– © $ varies by therapy. Antimetabolite. Serious: Bone marrow suppression, hepatotoxicity, pancreatitis, peripheral neuropathy, "cytarabine syndrome" (fever, myalgia, bone pain, occasional chest pain, maculopapular rash, conjunctivitis, and malaise). Neurotoxicity. Chemical arachnoiditis (N/V, headache, and fever) with Depo-Cyt. Frequent: Bone marrow suppression, N/V, diarrhea, rash.

> **Nursing Implications** Should be injected only by a physician experienced in chemotherapies. Assess for all allergies, bone marrow or blood disorders, liver disease, kidney disease, and gout. Close and constant monitoring during drug administration. Report serious side effects such as weakness, bruising, bleeding, vision problems, eye pain, cough or breathing problems, urinary problems, black or bloody stools, unusual behavior or thoughts. Teach pt to avoid contact sports, sharp razors. Check injection site for thrombophlebitis. Assess for immunosuppression such as viral, bacterial, parasitic or fungal infections. Nausea and vomiting are most frequent side effects. Harmful to fetus.

Cytoprotective Agents

MESNA   (***Mesnex, ✦ Uromitexan***) ▶plasma ♀B ▶– © $ varies by therapy. Trade only: Tabs 400 mg, scored. Cytoprotective. Serious: Hypersensitivity. Frequent: Bad taste in mouth.

> Nursing Implications The dosage of this medication must be administered consistently– timing of dosage must be exact. Patients need to be observed for bladder hemorrhage when taking this medication.

PALIFERMIN   (***Kepivance***) ▶plasma ♀C ▶? © $ varies by therapy.   Cytoprotective, human keratinocyte growth factor. Serious: Fever. Frequent: Rash, erythema, edema, pruritus, oral/perioral dysesthesia, tongue discoloration or thickening, alteration of taste.

> Nursing Implications Patients need to be monitored for rash and oral changes. Patients should be assessed for alterations in taste during treatment with this medication.

Immunomodulators

RITUXIMAB   (***Rituxan***) ▶Not metabolized ♀C ▶– © $ varies by therapy.   Rituximab is a chimeric monoclonal antibody that binds to the antigen CD20, a hydrophobic transmembrane protein found on the surface of B-cell precursors and mature B-lymphocytes, which mediates cell lysis. Serious: Fatal infusion reactions, hepatitis, hepatic failure, tumor lysis syndrome, severe mucocutaneous reactions, cardiac arrhythmias, nephrotoxicity, bowel obstruction and perforation, hypersensitivity, bone marrow suppression, infection. Frequent: Bone marrow suppression, infection.

> Nursing Implications Do not vaccinate with viral vaccines following use of Rituxan. Do not breastfeed until there are nonexistent levels of medication present in the system. Child-bearing women should be advised to use contraceptives during 12 months of Rituxan treatment to protect the fetus from untoward effects. Patients should read and acknowledge the patient information pamphlet before treatment sessions. Periodically check CBC and platelet counts. Patients can experience signs and symptoms of chills, shakes, fever, hives, sneezing, itching, throat irritations, swelling, and cough within 24 h of the first Rituxan infusion. Other common side effects are nausea, headaches, joint aches, and upper respiratory infections. Physician must be notified of these side effects as well as any signs and symptoms of infection, flu-like symptoms, abdominal pain, skin reactions, sores, blisters, ulcers, and peeling skin.

Mitotic Inhibitors

DOCETAXEL   (***Taxotere***) ▶L ♀D ▶– © $ varies by therapy.   Mitotic Inhibitor. Serious: Hypersensitivity/anaphylaxis, cutaneous events, edema, neutropenia, rash, erythema of the extremities, nail hypo- or hyperpigmentation, hepatotoxicity, paresthesia/dysesthesia. Frequent: Rash, N/V, diarrhea, bone marrow suppression.

> Nursing Implications Administer by central or peripheral IV infusion ONLY. Should be administered only by physician experienced in immunosuppressive therapies and in a proper facility. Patient should receive only once to prevent hypersensitivity. Discard if particulate matter is in solution. Reconstituted solution may be kept for 24 hours only, then discard. Monitor patient for the following adverse events; viral infections, fever, GI symptoms, low BP, insomnia, anemia, symptoms of metabolic disorders such as hyperkalemia, hyperglycemia; headache, tremors and difficulties breathing. Teach/inform patient about the risks of immunosuppressive therapy.

PACLITAXEL   (***Taxol, Abraxane, Onxol***) ▶L ♀D ▶– © $ varies by therapy.   Mitotic inhibitor. Serious: Anaphylaxis, bone marrow suppression, cardiac conduction abnormalities, peripheral neuropathy. Frequent: Bone marrow suppression, peripheral neuropathy, hypotension, mucositis, N/V.

> Nursing Implications Administer by IV infusion once q 3 weeks. Gloves must be worn during preparation and administration. Advise patient that hair loss will occur, to protect scalp from sun exposure, cut hair short, and be gentle with daily hair-care routine. Advise patient to contact provider if fever over 100.4°F occurs and to take precautions to prevent infections. Prepare pts for most common adverse reactions such as infections, GI disturbances, anemia, fatigue, abnormal ECG, and neuropathies.

If numbness, tingling, or burning in extremities; fatigue; weakness; or joint or muscle pain occurs, report to provider. Teach pts that redness or sores may appear in the mouth or on the lips, usually a few days after first treatment. These resolve within about 1 week. Encourage light exercise, increased fluids, small meals, and plenty of rest. Monitor for upset stomach, diarrhea, and irritation at the injection site. Notify provider if patient experiences dizziness, fainting, or shortness of breath. CBC, complete chemistry profile, and liver function studies need to be performed periodically on patients taking this medication. The elderly are more sensitive to this medication. This medication is also teratogenic and should not be used in pregnancy.

Platinum-Containing Agents

CARBOPLATIN   (*Paraplatin*) ▶K ♀D ▶– © $ varies by therapy.   Alkylating agent. Serious: Bone marrow suppression, peripheral neuropathy, anaphylaxis, nephrotoxicity. Frequent: Bone marrow suppression, N/V, increased LFTs. Possible: alopecia, dehydration, mucositis.

> Nursing Implications Follow manufacturer's instructions for infusion via IV. Do not use in patients allergic to this drug or similar medications. Do not use in patients experiencing bone marrow suppression or severe bleeding. Use cautiously in patients with renal or liver dysfunction, a weak immune system, or those who have taken carboplatin before. Monitor for pale skin, shortness of breath, irregular heartbeat, bruising, unusual bleeding, flu-like symptoms, sores in mouth or throat, ongoing vomiting, stomach pain, yellowing of skin or eyes, numbness or tingling in extremities, hearing or vision problems, skin changes at the injection site, and low magnesium levels. Promote avoidance of crowds and people with infections. Promote regular visits to provider for monitoring.

OXALIPLATIN   (*Eloxatin*) ▶LK ♀D ▶– © $ varies by therapy.   Alkylating agent. Serious: Bone marrow suppression, anaphylaxis, neuropathy, pulmonary fibrosis. Frequent: N/V, diarrhea.

> Nursing Implications Administer by IV injection. Monitor for severe allergic reaction/anaphylaxis. Assess pt for blood or bone marrow disorders, kidney or nerve problems. Assess pt for allergy to drugs containing platinum. Caution pt not to drive or engage in activities requiring clear vision until used to drug. Teach pt to call prescriber if experiencing numbness or burning pain, problems with tongue, swallowing, or speech; hypersensitivity to cold; flu-like symptoms; thirst; dry mouth; decreased urination; vision problems; oral white patches; bruising/bleeding or weakness; chest, jaw, or eye pain. Observe pts for signs and symptoms of depression and for leg calf pain. Neuropathies can develop. Teach pt not to chew on ice chips, to comply with blood tests, and to avoid other people to prevent infections. Toxic levels of this medication can result in pulmonary fibrosis and hepatotoxicity. This medication is teratogenic.

Other

ARSENIC TRIOXIDE   (*Trisenox*) ▶L ♀D ▶– © $ varies by therapy. Serious: APL differentiation syndrome: fever, dyspnea, weight gain, pulmonary infiltrates, and pleural/pericardial effusions, with or without leukocytosis. QT prolongation, tachycardia, AV block, torsade de pointes, hyperleukocytosis. Frequent: Hypotension, N/V, diarrhea, hyperglycemia, fever, fatigue, dermatitis, nausea, electrolyte abnormalities.

> Nursing Implications When on Trisenox, the heart rate should be monitored due to sometimes fatal changes in heart rate. Patients on Trisenox plus diuretics should have their heart rates even more closely monitored. Before starting and during Trisenox use, labs inclusive of an ECG, blood electrolyte levels, and blood creatinine levels should be done. This medication lowers the body's ability to fight infection. This medication may elevate blood sugar levels, so diabetic patients should be advised to monitor blood sugar levels more closely. This medication is found in breastmilk and is also teratogenic.

IRINOTECAN   (*Camptosar*) ▶L ♀D ▶– © $ varies by therapy.   Topoisomerase inhibitor. Serious: Severe diarrhea, dehydration, bone marrow suppression, orthostatic hypotension, colitis/ileus, hypersensitivity, pancreatitis. Frequent: Diarrhea, bone marrow suppression, alopecia, N/V, rhinitis, salivation, lacrimation, miosis. Myocardial ischemic events, elevated serum transaminases, hiccups, and megacolon have also occurred.

Nursing Implications This medication is contraindicated in patients who are lactating or pregnant. This medication must be utilized cautiously in patients with bone marrow suppression and severe diarrhea. A CBC must be obtained prior to each administration of this medication. Patients need to be advised to utilize contraceptives. Patients need to report any signs of infection and diarrhea to provider. Patients should be educated to avoid crowded areas or people with known infections. Patients should be advised to eat frequent, small meals.

RASBURICASE (*Elitek*, ✚ *Fasturtec*) ▶L ♀C ▶– © $$$$$ Catalyzes enzymatic oxidation of uric acid into an inactive and soluble metabolite. Serious: Anaphylaxis, hemolysis, methemoglobinemia, acute renal failure, arrhythmia, cardiac failure, cardiac arrest, cellulitis, cerebrovascular disorder, chest pain, convulsions, dehydration, ileus, infection, intestinal obstruction, hemorrhage, myocardial infarction, paresthesia, pancytopenia, pneumonia, pulmonary edema, pulmonary hypertension, retinal hemorrhage, rigors, thrombosis, and thrombophlebitis. Frequent: Fever, neutropenia with fever, respiratory distress, sepsis, neutropenia, mucositis, vomiting, nausea, headache, abdominal pain, constipation, diarrhea, rash.

Nursing Implications For IV infusion into bag only, NOT for bolus injection into line. Swirl when mixing, do not shake. Check for particulate matter or discoloration and discard if present. Do not use line filters. Store at 36 to 46° F but do not freeze. Monitor for severe allergic reaction which can occur at any time during treatment: breathing difficulties, low BP, chest pain, rash, and shock. Assess for adverse reactions of nausea and vomiting, fever, headache, GI symptoms, rash, abdominal pain, and pharyngolaryngeal pain. Contraindicated for African American or Mediterranean pts with G6PD deficiency.

OPHTHALMOLOGY

Non-Steroidal Anti-Inflammatories

KETOROLAC—OPHTHALMIC (*Acular, Acular LS*) 1 gtt in each affected eye four times per day. ▶L ♀C ▶? © $$$$ Generic/Trade: Soln (Acular LS) 0.4% (5 mL). Trade only: Acular 0.5% (3, 5, 10 mL), preservative-free Acular 0.45% unit dose (0.4 mL). Blocks prostaglandin synthesis by inhibiting cyclooxygenase. Frequent: Transient stinging/burning. Severe: Keratitis, corneal thinning, erosion, ulceration, perforation.

Nursing Implications Topical administration by eye gtt. Monitor pt for red conjunctiva, eye edema, pain, and headache. Call prescriber if severe burning, pain, light sensitivity, drainage, or white patches appear on eye. Corneal erosion or perforation may occur. Assess pt for previous sensitivity to NSAIDs, and if present consult with prescriber.

Other Ophthalmologic Agents

CYCLOSPORINE—OPHTHALMIC (*Restasis*) 1 gtt in each eye q 12 h. ▶Minimal absorption ♀C ▶? © $$$$ Trade only: Emulsion 0.05% (0.4 mL single-use vials). Immunomodulator and anti-inflammatory. Frequent: Ocular burning.

Nursing Implications Not recommended for ages 16 yr or younger or patients with active ocular infections. Ocular burning, pain, stinging, discharge, foreign body sensation, conjuctival hyperemia, blurring, and pruritus are common side effects of this medication. Contact lenses may be placed back in eye after 15 minutes of use. Patients should be advised to wash their hands prior to instillation of this medication and after use. This medication should be used at the same time each day.

PSYCHIATRY

Antidepressants—Heterocyclic Compounds

AMITRIPTYLINE (*Elavil*) Depression: Start 25 to 100 mg PO at bedtime; gradually increase to usual effective dose of 50 to 300 mg/day. Primarily inhibits serotonin reuptake. Demethylated to nortriptyline, which primarily inhibits norepinephrine reuptake. Suicidality. ▶L ♀D ▶– © $$ Generic: Tabs 10, 25, 50, 75, 100, 150 mg. Elavil brand name no longer available; has been retained in this entry for name recognition purposes only. Serotonin/norepinephrine reuptake inhibitor. Serious: Atrial/ventricular arrhythmias, seizures, MI, CHF, stroke. Frequent: Drowsiness, dry mouth, constipation, nausea, orthostatic hypotension, dizziness, confusion, urinary retention, sexual dysfunction.

> Nursing Implications Follow dosage directions for entire course of therapy. Do not use in patients allergic to amitriptyline or with a recent history of heart attack. Do not use with MAO inhibitor drugs. Use cautiously in patients with a history of heart problems, bipolar disorder, schizophrenia, mental illness, diabetes, overactive thyroid, glaucoma, or urination problems. Notify prescriber immediately if patient experiences any changes in mood, or reports having depressed or suicidal thoughts. Promote gradual decrease in dosage until therapy is completed. Avoid stopping therapy suddenly.

CLOMIPRAMINE (*Anafranil*) OCD: Start 25 mg PO at bedtime; gradually increase to usual effective dose of 150 to 250 mg/day. Max 250 mg/day. Primarily inhibits serotonin reuptake. Suicidality. ▶L ♀C ▶+ © $$$ Generic/Trade: Caps 25, 50, 75 mg. Serotonin/norepinephrine reuptake inhibitor. Serious: Atrial/ventricular arrhythmias, seizures, MI, CHF, stroke. Frequent: Drowsiness, dry mouth, constipation, nausea, orthostatic hypotension, dizziness, confusion, urinary retention, sexual dysfunction.

> Nursing Implications Administer with food. Do not use in patients who have recently suffered a heart attack, or those on MAO inhibitor drugs. Monitor for behavior or mood changes, depression, suicidal thoughts, anxiety, panic attacks, or restlessness. Gradually reduce dosage over time, do not stop suddenly. Notify provider immediately if patient experiences chest pain, nausea, sweating, headache, imbalance, fever, confusion, pale skin, unusual bleeding, or increased urination.

NORTRIPTYLINE (*Aventyl, Pamelor*) Depression: Start 25 mg PO given once daily or divided two to four times per day. Usual effective dose is 75 to 100 mg/day, max 150 mg/day. Primarily inhibits norepinephrine reuptake. Suicidality. ▶L ♀D ▶+ © $$$ Generic/Trade: Caps 10, 25, 50, 75 mg. Oral soln 10 mg/5 mL. Norepinephrine/serotonin reuptake inhibitor. Serious: Atrial/ventricular arrhythmias, seizures, MI, CHF, stroke. Frequent: Drowsiness, dry mouth, constipation, nausea, orthostatic hypotension, dizziness, confusion, urinary retention, sexual dysfunction.

> Nursing Implications Observe patients for severe allergic reactions such as hives, urticaria, shortness of breath, tightness in the chest, and swelling of the mouth, face, lips, or tongue. Other medications and alcohol should not be taken when patients are on this medication. Observe for signs and symptoms of mental or mood changes (eg, increased anxiety, mood swings, agitation, irritability, nervousness, restlessness, panic attacks). Patients need to be observed closely for increased risk of suicide ideation and action, especially children, adolescents, and young adults, when they are taking this medication. Patients may report decreased libido when on this medication. This medication must be utilized cautiously in the elderly.

Antidepressants—Selective Serotonin Reuptake Inhibitors (SSRIs)

CITALOPRAM (*Celexa*) Depression: Start 20 mg PO daily. May increase after 1 or more weeks to max 40 mg PO daily or 20 mg daily if older than 60 yo. Suicidality. ▶LK ♀C but – in third trimester ▶– © $$$ Generic/Trade: Tabs 10, 20, 40 mg. Oral soln 10 mg/5 mL. Generic only: Orally disintegrating tabs 10, 20, 40 mg. Selective serotonin reuptake inhibitor. Serious: Suicidality, serotonin syndrome, neuroleptic malignant syndrome, abnormal bleeding, withdrawal reactions, increased QTc interval. Frequent: N/V, diarrhea, insomnia, drowsiness, headache, sexual dysfunction, dry mouth, anorexia, anxiety, nervousness.

> Nursing Implications Schedule medication at same time each day. Use cautiously in patients with renal or liver dysfunction, seizures, bipolar disorder, or history of depression and suicidal thoughts. Do not administer in conjunction with MAO inhibitor drugs. Monitor for behavior or mood changes, depression, suicidal thoughts, anxiety, panic attacks, or restlessness. Promote completion of entire course of therapy. Promote seeking emergency medical help in case of allergic reaction. Refer to manufacturer's list of drug interactions.

ESCITALOPRAM (*Lexapro*, ✦ *Cipralex*) Depression—generalized anxiety disorder, adults, and age 12 yo or older: Start 10 mg PO daily; max 20 mg/day. Suicidality. ▶LK ♀C but–in 3rd trimester ▶– © $$$ Generic/Trade: Tabs 5, 10, 20 mg. Trade only: Oral soln 1 mg/mL. Selective serotonin reuptake inhibitor. Serious: Suicidality, serotonin syndrome, abnormal bleeding, withdrawal reactions. Frequent: Insomnia, ejaculatory disorders, nausea, sweating, fatigue, somnolence.

> **Nursing Implications** Administer tablet or solution by mouth. Do not give to patients on MAOI inhibitors or who might be pregnant. May increase GI bleeding if patients are also taking aspirin or non-steroidal inflammatory drugs. Teach patient to recognize and report side effects especially: suicidal thinking, worsening depression, restlessness, anxiety, hostility, impulsiveness, panic attacks or sleeping difficulties. Drug may cause QT prolongation so caution patient to report any cardiac symptoms. Caution patient not to abruptly stop taking the drug as it must be weaned and not to drive or use machinery until used to drug.

FLUOXETINE (*Prozac, Prozac Weekly, Sarafem*) Depression, OCD: Start 20 mg PO q am; usual effective dose is 20 to 40 mg/day, max 80 mg/day. Depression, maintenance: 20 to 40 mg/day (standard-release) or 90 mg PO once a week (Prozac Weekly) starting 7 days after last standard-release dose. Bulimia: 60 mg PO daily; may need to titrate slowly, over several days. Panic disorder: Start 10 mg PO q am; titrate to 20 mg/day after 1 week, max 60 mg/day. Premenstrual dysphoric disorder (Sarafem): 20 mg PO daily, given either throughout the menstrual cycle or for 14 days prior to menses; max 80 mg/day. Doses greater than 20 mg/day can be divided two times per day (in morning and at noon). Bipolar depression, olanzapine plus fluoxetine: Start 5 mg olanzapine plus 20 mg fluoxetine daily in the evening. Increase to usual range of 5 to 12.5 mg olanzapine plus 20 to 50 mg fluoxetine as tolerated. Treatment-resistant depression, olanzapine plus fluoxetine: Start 5 mg olanzapine plus 20 mg fluoxetine daily in the evening. Increase to usual range of 5 to 20 mg olanzapine plus 20 to 50 mg fluoxetine as tolerated. Suicidality, many drug interactions. ▶L ♀C but – in 3rd trimester ▶– © $$$ Generic/Trade: Tabs 10 mg. Caps 10, 20, 40 mg. Oral soln 20 mg/5 mL. Caps (Sarafem) 10, 20 mg. Trade only: Tabs (Sarafem) 10, 15, 20 mg. Caps delayed-release (Prozac Weekly) 90 mg. Generic only: Tabs 20, 40 mg. Selective serotonin reuptake inhibitor. Serious: Suicidality, serotonin syndrome, neuroleptic malignant syndrome, SIADH, abnormal bleeding, withdrawal reactions, hypoglycemia. Frequent: N/V, diarrhea, insomnia, drowsiness, headache, sexual dysfunction, dry mouth, anorexia, anxiety, nervousness.

> **Nursing Implications** May cause suicidal behavior in children and adolescents. Discontinue drug 5 weeks before giving MAO inhibitors. Give before 2 pm to avoid insomnia. Monitor for anxiety, insomnia, agitation, seizures, suicidal ideas, chest pain and heart arrhythmias, disturbed vision, GI symptoms and loss of appetite, sexual dysfunction, frequent urination and painful periods, hypoglycemia, breathing problems, and skin rashes. Teach pt to report depression or suicidal thoughts, to eat frequent, small meals and drink adequate fluids. Drug may not take effect for 4 weeks.

PAROXETINE (*Paxil, Paxil CR, Pexeva*) Depression: Start 20 mg PO q am, max 50 mg/day. Depression, controlled-release: Start 25 mg PO q am, max 62.5 mg/day. OCD: Start 10 to 20 mg PO q am, max 60 mg/day. Social anxiety disorder: Start 10 to 20 mg PO q am, max 60 mg/day. Social anxiety disorder, controlled-release: Start 12.5 mg PO q am, max 37.5 mg/day. Generalized anxiety disorder: Start 20 mg PO q am, max 50 mg/day. Panic disorder: Start 10 mg PO q am, increase by 10 mg/day at intervals of 1 week or more to usual effective dose of 10 to 60 mg/day; max 60 mg/day. Panic disorder, controlled-release: Start 12.5 mg PO q am, max 75 mg/day. Post-traumatic stress disorder: Start 20 mg PO q am, max 50 mg/day. Premenstrual dysphoric disorder (PMDD), continuous dosing: Start 12.5 mg PO q am (controlled-release); may increase dose after 1 week to max 25 mg q am. PMDD, intermittent dosing (given for 2 weeks prior to menses): 12.5 mg PO q am (controlled-release), max 25 mg/day. Suicidality, many drug interactions. ▶LK ♀D ▶? © $$$ Generic/Trade: Tabs 10, 20, 30, 40 mg. Oral susp 10 mg/5 mL. Controlled-release tabs 12.5, 25 mg. Trade only: (Paxil CR) 37.5 mg. Selective serotonin reuptake inhibitor. Serious: Suicidality, serotonin syndrome, SIADH, hyponatremia, abnormal bleeding, withdrawal reactions. Frequent: Asthenia, nausea, diarrhea, constipation, insomnia, drowsiness, sexual dysfunction, dry mouth, anorexia, nervousness, sweating, dizziness, tremor.

> **Nursing Implications** Patients need to be aware of severe allergic reactions (rash; hives; itching; difficulty breathing; tightness in the chest; swelling of the mouth, face, lips, or tongue) that may develop when taking this medication. Patients need to be advised to take this medication for a minimum of 3 to 4 weeks in order to achieve the desired effect. Patients need to consult their healthcare provider should they have any problems taking this medication. The main side effects to this medication are mental confusion, agitation, and drowsiness. This medication also causes decreased sexual libido. Patients need to be educated that this medication should not be abruptly discontinued with the exception of an acute allergic reaction. This medication should be weaned down gradually when one wants to stop taking this medication.

SERTRALINE   (**Zoloft**) Depression, OCD: Start 50 mg PO daily; usual effective dose is 50 to 200 mg/day, max 200 mg/day. Panic disorder, post-traumatic stress disorder, social anxiety disorder: Start 25 mg PO daily, max 200 mg/day. PMDD, continuous dosing: Start 50 mg PO daily, max 150 mg/day. PMDD, intermittent dosing (given for 14 days prior to menses): Start 50 mg PO daily for 3 days, then increase to 100 mg/day. Suicidality. ▶LK ♀C but – in third trimester ▶+ © $$$ Generic/Trade: Tabs 25, 50, 100 mg. Oral concentrate 20 mg/mL (60 mL). Selective serotonin reuptake inhibitor. Serious: Suicidality, serotonin syndrome, neuroleptic malignant syndrome, SIADH, hyponatremia, abnormal bleeding, withdrawal symptoms. Frequent: N/V, diarrhea, insomnia, drowsiness, headache, sexual dysfunction, dry mouth, anorexia, anxiety, nervousness.

> **Nursing Implications** Zoloft should not be taken within 14 days of taking linezolid, MAOIs, or St. John's wort. Do not take Zoloft with astemizole, fenfluramine derivatives, nefazodone, pimozide, serotonin-norepinephrine reuptake inhibitors, sibutramine, terfenadine, thioridazine, or tryptophan. If there is a history of GI or heart problems or a family history of mental mood issues, Zoloft should not be used. Alcohol and other CNS depressants should be avoided when taking Zoloft. There is a higher incidence of suicidal ideation and action in adolescent patients taking this medication. Adolescents have to be assessed frequently for suicide ideation. Observe patients for serotonin syndrome, which can be a fatal condition. Signs and symptoms of this condition include agitation, confusion, hallucinations, coma, fever, cardiac dysrhythmias, tremor, excessive sweating, nausea, vomiting, and diarrhea. Observe patients for neuroleptic malignant syndrome (NMS), which also can be fatal. Signs and symptoms of this medication include fever and muscle stiffness. Emergency medical care must be sought should these conditions result.

Antidepressants—Serotonin-Norepinephrine Reuptake Inhibitors (SNRIs)

VENLAFAXINE   (**Effexor, Effexor XR**) Depression/anxiety: Start 37.5 to 75 mg PO daily (Effexor XR) or 75 mg/day divided two to three times per day (Effexor). Usual effective dose is 150 to 225 mg/day, max 225 mg/day (Effexor XR) or 375 mg/day (Effexor). Generalized anxiety disorder: Start 37.5 to 75 mg PO daily (Effexor XR), max 225 mg/day. Social anxiety disorder: 75 mg PO daily (Effexor XR). Panic disorder: Start 37.5 mg PO daily (Effexor XR), may titrate by 75 mg/day at weekly intervals to max 225 mg/day. Suicidality, seizures, HTN. ▶LK ♀C but – in 3rd trimester ▶? © $$$$ Generic/Trade: Caps extended-release 37.5, 75, 150 mg. Tabs 25, 37.5, 50, 75, 100 mg. Generic only: Tabs extended-release 37.5, 75, 150, 225 mg. Serotonin and norepinephrine reuptake inhibitor; also a weak inhibitor of dopamine reuptake. Serious: Suicidality, mania/hypomania, seizures, hypertension, withdrawal symptoms, serotonin syndrome, neuroleptic malignant syndrome, interstitial lung disease and eosinophilic pneumonia, toxic epidermal necrolysis. Frequent: Drowsiness, dizziness, sexual dysfunction, anorexia, N/V, asthenia, nervousness, insomnia, diaphoresis, constipation, dry mouth, abnormal vision.

> **Nursing Implications** Observe patients for signs and symptoms of allergic reactions such as hives, urticaria, shortness of breath, tightness in the chest, unusual hoarseness, and swelling of the mouth, face, lips, or tongue. These medications may increase signs and symptoms of depression. Patients must be observed cautiously for suicidal ideation. Assess patients frequently for suicidal ideation and if they have a plan to commit suicide. Observe for other changes in behavior. Serotonin syndrome or neuroleptic malignant syndrome (NMS) – like reaction can result when patients are taking this medication. Monitor blood pressure to assess for elevation in systolic and diastolic blood pressure. Other medications that affect the neurological system should be used cautiously with careful monitoring of the patient.

Antidepressants—Other

BUPROPION   (**Wellbutrin, Wellbutrin SR, Wellbutrin XL, Aplenzin, Zyban, Buproban**) Depression: Start 100 mg PO two times per day (immediate-release tabs); can increase to 100 mg three times per day after 4 to 7 days. Usual effective dose is 300 to 450 mg/day, max 150 mg/dose and 450 mg/day. Sustained-release: Start 150 mg PO q am; may increase to 150 mg two times per day after 4 to 7 days, max 400 mg/day. Give last dose no later than 5 pm. Extended-release: Start 150 mg PO q am; may increase to 300 mg q am after 4 days, max 450 mg q am. Extended-release (Aplenzin): Start 174 mg PO q am; increase to target dose of 348 mg/day after 4 days or more. May increase to max dose of 522 mg/day after 4 weeks or more. Seasonal affective disorder: Start 150 mg of extended-release PO q am in autumn; can increase to 300 mg q am after 1 week, max 300 mg/day. In the spring, decrease to 150 mg/day for 2 weeks and then discontinue. Smoking cessation (Zyban, Buproban): Start 150 mg PO q am for 3 days, then increase to 150 mg PO two times per day for 7 to 12 weeks. Max 150 mg PO two times per day. Give last dose no later than 5 pm. Seizures, suicidality. ▶LK ♀C ▶– © $$$$ Generic/Trade (for depression, bupropion HCl): Tabs 75, 100 mg. Sustained-release tabs 100, 150, 200 mg. Extended-release tabs 150, 300 mg (Wellbutrin XL). Generic/Trade (Smoking cessation): Sustained-release tabs 150 mg (Zyban, Buproban). Trade only: Extended-release (Aplenzin, bupropion hydrobromide) tabs 174, 348, 522 mg. Norepinephrine and dopamine reuptake inhibitor. Serious: Suicidality, seizures, psychosis, HTN, Stevens-Johnson syndrome, rhabdomyolysis, hallucinations. Frequent: Headache, tremor, agitation, insomnia, diaphoresis, weight loss, dry mouth, nausea, constipation, dizziness.

> **Nursing Implications** Use cautiously in patients taking seizure medications such as Tegretol, Phenobarbital or Dilantin; or on antipsychotic drugs such as Mellaril, Haldol, or Risperidal. Read manufacturer list of drug interactions. Monitor for suicidal thoughts or unusual changes in behavior. Promote reporting of symptoms to provider such as agitation, dry mouth, insomnia, headache, nausea, constipation, and tremors.

TRAZODONE (*Desyrel, Oleptro*) Depression: Start 50 to 150 mg/day PO in divided doses; usual effective dose is 400 to 600 mg/day. Extended-release: Start 150 mg PO at bedtime. May increase by 75 mg/day q 3 days to max 375 mg/day. Insomnia: 50 to 150 mg PO at bedtime. ▶L ♀C ▶– © $ Trade only: Extended-release tabs (Oleptro) 150, 300 mg. Generic only: Tabs 50, 100, 150, 300 mg. Serotonin reuptake inhibitor and 5-HT2A receptor antagonist. Serious: Orthostatic hypotension, priapism, syncope. Frequent: Drowsiness, dizziness, nervousness, headache, tremor, fatigue, dry mouth, blurred vision.

> **Nursing Implications** Risk of suicidal thoughts or actions are higher in children, teenagers, and young adults. These individuals need to be assessed frequently for suicide ideation. Families and those providing care need to observe the patient closely and report to the prescribing healthcare provider any changes in behavior or if feelings of suicide or depression have increased. Patients need to be observed for serotonin syndrome and neuroleptic malignant syndrome, which are both life-threatening conditions. Emergency medical care must be sought immediately when signs and symptoms of these conditions occur.

Antimanic (Bipolar) Agents

LITHIUM (*Eskalith, Eskalith CR, Lithobid, ♦ Lithane*) Acute mania: Start 300 to 600 mg PO two to three times per day; usual effective dose is 900 to 1800 mg/day. Steady state is achieved in 5 days. Bipolar maintenance usually 900 to 1200 mg/day titrated to therapeutic trough level of 0.6 to 1.2 mEq/L. ▶K ♀D ▶– © $ Generic/Trade: Caps 300, Extended-release tabs 300, 450 mg. Generic only: Caps 150, 600 mg, Tabs 300 mg, Syrup 300 mg/5 mL. Unknown, may increase synthesis and release of serotonin and inhibit its reuptake. Serious: Seizures, ventricular arrhythmias, leukocytosis, hypothyroidism, renal failure, nephrogenic diabetes insipidus, coma, drug-induced parkinsonism. Frequent: Tremor, N/V, diarrhea, cramps, polyuria, polydipsia, rash, fatigue.

> **Nursing Implications** Administer tablet, capsule or syrup by mouth. Lithium may cause goiter therefore symptoms of hypothyroidism must be reported including: dry skin, hair loss, voice changes, increased mania or depression, swelling of lower extremities or neck, and sensitivity to cold. Patient must comply with periodic blood lithium blood level tests since high levels can cause nausea, muscle twitching, confusion, heart arrhythmias, vision changes, poor appetite, tremors, gait problems, seizures and coma. Teach patient to limit alcohol consumption and activities that cause sweating such as exercise, hot tubs, etc. Do not drive or operate machinery until effects of drugs are known. Dosage may need to be monitored more closely in elderly patients as they may have a greater sensitivity to the drug.

VALPROIC ACID—PSYCH (*Depakote, Depakote ER, Stavzor*, divalproex, *♦ Epiject, Epival, Deproic*) Mania: 250 mg PO three times per day (Depakote) or 25 mg/kg once daily (Depakote ER); max 60 mg/kg/day. Hepatotoxicity, drug interactions, reduce dose in the elderly. ▶L ♀D ▶+ © $$$$ Generic only: Syrup (Valproic acid) 250 mg/5 mL. Generic/Trade: Delayed-release tabs (Depakote) 125, 250, 500 mg. Extended-release tabs (Depakote ER) 250, 500 mg. Delayed-release sprinkle caps (Depakote) 125 mg. Trade only (Stavzor): Delayed-release caps 125, 250, 500 mg. Anticonvulsant; may increase GABA levels and modulate sodium channels. Serious: Hepatotoxicity, anaphylaxis, polycystic ovarian syndrome, bone marrow suppression, thrombocytopenia, pancreatitis, Stevens-Johnson syndrome, hyperammonemia, drug-induced parkinsonism. Frequent: N/V, diarrhea, dyspepsia, weight gain, CNS depression, drowsiness, dizziness, tremor, alopecia, rash, nystagmus.

> Nursing Implications   Liver failure resulting in death can occur; serious pancreatitis can occur. Closely monitor for seizures; regularly titrate drug blood levels; take with food; swallow extended-release capsules whole. Patient must report malaise, weakness, appetite, vomiting, jaundice. Drug must be weaned. Avoid alcohol. Review patient's other drugs and check regularly for interactions.

Antipsychotics—First Generation (Typical)

PERPHENAZINE   Start 4 to 8 mg PO three times per day or 8 to 16 mg PO two to four times per day (hospitalized patients), maximum 64 mg/day PO. Can give 5 to 10 mg IM q 6 h, maximum 30 mg/day IM. ▶LK ♀C ▶? © $$$ Generic only: Tabs 2, 4, 8, 16 mg. Oral concentrate 16 mg/5 mL. High-potency dopamine antagonist. Serious: Seizures, neuroleptic malignant syndrome, extrapyramidal side effects, tardive dyskinesia, QT prolongation, jaundice. Frequent: Drowsiness, nausea, dry mouth, constipation, urinary retention, hypotension, headache, hyperprolactinemia.

> Nursing Implications   This medication may cause twitching or uncontrollable movements of eyes, lips, tongue, face, arms, or legs; tremor (uncontrolled shaking); drooling; trouble swallowing; problems with balance or walking; feeling restless, jittery, or agitated; confusion; unusual thoughts or behavior; and feeling like "passing out." This medication may lower the seizure threshold, thus a patient will be more prone to seizures. Decreased night vision, tunnel vision, watery eyes, and photosensitivity may result when takng this medication. Nurses need to monitor renal and liver function. Patients need to be advised not to drink alcohol when taking this medication. Patients need to be educated to avoid exposure to sunlight or tanning beds.

Antipsychotics—Second Generation (Atypical)

LURASIDONE   (*Latuda*)   Start 40 mg PO daily. Effective dose range 40 to 120 mg/day, max 160 mg/day. Take with food. ▶K − ♀B ▶? © Trade only: Tabs 20, 40, 80, 120 mg. Dopamine-2/serotonin 2A antagonist Serious: Neuroleptic malignant syndrome, hyperglycemia, diabetes, tardive dyskinesia, hyperlipidemia, hyperprolactinemia, leukopenia, neutropenia, agranulocytosis, orthostatic hypotension, syncope. Frequent: Parkinsonism, akathisia, somnolence, nausea, agitation.

> Nursing Implications   Administer tablet with food. Patient may experience sleepiness, agitation, akatisia (inability to remain still), Parkinson-like symptoms and nausea. Not for use in elderly with dementia/psychosis. Assess patient per administration for kidney, liver disease, diabetes including family history, obesity, hypotension, seizures, swallowing problems and low WBC. Drug may cause tardive dyskinsia (a permanent condition), high blood sugar, high prolactin levels causing lactation, prolonged erection in males or Neuroleptic Malignant Syndrome which can cause death. Prescriber should be called immediately if any of the above symptoms occur. Patient should avoid strenuous activities that cause overheating since drug may interfere with sweating mechanism. Do not drive or operate machinery until effects of medication is known.

QUETIAPINE   (*Seroquel, Seroquel XR*)   Schizophrenia: Start 25 mg PO two times per day (regular tabs); increase by 25 to 50 mg two to three times per day on days 2 and 3, and then to target dose of 300 to 400 mg/day divided two to three times per day on day 4. Usual effective dose is 150 to 750 mg/day, max 800 mg/day. Schizophrenia, extended-release tabs: Start 300 mg PO daily in evening, increase by up to 300 mg/day at intervals of more than 1 day to usual effective range of 400 to 800 mg/day. Acute bipolar mania, monotherapy, or adjunctive: Start 50 mg PO two times per day on day 1, then increase to no higher than 100 mg two times per day on day 2, 150 mg two times per day on day 3, and 200 mg two times per day on day 4. May increase prn to 300 mg two times per day on day 5 and 400 mg two times per day thereafter. Usual effective dose is 400 to 800 mg/day. Acute bipolar mania, monotherapy or adjunctive, extended-release: Start 300 mg PO evening of day 1, 600 mg day 2, and 400 to 800 mg/day thereafter. Bipolar depression, regular and extended-release: 50 mg PO at bedtime on day 1, 100 mg at bedtime day 2, 200 mg at bedtime day 3, and 300 mg at bedtime day 4. May increase prn to 400 mg at bedtime on day 5 and 600 mg at bedtime on day 8. Bipolar maintenance: Continue dose required to maintain remission. Major depressive disorder, adjunctive to antidepressants, extended-release: Start 50 mg evening of day 1, may increase to 150 mg on day 3. Max 300 mg/day. Eye exam for cataracts recommended q 6 months. ▶LK ♀C ▶– © $$$$$ Trade only: Tabs 25, 50, 100, 200, 300, 400 mg. Extended-release tabs 50, 150, 200, 300, 400 mg. Dopamine receptor antagonist; 5-HT2A receptor antagonist. Serious: Seizures, orthostatic hypotension, syncope, hyperglycemia, diabetes, dyslipidemia, neuroleptic malignant syndrome, QT prolongation, suicidal thinking/behavior. Frequent: Drowsiness, weight gain, nausea, dry mouth, constipation, dizziness.

> **Nursing Implications** Administer PO by tab. Monitor for severe allergic reaction/anaphylaxis. May cause death if given to elderly pts experiencing dementia-related psychosis. May increase risk of suicide in depressed patients. Teach family/caregivers to watch for suicidal potential, and changes in behavior and report to prescriber. Most common adverse reactions are headache, dry mouth, sleepiness, agitation, and dizziness. GI disturbances, elevated HR, and extrapyramidal symptoms may occur. Teach family to report dystonia including muscle spasms, swallowing and breathing difficulties, and involuntary protrusion of tongue. Caution in use with other drugs that act on CNS and with drugs known to cause electrolyte imbalance or an increase in the QT interval of the heart.

Anxiolytics/Hypnotics—Benzodiazepines—Long Half-Life (25 to 100 h)

CLONAZEPAM (*Klonopin, Klonopin Wafer, ✦ Rivotril, Clonapam*) Panic disorder: Start 0.25 to 0.5 mg PO two to three times per day, max 4 mg/day. Half-life 18 to 50 h. Epilepsy: Start 0.5 mg PO three times per day. Max 20 mg/day. ▶LK ♀D ▶– ©IV $ Generic/Trade: Tabs 0.5, 1, 2 mg. Orally disintegrating tabs (approved for panic disorder only) 0.125, 0.25, 0.5, 1, 2 mg. Enhances actions of GABA. Serious: Respiratory depression, CNS depression, dependence, withdrawal reactions, seizures. Frequent: Sedation, fatigue, ataxia, memory impairment, depression, confusion, nausea, constipation, dry mouth, rash.

ANTIPSYCHOTIC RELATIVE ADVERSE EFFECTS[a]

Generation	Antipsychotic	Anticholinergic	Sedation	Hypotension	EPS	Weight Gain	Diabetes/Hyperglycemia	Dyslipidemia
1st	chlorpromazine	+++	+++	++	++	++	?	?
1st	fluphenazine	++	+	+	++++	++	?	?
1st	haloperidol	+	+	+	++++	++	0	?
1st	loxapine	++	+	+	++	+	?	?
1st	molindone	++	++	+	++	+	?	?
1st	perphenazine	++	++	+	++	+	+/?	?
1st	pimozide	+	+	+	+++	?	?	?
1st	thioridazine	++++	+++	+++	+	+++	+/?	?
1st	thiothixene	+	++	++	+++	++	?	/
1st	trifluoperazine	++	+	+	+++	++	?	?
2nd	aripiprazole	++	+	0	0	0/+	0	0
2nd	asenapine	+	+	++	++	+	?	?
2nd	clozapine	++++	+++	+++	0	+++	+	+
2nd	iloperidone	++	+	+++	+	++	?	?
2nd	olanzapine	+++	++	+	0[b]	+++	+	+
2nd	paliperidone	+	+	++	++	++	?	?
2nd	risperidone	+	++	+	+[b]	++	?	?
2nd	quetiapine	+	+++	++	0	++	?	?
2nd	ziprasidone	+	+	0	0	0/+	0	0

[a]Risk of specific adverse effects is graded from 0 (absent) to ++++ (high). ? = Limited or inconsistent comparative data.
[b]Extrapyramidal symptoms (EPS) are dose-related and are more likely for risperidone greater than 6 to 8 mg/day, olanzapine greater than 20 mg/day. Akathisia risk remains unclear and may not be reflected in these ratings. There are limited comparative data for aripiprazole iloperidone, paliperidone, and asenapine relative to other second-generation antipsychotics.

References: Goodman & Gilman 11e p461-500, *Applied Therapeutics* 8e p78, APA schizophrenia practice guideline, *Psychiatry Q* 2002; 73:297, *Diabetes Care* 2004;27:596, *Pharmacotherapy. A Pathophysiologic Approach*, 8. pg 1158, 2011.

> **Nursing Implications** Take with 8 ounces of water. Instruct patient to allow tab to dissolve on tongue. Do not use in patients with severe liver disease or patients allergic to this drug and other benzodiazepines. Use cautiously in patients with liver or kidney disease, glaucoma, breathing disorders, history of depression or suicidal thoughts, or history of alcohol and drug addiction. Promote seeking emergency medical help if allergic reaction symptoms occur. Administer largest dose at bedtime to avoid daytime sedation. Taper by 0.25 mg every 3 days to decrease signs and symptoms of withdrawal. Some patients may require longer taper period (months). Institute seizure precautions for patients on initial therapy or undergoing dose manipulations.

DIAZEPAM (*Valium, Diastat, Diastat AcuDial, Diazepam Intensol, ✦ Vivol, E Pam, Diazemuls*) Active seizures: 5 to 10 mg IV q 10 to 15 min to max 30 mg, or 0.2 to 0.5 mg/kg rectal gel PR. Skeletal muscle spasm, spasticity related to cerebral palsy, paraplegia, athetosis, "stiff man syndrome": 2 to 10 mg PO/PR three to four times per day. Anxiety: 2 to 10 mg PO two to four times per day. Half-life 20 to 80 h. Alcohol withdrawal: 10 mg PO three to four times per day for 24 h then 5 mg PO three to four times per day prn. ▶LK ♀D ▶– ©IV $ Generic/Trade: Tabs 2, 5, 10 mg. Generic only: Oral soln 5 mg/5 mL. Oral concentrate (Intensol) 5 mg/mL. Trade only: Rectal gel (Diastat) 2.5, 5, 10, 15, 20 mg. Rectal gel (Diastat AcuDial) 10, 20 mg. Enhances actions of GABA, skeletal muscle relaxant. Serious: Respiratory depression, oversedation, dependence, withdrawal reactions, cardiovascular collapse (parenteral), vascular impairment or venous thrombosis (IV only), seizures. Frequent: Sedation, ataxia, CNS stimulation, depression, N/V, constipation or diarrhea, confusion, tinnitus, blurred vision.

> **Nursing Implications** Avoid alcohol; wean drug/never stop abruptly; avoid driving until effects of drug are known. If IV administer slowly and force bed rest; provide ambulation support for elderly; Avoid use in elderly pts if possible.

Anxiolytics/Hypnotics—Benzodiazepines—Medium Half-Life (10 to 15 h)

NOTE: *To avoid withdrawal, gradually taper when discontinuing after prolonged use. Sedative-hypnotics have been associated with severe allergic reactions and complex sleep behaviors including sleep driving. Use caution and discuss with patients.*

LORAZEPAM (*Ativan*) Anxiety: 0.5 to 2 mg IV/IM/PO q 6 to 8 h, max 10 mg/day. Half-life 10 to 20 h. Status epilepticus: Adult: 4 mg IV over 2 min; may repeat in 10 to 15 min. Status epilepticus: Peds: 0.05 to 0.1 mg/kg (max 4 mg) IV over 2 to 5 min; may repeat 0.05 mg/kg once in 10 to 15 min. ▶LK ♀D ▶– ©IV $ Generic/Trade: Tabs 0.5, 1, 2 mg. Generic only: Oral concentrate 2 mg/mL. Enhances actions of GABA. Serious: Cardiovascular collapse, hypotension, apnea (parenteral), respiratory depression, dependence, withdrawal syndrome. Frequent: Drowsiness, dizziness, ataxia, headache, confusion, memory problems, depression, paradoxical CNS stimulation.

> **Nursing Implications** Administer tablet with 8 oz of water only; do not administer with, or just after, a meal. Do not crush, chew or break tablet. Do not use in patients allergic to zolpidem. Use cautiously in patients with lactose intolerance, history of renal or liver dysfunction, lung disease or breathing problems, myasthenia gravis, history of depression or suicidal thoughts, or history of drug or alcohol addiction. Notify provider immediately if symptoms such as stomach pain, cramps, nausea, vomiting, anxiety, tremors and seizure occur. Teach patient to refrain from drinking alcohol and driving. Notify provider immediately if memory loss occurs.

TEMAZEPAM (*Restoril*) 7.5 to 30 mg PO at bedtime. Half-life 8 to 25 h. ▶LK ♀X ▶– ©IV $ Generic/Trade: Caps 7.5, 15, 22.5, 30 mg. Enhances actions of GABA. Serious: Respiratory depression, dependence, withdrawal reactions, seizures. Frequent: Sedation, fatigue, ataxia, memory impairment, depression, confusion, nausea, constipation, dry mouth, rash.

> **Nursing Implications** Administer tablet by mouth 30 minutes before bedtime. Avoid use with alcohol or drugs that promote drowsiness. Teach patient that medication may cause excessive sleepiness/drowsiness, headache, depression and loss of orientation. Patient should not drive or operate machinery until effects of medication is known. Drug needs to be weaned; stopping drug suddenly may cause seizures, tremors, muscle pain, vomiting, excessive sweating, or feelings of lack of self-worth.

Anxiolytics/Hypnotics—Benzodiazepines—Short Half-Life (Less than 12 h)

NOTE: *To avoid withdrawal, gradually taper when discontinuing after prolonged use. Sedative-hypnotics have been associated with severe allergic reactions and complex sleep behaviors including sleep driving. Use caution and discuss with patients.*

OXAZEPAM (*Serax*) 10 to 30 mg PO three to four times per day. Half-life 8 h. ▶LK ♀D ▶– ©IV $$$ Generic/Trade: Caps 10, 15, 30 mg. Trade only: Tabs 15 mg. Enhances actions of GABA. Serious: Respiratory depression, dependence, withdrawal reactions, seizures. Frequent: Sedation, fatigue, ataxia, memory impairment, depression, confusion, nausea, constipation, dry mouth, rash.

> Nursing Implications Patients need to be made aware that this medication may be habit forming. This is a controlled dangerous substance. Patients should be advised not to drink alcohol when taking this medication as the effects of this medication can be potentiated. Other medications that have a similar effect on the central nervous system should be avoided. The most dangerous side effect is grand mal seizures when patients are withdrawing from this medication. The most common side effects of this medication are drowsiness, dizziness, amnesia or forgetfulness, trouble concentrating, slurred speech, swelling, and headache.

Anxiolytics/Hypnotics—Other

ZOLPIDEM (*Ambien, Ambien CR, Zolpimist, Edluar*) Adult: Insomnia: Standard tabs: 10 mg PO at bedtime. For age older than 65 yo or debilitated: 5 mg PO at bedtime. Oral spray: 10 mg PO at bedtime. For age older than 65 yo or debilitated: 5 mg PO at bedtime. Controlled-release tabs: 12.5 mg PO at bedtime. For age older than 65 yo or debilitated: Give 6.25 mg PO at bedtime. Do not use for benzodiazepine or alcohol withdrawal. ▶L ♀C ▶+ ©IV $$$$ Generic/Trade: Tabs 5, 10 mg. Trade only: Controlled-release tabs 6.25, 12.5 mg, oral spray 5 mg/actuation (Zolpimist), sublingual tab 5, 10 mg (Edluar). Selective GABA-benzodiazepine omega-1 agonist. Serious: Sleep driving, abnormal thinking, behavioral changes, depression, suicidal ideation, hallucinations, anaphylaxis. Frequent: Drowsiness, dizziness, nausea, headache, nervousness, decreased daytime recall.

> Nursing Implications Assess for all allergies especially to benzodiazepines, kidney and liver disease, glaucoma, breathing problems, mood disorders, or alcohol abuse. Teach pt to avoid driving, operating machinery, or any complex activities until used to drug. Monitor for development of confusion, depression, suicidal thoughts, agitation/hostility, hallucinations, fainting, vision problems, GI symptoms including increased bilirubin, rashes, alopecia, and blood disorders. Should not be used in pts with primary depression or psychosis. Teach pt that dependence is possible; drug should be weaned. Use zolpidem cautiously when patients are also on CNS depressants, azole antifungal agents, flumazenil, rifamycins, and ritonavir. It is important to educate the patient about lifestyle changes to improve sleep such as the avoidance of caffeine and nicotine, maintaining a quiet and dark environment, relaxation techniques, and warm baths. Patients should be advised not to take this medication unless they are planning to obtain 7 to 8 h of sleep. It is important not to use alcohol or other CNS depressants when taking this medication. Should not be given to breastfeeding mothers.

Drug-Dependence Therapy

VARENICLINE (*Chantix*) Smoking cessation: Start 0.5 mg PO daily for days 1 to 3, then 0.5 mg two times per day days 4 to 7, then 1 mg two times per day thereafter. Take after meals with full glass of water. Start 1 week prior to cessation and continue for 12 weeks or patient may start the drug and stop smoking between days 8 and 35 or treatment. ▶K ♀C ▶? © $$$$ Trade only: Tabs 0.5, 1 mg. Nicotinic acetylcholine receptor agonist. Serious: Depression, suicidal thoughts, aggression, erratic behavior, MI, stroke, angina. Frequent: N/V, drowsiness, dreaming disturbances, insomnia, headache, abnormal dreams, constipation.

> Nursing Implications Begin taking 1 week prior to last designated date for smoking. Administer with 8 ounces of water and after a meal. Use cautiously in patients with history of kidney disease or mental illness. Promote caution while driving or using heavy machinery. Promote notifying provider and stoppage of drug if patient experiences mood or behavior changes or thoughts of suicide. Monitor for fever, sore throat, headache, rash, and blistering of skin. Discuss drug interactions with provider.

Stimulants/ADHD/Anorexiants

METHYLPHENIDATE (*Ritalin, Ritalin LA, Ritalin SR, Methylin, Methylin ER, Metadate ER, Metadate CD, Concerta, Daytrana,* ✦ *Biphentin*) ADHD/narcolepsy: 5 to 10 mg PO two to three times per day or 20 mg PO q am (sustained and extended-release), max 60 mg/day. Or 18 to 36 mg PO q am (Concerta), max 72 mg/day. Avoid evening doses. Monitor growth and use drug holidays when appropriate. ▶LK ♀C ▶? ©II

BODY MASS INDEX* (Heights are in feet and inches; weights are in pounds)

BMI	Class	4' 10"	5' 0"	5' 4"	5' 8"	6' 0"	6' 4"
<19	Underweight	<91	<97	<110	<125	<140	<156
19–24	Healthy weight	91–119	97–127	110–144	125–163	140–183	156–204
25–29	Overweight	120–143	128–152	145–173	164–196	184–220	205–245
30–40	Obese	144–191	153–204	174–233	197–262	221–293	246–328
>40	Very Obese	>191	>204	>233	>262	>293	>328

*BMI = kg/m² = (wt in pounds)(703)/(height in inches)². Anorectants appropriate if BMI ≥30 (with comorbidities ≥27); surgery an option if BMI >40 (with comorbidities 35–40). www.nhlbi.nih.gov

$$ Trade only: Tabs 5, 10, 20 mg (Ritalin, Methylin, Metadate). Tabs extended-release 10, 20 mg (Methylin ER, Metadate ER). Tabs extended-release 18, 27, 36, 54 mg (Concerta). Caps extended-release 10, 20, 30, 40, 50, 60 mg (Metadate CD) May be sprinkled on food. Tabs sustained-release 20 mg (Ritalin SR). Caps extended-release 10, 20, 30, 40 mg (Ritalin LA). Tabs chewable 2.5, 5, 10 mg (Methylin). Oral soln 5 mg/5 mL, 10 mg/5 mL (Methylin). Transdermal patch (Daytrana) 10 mg/9 h, 15 mg/9 h, 20 mg/9 h, 30 mg/9 h. Generic only: Tabs 5, 10, 20 mg, tabs extended-release 10, 20 mg, tabs sustained-release 20 mg. CNS stimulant, increases norepinephrine and dopamine. Serious: Sudden death, seizures, psychosis, hypertension, contact sensitization (Daytrana). Frequent: Appetite suppression, weight loss, insomnia, nervousness, N/V, dizziness, palpitations, tachycardia, headache.

> Nursing Implications Do not crush extended-release tabs; give in cool, semisolid food; if using patch apply to clean, dry hip area; should be given before bedtime to prevent insomnia; carefully monitor for CNS side effects including tics, for rises or a drop in BP, for blurred vision, GI symptoms, and skin eruptions. Child's wt and growth pattern should be carefully monitored in long-term use treatment. Watch for drug interactions especially with drinks, drugs, or herbs that contain caffeine. Monitor pulse, BP, and respiration before and periodically during treatment. This medication can produce false states of euphoria and well being. Observe patients for recurring depression and frequent periods of rest after the medication effects wear off. Ritalin has high abuse and dependency potential. ADHD pts: Check impulse control, interactions with other individuals, and assess patients for attention span. Treatment can be interrupted at intervals to decide if symptoms could be tolerated with continuation of therapy. Observe and document episode frequency with narcolepsy. Monitor CBC and platelet counts with patients receiving prolonged treatment/therapy.

MODAFINIL   (*Provigil, ✦ Alertec*) Narcolepsy and sleep apnea/hypopnea: 200 mg PO q am. Shift work sleep disorder: 200 mg PO 1 h before shift. ▶L ♀C ▶? ©IV $$$$$ Trade only: Tabs 100, 200 mg. Wake-promoting agent; CNS stimulant. Serious: Rash, Stevens-Johnson syndrome, multi-organ hypersensitivity, leukopenia, psychosis, mania, suicidal ideation, aggression. Frequent: Insomnia, nausea, headache, nervousness, anxiety.

> Nursing Implications Medication should be used cautiously with cardiac disease patients. This includes chest pain, ventricular hypertrophy (left side), ischemic ECG changes, mitral valve prolapse, unstable agina, recent MI, and dysrhythmias. This medication is a controlled substance and may cause dependency and addiction. Patients on hormonal birth control products need to be advised to use alternative and additional birth control methods. Serious fatal reactions such as Stevens-Johnson syndrome may occur with this medication.

PULMONARY

Beta Agonists—Short-Acting

ALBUTEROL   (*AccuNeb, Ventolin HFA, Proventil HFA, ProAir HFA, VoSpire ER, ✦ Airomir, Asmavent, salbutamol*) MDI: 2 puffs q 4 to 6 h prn. Soln: 0.5 mL of 0.5% soln (2.5 mg) nebulized three to four times per day. One 3 mL unit dose (0.083%) nebulized three to four times per day. Caps for inhalation: 200 to 400 mcg q 4 to 6 h. Tabs: 2 to 4 mg PO three to four times per day or extended-release 4 to 8 mg PO q 12 h up to 16 mg PO q 12 h. Peds: 0.1 to 0.2 mg/kg/dose PO three times per day up to 4 mg three times per day for age 2 to 5 yo, 2 to 4 mg or extended-release 4 mg PO q 12 h for age 6 to 12 yo. Prevention of exercise-induced bronchospasm: MDI: 2 puffs 10 to 30 min before exercise. ▶L ♀C ▶? © $$ Trade only: MDI

90 mcg/actuation, 200 metered doses/canister. "HFA" inhalers use hydrofluoroalkane propellant instead of CFCs but are otherwise equivalent. Generic/Trade: Soln for inhalation 0.021% (AccuNeb), 0.042% (AccuNeb), and 0.083% in 3 mL vials, 0.5% (5 mg/mL) in 20 mL with dropper. Tabs extended-release 4, 8 mg (VoSpire ER). Generic only: Syrup 2 mg/5 mL. Tabs immediate-release 2, 4 mg. Short-acting beta agonist bronchodilator. Serious: Hypersensitivity, paradoxical bronchospasm. Frequent: Palpitations, tachycardia, hypokalemia, tremor, lightheadedness, nervousness, headache, and nausea.

> Nursing Implications Use cautiously in patients with history of heart disease, high blood pressure, congestive heart failure, seizure disorders, diabetes, or overactive thyroid. Notify provider immediately if symptoms appear such as nervousness, headache, tremors, dry mouth, chest pain, rapid heart rate, pain in arm or shoulder, nausea, sweating, dizziness, seizure, or fainting.

LEVALBUTEROL (*Xopenex, Xopenex HFA*) MDI 2 puffs q 4 to 6 h prn. Nebulizer 0.63 to 1.25 mg q 6 to 8 h. Peds: 0.31 mg nebulized three times per day for age 6 to 11 yo. ▶L ♀C ▶? © $$$ Generic/Trade: Soln for inhalation 0.31, 0.63, 1.25 mg in 3 mL and 1.25 mg in 0.5 mL unit-dose vials. Trade only: HFA MDI 45 mcg/actuation, 15 g 200/canister. "HFA" inhalers use hydrofluoroalkane propellant. Short-acting beta agonist bronchodilator. Serious: Hypersensitivity, paradoxical bronchospasm, arrhythmias. Frequent: Palpitations, tachycardia, hypokalemia, tremor, lightheadedness, nervousness, headache, and nausea.

> Nursing Implications Administered by inhalation through nebulizer. Check solution and do not use if discolored or containing particles. If concentrated solution used, dilute with sterile saline. Teach patient proper preparation, inhalation and cleaning techniques. Only mix with other drugs in nebulizer as directed by prescriber. Teach patient to immediately report symptoms of anxiety, irregular/rapid HR, cramps in legs, weakness, chest pain or increased breathing problems. Assess for cardiac disease including high BP, arrhythmias; history of seizures, hyperthyroidism, diabetes or kidney disease and report to prescriber. Do not drive or operate machinery until used to drug. Elderly may be more sensitive and prone to side effects on the heart. Carefully assess all other medications patient is taking for possible drug interactions.

Combinations

ADVAIR (fluticasone—inhaled + salmeterol, *Advair HFA*) Asthma: DPI: 1 puff two times per day (all strengths). MDI: 2 puffs two times per day (all strengths). COPD: DPI: 1 puff two times per day (250/50 only). ▶L ♀C ▶? © $$$$$ Trade only: DPI: 100/50, 250/50, 500/50 mcg fluticasone/salmeterol per actuation; 60 doses/DPI. Trade only (Advair HFA): MDI 45/21, 115/21, 230/21 mcg fluticasone/salmeterol per actuation; 120 doses/canister. Anti-inflammatory/long-acting beta agonist bronchodilator combination. Serious: Hypersensitivity, anaphylaxis, paradoxical bronchospasm, Churg-Strauss syndrome. Frequent: Thrush, dysphonia, pharyngitis, palpitations, tachycardia, tremor, lightheadedness, nervousness, headache, nausea.

> Nursing Implications Promote reporting of symptoms to provider, such as headache, dizziness, muscle or bone pain, nausea, nervousness, sore throat, shakiness, and vomiting. Monitor and report severe symptoms such as difficulty breathing, fever, behavioral changes, chest pain, vision changes, numbness or tingling in hands and feet, seizures, and cramps. Promote rinsing and cleaning of mouth and teeth after dosage to prevent occurrence of thrush. Inhaler use instruction. Date canister when first used.

PREDICTED PEAK EXPIRATORY FLOW (liters/min)   *Am Rev Resp Dis* 1963; 88:644

Age (yo)	Women (height in inches)					Men (height in inches)					Child (height in inches)	
	55"	60"	65"	70"	75"	60"	65"	70"	75"	80"		
20	390	423	460	496	529	554	602	649	693	740	44"	160
30	380	413	448	483	516	532	577	622	664	710	46"	187
40	370	402	436	470	502	509	552	596	636	680	48"	214
50	360	391	424	457	488	486	527	569	607	649	50"	240
60	350	380	412	445	475	463	502	542	578	618	52"	267
70	340	369	400	432	461	440	477	515	550	587	54"	293

Inhaled Steroids

NOTE: *See Endocrine—Corticosteroids when oral steroids necessary.*

FLUTICASONE—INHALED (*Flovent HFA, Flovent Diskus*) 2 to 4 puffs two times per day. ▶L ♀C ▶?
© $$$$ Trade only: HFA MDI: 44, 110, 220 mcg/actuation 120/canister. DPI (Diskus): 50, 100, 250 mcg/actuation delivering 44, 88, 220 mcg respectively. Steroidal anti-inflammatory. Serious: Adrenal suppression (high dose), anaphylaxis, Churg-Strauss syndrome, bronchospasm. Frequent: Thrush, dysphonia, pharyngitis, headache.

> **Nursing Implications** Assess pt for history of allergies, current and past infections such as TB and herpes; eye disorders, bone loss, and liver disease. Teach pt to wash hands before treatment to prevent infection spread and to avoid persons with infections. In pts also receiving chronic oral corticosteroid therapy with Flovent, carefully monitor for signs of asthma instability and adrenal insufficiency. Teach pt to avoid spraying near eyes, shake well before use, and store at room temp.

INHALED STEROIDS: ESTIMATED COMPARATIVE DAILY DOSES*

Adults and Children older than 12 yo				
Drug	**Form**	**Low Dose**	**Medium Dose**	**High Dose**
beclomethasone HFA MDI	40 mcg/puff	2–6 puffs/day	6–12 puffs/day	>12 puffs/day
	80 mcg/puff	1–3 puffs/day	3–6 puffs/day	>6 puffs/day
budesonide DPI	90 mcg/dose	2–6 inhalations/day	6–13 inhalations/day	>13 inhalations/day
	180 mcg/dose	1–3 inhalations/day	3–7 inhalations/day	>7 inhalations/day
budesonide	soln for nebs	—	—	—
flunisolide HFA MDI	80 mcg/puff	4puffs/day	5–8 puffs/day	>8 puffs/day
fluticasone HFA MDI	44 mcg/puff	2–6 puffs/day	6–10 puffs/day	>10 puffs/day
	110 mcg/puff	1–2 puffs/day	2–4 puffs/day	>4 puffs/day
	220 mcg/puff	1 puffs/day	1–2 puffs/day	>2 puffs/day
fluticasone DPI	50 mcg/dose	2–6 inhalations/day	6–10 inhalations/day	>10 inhalations/day
	100 mcg/dose	1–3 inhalations/day	3–5 inhalations/day	>5 inhalations/day
	250 mcg/dose	1 inhalation/day	2 inhalations/day	>2 inhalations/day
mometasone DPI	220 mcg/dose	1 inhalations/day	2 inhalations/day	>2 inhalations/day
CHILDREN (age 5 to 11 yo)				
Drug	**Form**	**Low Dose**	**Medium Dose**	**High Dose**
beclomethasone HFA MDI	40 mcg/puff	2–4 puffs/day	4–8 puffs/day	>8 puffs/day
	80 mcg/puff	1–2 puffs/day	2–4 puffs/day	>4 puffs/day
budesonide DPI	90 mcg/dose	2–4 inhalations/day	4–9 inhalations/day	>9 inhalations/day
	180 mcg/dose	1–2 inhalations/day	2–4 inhalations/day	>4 inhalations/day
budesonide	soln for nebs	0.5 mg	1 mg	2 mg
		0.25–0.5 mg	>0.5–1 mg	>1 mg
		(0–4 yo)	(0–4 yo)	(0–4 yo)
flunisolide HFA MDI	80 mcg/puff	2 puffs/day	4 puffs/day	≥8 puffs/day
fluticasone HFA MDI (0–11 yo)	44 mcg/puff	2–4 puffs/day	4–8 puffs/day	>8 puffs/day
	110 mcg/puff	1–2 puff/day	2–3 puffs/day	>4 puffs/day
	220 mcg/puff	n/a	1–2 puffs/day	>2 puffs/day
fluticasone DPI	50 mcg/dose	2–4 inhalations/day	4–8 inhalations/day	>8 inhalations/day
	100 mcg/dose	1–2 inhalations/day	2–4 inhalations/day	>4 inhalations/day
	250 mcg/dose	n/a	1 inhalation/day	>1 inhalation/day
mometasone DPI	220 mcg/dose	n/a	n/a	n/a

*HFA = Hydrofluoroalkane (propellant). MDI = metered dose inhaler. DPI = dry powder inhaler.
Reference: http://www.nhlbi.nih.gov/guidelines/asthma/asthsumm.pdf

INHALER COLORS (Body then cap—Generics may differ)

Inhaler	Colors	Inhaler	Colors
Advair	purple	Maxair Autohaler	white/white
Advair HFA	purple/light purple	ProAir HFA	red/white
Aerobid-M	grey/green	Proventil HFA	yellow/orange
Aerospan	purple/grey		
Alupent	clear/blue	Pulmicort	white/brown
Alvesco		QVAR	
80 mcg	brown/red	40 mcg	beige/grey
160 mcg	red/red	80 mcg	mauve/grey
Asmanex	white/pink	Serevent Diskus	green
Atrovent HFA	clear/green		
Combivent	clear/orange	Spiriva	grey
Flovent HFA	orange/peach	Ventolin HFA	light blue/navy
Foradil	grey/beige	Xopenex HFA	blue/red

Leukotriene Inhibitors

MONTELUKAST (*Singulair*) Adults: 10 mg PO daily in the evening. Chronic asthma, allergic rhinitis: Give 5 mg PO daily for age 6 to 14 yo, give 4 mg (chew tab or oral granules) PO daily for age 2 to 5 yo. Asthma age 12 to 23 mo: 4 mg (oral granules) PO daily. Allergic rhinitis age 6 to 23 mo: 4 mg (oral granules) PO daily. Prevention of exercise-induced bronchoconstriction: 10 mg PO 2 h before exercise. ▶L ♀B ▶? © $$$$ Trade only: Tabs 10 mg. Oral granules 4-mg packet, 30/box. Chewable tabs (cherry flavored) 4, 5 mg. Leukotriene receptor antagonist. Serious: Churg-Strauss syndrome, hepatitis, anaphylaxis, angioedema, erythema nodosum, suicidal thinking, pancreatitis. Frequent: Headache, dyspepsia.

> Nursing Implications Observe for signs and symptoms of severe allergic reactions such as hives, urticaria, shortness of breath, tightness in the chest, unusual hoarseness, and swelling of the mouth, face, lips, or tongue; this medication is contraindicated if the patient experiences a hypersensitivity reaction. Cautiously use in acute asthma attacks. Lower doses may be required for hepatic impairment. Patients should be advised not to drink alcohol while on this medication. This medication may cause mental status and changes in moods inclusive of suicidal thoughts or actions.

Other Pulmonary Medications

DORNASE ALFA (*Pulmozyme*) Cystic fibrosis: 2.5 mg nebulized one to two times per day. ▶L ♀B ▶? © $$$$$ Trade only: Soln for inhalation: 1 mg/mL in 2.5 mL vials. Mucolytic. Serious: None. Frequent: Voice alteration, pharyngitis, laryngitis, and rash.

> Nursing Implications Administer by inhalation through nebulizer. Do not mix with other drugs in nebulizer. Refrigerate until used and keep out of strong light. Call prescriber if fever, breathing problems, or chest pain occurs. Mild rash and rhinitis may also occur.

IPRATROPIUM—INHALED (*Atrovent, Atrovent HFA*) 2 puffs four times per day, or one 500 mcg vial neb three to four times per day. Contraindicated with soy or peanut allergy (Atrovent MDI only). ▶Lung ♀B ▶? © $$$$ Trade only: Atrovent HFA MDI: 17 mcg/actuation, 200/canister. Generic/Trade: Soln for nebulization: 0.02% (500 mcg/vial) in unit dose vials. Short-acting anticholinergic bronchodilator. Serious: Anaphylaxis, angioedema. Frequent: Dry mouth, blurred vision.

> Nursing Implications If used concurrently with other inhaled meds, wait 5 mins between medications. See drug insert for recommended guidelines for inhalation/nebulization. Date canister when first used. Each canister contains 200 inhalations. Keep canister away from heat and flame

TIOTROPIUM (*Spiriva*) COPD: Handihaler: 18 mcg inhaled daily. ▶K ♀C ▶– © $$$$ Trade only: Caps for oral inhalation 18 mcg. To be used with "Handihaler" device only. Packages of 5, 30, 90 caps with Handihaler device. Long-acting anticholinergic bronchodilator. Serious: Anaphylaxis, angioedema, paradoxical bronchospasm, QT prolongation. Frequent: Dry mouth, cough.

Nursing Implications See recommended instructions for administration of inhalation medications. Capsule should only be used with inhaler. Never take by mouth. Will only work with inhaler provided.

TOXICOLOGY

Toxicology

ACETYLCYSTEINE   (*N-acetylcysteine, Mucomyst, Acetadote*, ✦*Parvolex*) Contrast nephropathy prophylaxis: 600 mg PO two times per day on the day before and on the day of contrast. Acetaminophen toxicity: Mucomyst: Loading dose 140 mg/kg PO or NG, then 70 mg/kg q 4 h for 17 doses. May be mixed in water or soft drink diluted to a 5% soln. Acetadote (IV): Loading dose 150 mg/kg in 200 mL of D5W infused over 60 min; maintenance dose 50 mg/kg in 500 mL of D5W infused over 4 h followed by 100 mg/kg in 1000 mL of D5W infused over 16 h. ▶L ♀B ▶? © $$$$ Generic/Trade: Soln 10%, 20%. Trade only: IV (Acetadote). Directly combines with the toxic acetaminophen metabolite as a glutathione substitute. Antioxidant believed to attenuate ischemic renal failure. Serious: Hypersensitivity, anaphylaxis, angioedema, bronchoconstriction, chest tightness. Frequent: Nausea, vomiting, disagreeable odor, generalized urticaria, rash, stomatitis, fever, rhinorrhea, drowsiness, clamminess, pruritus, tachycardia, hypertension, hypotension.

Nursing Implications If used for asthmatics check airway frequently for secretions and suction if necessary. If vomiting occurs, check on the need for additional dose post-vomiting. Bronchospasm can occur unpredictably and can cause death. If used with asthmatics check airway frequently and suction if necessary. Discontinue if allergic symptoms occur (eg, urticaria). If used as an antidote to acetaminophen, vomiting may be pronounced, and there is an increased risk of upper GI hemorrhage in pts with esophageal varices. Carefully assess time of acetaminophen ingestion and if extended-release type. Blood serum acetaminophen levels may be inaccurate if less than 4 h post-ingestion or less than 8 h post-ingestion of an extended-release preparation. Previously open vials should be discarded. Do not put drug in a "hot" nebulizer; clean nebulizer soon after use; do not mix with antibiotics. Refrigerate unused sterile soln to guard from contamination.

UROLOGY

Benign Prostatic Hyperplasia

ALFUZOSIN   (*UroXatral*, ✦*Xatral*) 10 mg PO daily after a meal. ▶KL ♀B ▶– © $$$$ Generic/Trade: Tab extended-release 10 mg. Selective alpha-1 receptor antagonist that increases urinary flow rate. Serious: Postural hypotension, chest pain, priapism, angioedema. Frequent: Dizziness, headache.

Nursing Implications Do not take UroXatral with alpha-blockers such as Hytrin, azole antifungals, HIV protease inhibitors, macrolide antibiotics, nefazodone, or telithromycin. Patients with liver issues, taking medicine for high blood pressure; a history of dizziness, lightheadedness, or fainting; planning eye surgery; low blood pressure; liver problems; kidney problems; other prostate gland problems; cancer; or a family history of heart problems should not take his medicine. Patients should be advised to take this medication with food and at the same meal every day. The tab should be swallowed whole. Patients should be educated not to use alcohol while on this medication and to avoid excessive heat.

FINASTERIDE   (*Proscar, Propecia*) Proscar: 5 mg PO daily alone or in combination with doxazosin to reduce the risk of symptomatic progression of BPH. Androgenetic alopecia in men: Propecia: 1 mg PO daily. ▶L ♀X ▶– © $$$ Generic/Trade: Tabs 1 mg (Propecia), 5 mg (Proscar). 5-alpha reductase inhibitor that decreases conversion of testosterone into dihydrotestosterone. Serious: Hypersensitivity, swelling of lips and face, breast cancer (long-term treatment), depression. Frequent: Impotence, decreased libido, decreased ejaculatory volume, testicular pain, rash, pruritus.

Nursing Implications Administer once daily with or without meals.

ANTIDOTES

Toxin	Antidote/Treatment	Toxin	Antidote/Treatment
acetaminophen	N-acetylcysteine	digoxin	dig immune Fab
TCAs	sodium bicarbonate	ethylene glycol	fomepizole
arsenic, mercury	dimercaprol (BAL)	heparin	protamine
benzodiazepine	flumazenil	iron	deferoxamine
beta blockers	glucagon	lead	BAL, EDTA, succimer
calcium channel blockers	calcium chloride, glucagon	methanol	fomepizole
		methemoglobin	methylene blue
cyanide	cyanide antidote kit, Cyanokit (hydroxocobalamin)	opioids/opiates	naloxone
		organophosphates	atropine+pralidoxime
		warfarin	vitamin K, FFP

TAMSULOSIN   (*Flomax*) 0.4 mg PO daily, 30 min after a meal. Maximum 0.8 mg/day. ▶LK ♀B ▶– ©
$$$$ Generic/Trade: Caps 0.4 mg. Selective alpha-1 receptor antagonist that increases urinary flow rate. Serious: Arrhythmia, orthostatic hypotension, chest pain. Frequent: Dizziness, headache, fatigue, somnolence, edema, dyspnea, asthenia, diarrhea, dyspepsia, dry mouth, nausea, palpitations, blurred vision, abnormal ejaculation.

> Nursing Implications Observe for severe allergic reactions including hives, swelling, itching, and difficulty breathing. In other severe cases blurry vision, shortness of breath, irregular heart beat, fever, and red or peeling skin can occur. Patients should be advised not to drink alcohol when taking this medication. Male patients should be advised that priapism (sustained penile erection) may be a side effect of this medication.

Bladder Agents—Anticholinergics and Combinations

OXYBUTYNIN   (*Ditropan, Ditropan XL, Gelnique, Oxytrol,* ✚ *Oxybutyn, Uromax*) Bladder instability: 2.5 to 5 mg PO two to three times per day, max 5 mg PO four times per day. Extended-release tabs: 5 to 10 mg PO daily, increase 5 mg/day q week to 30 mg/day. Oxytrol: 1 patch twice a week on abdomen, hips, or buttocks. Gelnique: Apply gel once daily to abdomen, upper arms/shoulders, or thighs. ▶LK ♀B ▶? © $ Generic/Trade: Tabs 5 mg. Syrup 5 mg/5 mL. Tabs extended-release 5, 10, 15 mg. Trade only: Transdermal patch (Oxytrol) 3.9 mg/day. Gelnique 3%, 10% gel, 1 g unit dose. Anticholinergic that exerts direct antispasmodic effects and inhibits muscarinic effects on smooth muscle. Serious: Heat stroke, hallucinations, QT prolongation, angioedema. Frequent: Somnolence, headache, dizziness, agitation, confusion, dry mouth, constipation, diarrhea, nausea, dyspepsia, blurred vision, dry eyes, asthenia, pain, rhinitis, urinary tract infection, application site reaction.

> Nursing Implications The most common side effects of this medication are belching, diarrhea, acid indigestion, and decreased sweating inclusive of dryness of the eyes, mouth, nose, and throat. Patients need to be observed for abdominal signs and symptoms. This medication should be taken with water on an empty stomach. There is an additive effect if alcohol or other CNS depressants are utilized—these medications should be avoided. Medications for allergies (eg, antihistamines) and medications for hay fever and colds should be avoided when patients are on this medication.

Bladder Agents—Other

PENTOSAN   (*Elmiron*) ▶LK ♀B ▶? © $$$$$ Trade only: Caps 100 mg. Heparin-like molecule that adheres to bladder wall mucosa and exerts anticoagulant and fibrinolytic effects and prevents irritation by buffering cell permeability. Serious: Thrombocytopenia, bleeding. Frequent: Alopecia, headache, rash, nausea, abdominal pain.

> Nursing Implications Thins blood; monitor for blood in stools, bleeding gums, bruising, nosebleed, coffee ground vomit. Lesser GI symptoms may also occur. Use cautiously if patient is pregnant, taking aspirin or anticoagulants, having surgery including dental surgery, has had an aneurysm, has an intestinal blockage, has low platelets, or has liver or spleen disorders.

Erectile Dysfunction

SILDENAFIL (**Viagra, Revatio**) Start 50 mg PO 0.5 to 4 h prior to intercourse. Max 1 dose/day. Usual effective range is 25 to 100 mg. Start at 25 mg if for age 65 yo or older or liver/renal impairment. Contraindicated with nitrates. ▶LK ♀B ▶– © $$$$ Trade only (Viagra): Tabs 25, 50, 100 mg. Unscored tab but can be cut in half. Selectively inhibits phosphodiesterase-5 resulting in enhanced relaxation of penile arteries and corpus cavernosal smooth muscle; enhances erectile function by increasing penile blood flow. Relaxes pulmonary vascular smooth muscle cells resulting in vasodilation of the pulmonary vascular bed. Serious: MI, CVA, hypotension, syncope, cerebral thrombosis, retinal hemorrhage, vision loss (nonarteritic ischemic optic neuropathy). Frequent: Headache, flushing, dyspepsia, abnormal vision.

> Nursing Implications Observe for signs and symptoms of severe allergic reactions (rash; hives; itching; difficulty breathing; tightness in the chest; swelling of the mouth, face, lips, or tongue). Do not prescribe if a patient is currently using nitrate medications for chest pain and heart problems/conditions. Taking Revatio with a nitrate medication can cause a severe and sudden decrease in blood pressure. Patients should avoid alcohol when taking this medication. May increase the risk of heart-related and other side effects such as chest, shoulder, neck, and jaw pain; paresthesia; dizziness; fainting, and vision changes.

INDEX

APPENDIX

ADULT EMERGENCY DRUGS (selected)

ALLERGY	diphenhydramine (*Benadryl*): 25 to 50 mg IV/IM/PO. epinephrine: 0.1 to 0.5 mg IM/SC (1:1000 solution), may repeat after 20 minutes. methylprednisolone (*Solu-Medrol*): 125 mg IV/IM.
HYPERTENSION	esmolol (*Brevibloc*): 500 mcg/kg IV over 1 minute, then titrate 50 to 200 mcg/kg/min. fenoldopam (*Corlopam.*): Start 0.1 mcg/kg/min, titrate up to 1.6 mcg/kg/min. labetalol: Start 20 mg slow IV, then 40 to 80 mg IV q10 min prn up to 300 mg total cumulative dose. nitroglycerin: Start 10 to 20 mcg/min IV infusion, then titrate prn up to 100 mcg/min. nitroprusside (*Nitropress*): Start 0.3 mcg/kg/min IV infusion, then titrate prn up to 10 mcg/kg/min.
DYSRHYTHMIAS / ARREST	adenosine (*Adenocard*): PSVT (not A-fib): 6 mg rapid IV & flush, preferably through a central line or proximal IV. If no response after 1-2 minutes, then 12 mg. A third dose of 12mg may be given prn. amiodarone: V-fib or pulseless V-tach: 300 mg IV/IO; may repeat 150 mg just once. Life-threatening ventricular arrhythmia: Load 150 mg IV over 10 min, then 1 mg/min × 6 h, then 0.5 mg/min × 18 h. atropine: 0.5 to 1 mg IV, repeat q 3-5 minutes prn to maximum of 3 mg. diltiazem (*Cardizem*): Rapid A-fib: bolus 0.25 mg/kg or 20 mg IV over 2 min. May repeat 0.35 mg/kg or 25 mg 15 min after 1st dose. Infusion 5-15 mg/h. epinephrine: 1 mg IV/IO q 3-5 minutes for cardiac arrest. [1:10,000 solution]. lidocaine (*Xylocaine*): Load 1 mg/kg IV, then 0.5 mg/kg q 8-10 min prn to max 3 mg/kg. Maintenance 2 g in 250 mL D5W (8 mg/mL) at 1 to 4 mg/min drip (7-30 mL/h).
PRESSORS	dobutamine: 2 to 20 mcg/kg/min. 70 kg: 5 mcg/kg/min with 1 mg/mL concentration (eg, 250 mg in 250 mL D5W) = 21 mL/h. dopamine: Pressor: Start at 5 mcg/kg/min, increase prn by 5 to 10 mcg/kg/min increments at 10 min intervals, max 50 mcg/kg/min. 70 kg: 5 mcg/kg/min with 1600 mcg/mL concentration (eg, 400 mg in 250 mL D5W) = 13 mL/h. Doses in mcg/kg/min: *2-4* = (traditional renal dose, apparently <2 ineffective) dopaminergic receptors; *5-10*= (cardiac dose) dopaminergic and beta1 receptors; *>10* = dopaminergic, beta1, and alpha1 receptors. norepinephrine (*Levophed*): 4 mg in 500 mL D5W (8 mcg/mL), start 8 to 12 mcg/min (1 to 1.5 mL/h), usual dose once BP is stabilized 2 to 4 mcg/min. 22.5 mL/h = 3 mcg/min. phenylephrine: 20 mg in 250 mL D5W (80 mcg/mL), start 100 to 180 mcg/min (75 to 135 mL/h), usual dose once BP is stabilized 40 to 60 mcg/min (30 to 45 mL/h).
INTUBATION	etomidate (*Amidate*): 0.3 mg/kg IV. methohexital (*Brevital*): 1 to 1.5 mg/kg IV. propofol (*Diprivan*): 2.0 to 2.5 mg/kg IV. rocuronium (*Zemuron*): 0.6 to 1.2 mg/kg IV. succinylcholine (*Anectine, Quelicin*): 0.6 to 1.1 mg/kg IV. Peds (<5 yo): 2 mg/kg IV. thiopental: 3 to 5 mg/kg IV.
SEIZURES	diazepam (*Valium*): 5 to 10 mg IV, or 0.2 to 0.5 mg/kg rectal gel up to 20 mg PR. fosphenytoin (*Cerebyx*): Load 15 to 20 mg "phenytoin equivalents" (PE)/ kg IV, no faster than 100 to 150 mg PE/min. lorazepam (Ativan): Status epilepticus: 4 mg IV over 2 min, may repeat in 10-15 min. Anxiolytic/sedation: 0.04 to 0.05 mg/kg IV/IM; usual dose 2 mg, max 4 mg. phenobarbital: Status epilepticus: 15 to 20 mg/kg IV load; may give additional 5 mg/kg doses q 15-30 mins to max total dose of 30 mg/kg. phenytoin (*Dilantin*): 15 to 20 mg/kg up to 1000mg IV no faster than 50 mg/min.

CARDIAC DYSRHYTHMIA PROTOCOLS (for adults and adolescents)

Chest compressions ~100/min. Ventilations 8-10/min if intubated; otherwise 30:2 compression/ventilation ratio. Drugs that can be administered down ET tube (use 2–2.5 × usual dose): epinephrine, atropine, lidocaine, naloxone, vasopressin*.

V-Fib, Pulseless V-Tach
Airway, oxygen, CPR until defibrillator ready
Defibrillate 360 J (old monophasic), 120–200 J (biphasic), or with AED
Resume CPR × 2 min (5 cycles)
Repeat defibrillation if no response
Vasopressor during CPR:
- Epinephrine 1 mg IV/IO q 3–5 minutes, or
- Vasopressin* 40 units IV to replace 1st or 2nd dose of epinephrine
Rhythm/pulse check every ~2 minutes
Consider antiarrhythmic during CPR:
- Amiodarone 300 mg IV/IO; may repeat 150 mg just once
- Lidocaine 1.0–1.5 mg/kg IV/IO, then repeat 0.5–0.75 mg/kg to max 3 doses or 3 mg/kg
- Magnesium sulfate 1–2 g IV/IO if suspect torsades de pointes

Asystole or Pulseless Electrical Activity (PEA)
Airway, oxygen, CPR
Vasopressor (when IV/IO access):
- Epinephrine 1 mg IV/IO q 3–5 min, or
- Vasopressin* 40 units IV/IO of replace 1st or 2nd dose to epinephrine
Consider atropine 1 mg IV/IO for asystole or slow PEA. Repeat q 3–5 min up to 3 doses.
Rhythm/pulse check every ~2 minutes
Consider 6 H's: hypovolemia, hypoxia, H+acidosis, hyper/ hypokalemia, hypoglycemia, hypothermia
Consider 5 T's: Toxins, tamponade-cardiac, tension pneumothorax, thrombosis (coronary or pulmonary), trauma

Bradycardia, <60 bpm and Inadequate Perfusion
Airway, oxygen, IV
Prepare for transcutaneous pacing; don't delay if advanced heart block
Consider atropine 0.5 mg IV; may repeat q 3–5 min to max 3 mg
Consider epinephrine (2–10 mcg/min) or dopamine(2–10mcg/kg/min)
Prepare for transvenous pacing

Tachycardia with Pulses
Airway, oxygen, IV
If unstable and heart rate >150 bpm, then synchronized cardioversion
If stable narrow-QRS (<120 ms):
- Regular: Attempt vagal maneuvers, If no success, adenosine 6 mg IV, then 12 mg prn (may repeat x 1)
- Irregular: Control rate with diltiazem or beta blocker (caution in CHF or severe obstructive disease).
If stable wide-QRS (>120 ms):
- Regular and suspect V-tach: Amiodarone 150 mg IV over 10 min; repeat prn to max 2.2 g/24 h. Prepare for elective synchronized cardioversion.
- Regular and suspect SVT with aberrancy: adenosine as per narrow-QRS above.
- Irregular and A-fib: Control rate with diltiazem or beta blocker (caution in CHF/ severe obstructive pulmonary disease).
- Irregular and A-fib with pre-excitation (WPW): Avoid AV nodal blocking agents; consider amiodarone 150 mg IV over 10 min,
- Irregular and torsades de pointes: magnesium 1–2 g IV load over 5–60 min, then infusion.

bpm=beats per minute; CPR=cardiopulmonary resuscitation; ET=endotracheal; IO=intraosseous; J=Joules; ms=milliseconds; WPW=Wolff-Parkinson-White. Sources: *Circulation* 2005; 112, suppl IV; *NEJM* 2008;359:21–30 (demonstrated no benefit over epinephrine and worse long-term neurological outcomes).

ANTIVIRAL DRUGS FOR INFLUENZA	Treatment* (Duration of 5 days)	Prevention (Duration of 7 to 10 days post-exposure)[†]
OSELTAMIVIR *(Tamiflu)*		
Adults and adolescents age 13 years and older		
	75 mg PO bid	75 mg PO once daily
Children, 1 year of age and older[‡]		
Body weight ≤15 kg	30 mg PO bid	30 mg PO once daily
Body weight >15 to 23 kg	45 mg PO bid	45 mg PO once daily
Body weight >23 to 40 kg	60 mg PO bid	60 mg PO once daily
Body weight >40 kg	75 mg PO bid	75 mg PO once daily
Infants, newborn to 11 months of age[‡,¶]		
Age 3 to 11 months old	3 mg/kg/dose PO bid	3 mg/kg/dose PO once daily
Age younger than 3 months old[§]	3 mg/kg/dose PO bid	Not for routine prophylaxis in infants <3 mo
ZANAMIVIR *(Relenza)***		
Adults and children (age 7 years and older for treatment, age 5 years and older for prophylaxis)		
	10 mg (two 5-mg inhalations) bid	10 mg (two 5-mg inhalations) once daily

Adapted from http://www.cdc.gov/mmwr/pdf/rr/rr6001.pdf
*Start treatment as soon as possible; benefit is greatest when started within 2 days of symptom onset. Consider longer treatment for patients who remain severely ill after 5 days of treatment.
[†]Duration is 10 days after household exposure, and 7 days after most recent known exposure in other situations. For long-term care facilities and hospitals, prophylaxis should last a minimum of 14 days and up to 7 days after the most recent known case was identified.
[‡]In July 2011, the concentration of Tamiflu suspension was changed from 12 mg/mL to 6 mg/mL. Tamiflu prescribing information contains instructions for pharmacists to compound a 6 mg/mL suspension when Tamiflu suspension is not available. The new Tamiflu suspension is provided with a 10 mL oral dispenser measured in mL rather than mg. Capsules can be opened and mixed with sweetened fluids to mask bitter taste. Make sure units of measure on dosing instructions match dosing device provided.
[¶]Oseltamivir is not FDA-approved for use in infants less than 1 year old. An Emergency Use Authorization for use in infants expired in June 2010.
[§]This dose is not intended for premature infants. Immature renal function may lead to slow clearance and high concentrations of oseltamivir in this age group.
**Zanamivir should not be used by patients with underlying pulmonary disease. Do not attempt to use *Relenza* in a nebulizer or ventilator; lactose in the formulation may cause the device to malfunction.
bid=two times per day.

NOTES

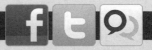